Associate's
SURVIVAL GUIDE

EDITED BY
Samuel M. Fassig, DVM, MA
CERTIFIED OD/SYSTEMS DESIGN

AAHA PRESS
LAKEWOOD, COLORADO

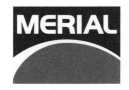

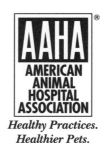

Healthy Practices.
Healthier Pets.

American Animal Hospital Association Press
12575 West Bayaud Avenue
Lakewood, Colordo 80228
800/252-2242 or 303/986-2800
www.aahanet.org

Printed in the United States of America

ISBN 9781583260595

Editor-in-Chief: Erin Landeck, MS, CPA
Design: Dianne Nelson
Cover Design: Elizabeth Lahey

Library of Congress Cataloging-in-Publication Data

On File

Associate's
Survival
Guide

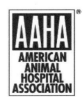

MERIAL

AAHA ®
AMERICAN
ANIMAL
HOSPITAL
ASSOCIATION

CONTENTS ◀

ix

CHAPTER 28: **SO YOU WANT TO BE THE BOSS**   319
Larry McCormick, DVM, MBA

► AUTHORS ◄

PROJECT EDITOR AND PRINCIPAL AUTHOR

SAMUEL M. FASSIG, DVM, MA,
  Certified OD/Systems Design
Director, Veterinary Business Resources
Fassig Farms Veterinary Services LLC
Chief Executive Officer
PCMR Foundation, Inc.
Boise, ID
208/841-2172
Fax: 208/562-1410
drsfassig@msn.com

Dr. Fassig is currently the Director of Veterinary Business Resources for General Fire & Casualty Company in Boise, Idaho, where he is involved with risk management, biosecurity, and product development. He interacts with congressional delegations at all levels of government, national agricultural and animal-oriented organizations, and principals of global reinsurance companies. He is regarded as an expert in biologics, biosecurity, and wound care and management. Dr. Fassig is internationally certified in organizational development and is certified by the Center for Food Security and Public Health as a trainer for agroterrorism and bioterrorism issues.

Dr. Fassig is past president of the American Association of Industrial Veterinarians (2000–2002), a former Board member of the American Academy of Veterinary Nutrition, a member of the Academy of Veterinary Consultants, and a charter member of Association of Veterinary Practice Management Consultants & Advisors. He is a member of the Idaho Veterinary Emergency Response Team (IVERT) and has been nominated to sit on the Idaho State Board of Veterinary Medicine.

Dr. Fassig's veterinary medical experience spans the military, clinical practice, academia, and the animal health pharmaceutical industry. Considered an expert on workplace dynamics, veterinary risk management, and the design and development of profit centers, Dr. Fassig is a nationally recognized speaker on business strategies. He has also served as the chief editor for several texts and professional journals and as the Director of Academic Affairs for three major animal health pharmaceutical companies.

As a practitioner, Dr. Fassig continues to focus his clinical career on animal athletes and animal production systems. Dr. Fassig also continues his consulting practice in southwest Idaho as the CEO of Fassig Farms Veterinary Services LLC and PCMR Foundation, Inc.

CONTRIBUTING AUTHORS

LINDA L. BLACK, EdD, LPC
Associate Professor of Counselor Education and
  Supervision
University of Northern Colorado
Campus Box 131—PPSY
Greeley, CO 80639
970/351-1638
Fax: 970/351-2625
linda.black@unco.edu

THOMAS E. CATANZARO, DVM, MHA, FACHE
Catanzaro & Associates, Inc.
Veterinary Practice Consultants®
18301 W. Colfax Ave., R-101
Golden, CO 80401
303/277-9800
Fax: 303/277-9888
cat9800@aol.com
www.v-p-c.com

ELIZABETH I. FASSIG, PsyD
Psychologist
Boise VA Medical Center
Boise, ID
elizabeth.fassig@med.va.gov

KAREN GENDRON, DVM
Owner
VIP Placement Service
167 Middle St.
West Newbury, MA 01985
978/363-2619
Fax: 978/363-2999
drgendron@comcast.net

CHARLOTTE LACROIX, DVM, Esq.
Veterinary Business Advisors, Inc
24 Coddington Road
Whitehouse Station, NJ 08889
908/534-8685
Fax: 908/534-8685
clacroix123@earthlink.net

LAUREL K. LAGONI, MS
Director, Emotional Support Resource Center
World by the Tail, Inc.
126 W. Harvard St., Suite 5
Ft. Collins, CO 80525
970/223-5590
Fax: 970/223-1226
llagoni@comcast.net
www.wbtt.com

LARRY MCCORMICK, DVM, MBA
Certified Business Appraiser
Simmons & Associates Mid-Atlantic
The McCormick Consultant Group
240 Miller Lane
Boalsburg, PA 16827
814/466-7084
Fax: 814/466-7233
lmccormick@tmccg.com
www.pvmc.net

LORRAINE MONHEISER LIST, CPA, MEd
Summit Veterinary Advisors, LLC
10390 W. Bradford Rd., Suite 110
Littleton, CO 80127
303/980-4000
Fax: 303/980-6900
lorraine@summitveterinaryadvisors.com
www.summitveterinaryadvisors.com

SHANNON PIGOTT, CVPM
Practice Consultant
American Animal Hospital Association
12575 W. Bayaud Ave.
Lakewood, CO 80228
210/240-1948
svpigott@aol.com

KERRY M. RICHARD, Esq.
Tobin, O'Connor, Ewing & Richard
5335 Wisconsin Ave. NW, Suite 700
Washington, DC 20015
202/362-5900
Fax: 202/362-5901
kmrichard@tobinoconnor.com
www.tobinoconnor.com

CARIN SMITH, DVM
Owner
Smith Veterinary Consulting
PO Box 698
Peshastin, WA 98847
www.smithvet.com

DEE STRBIAK, MS, LPC, CACIII, MAC
Director
Telesis
113 Ford St.
Golden, CO 80403
303/279-8081
Fax: 303/271-0592
d.strbiak@comcast.net

JAMES F. WILSON, DVM, JD
President
Priority Veterinary Consultants
16 S. Main St.
Yardley, PA 19067
215/321-9488
Fax: 215/321-7495
jwilson@pvmc.net
www.pvmc.net

▶ **PREFACE** ◀

> You can get everything in life you want if you will just help
> enough other people get what they want.
>
> — Zig Ziglar, REACHING THE TOP

You have arrived! Yahoo! Hooray! You've come through some demanding academic times to arrive at this point and, I imagine, you've been through quite a few emotional highs and lows. Many of you got here with your optimism and passion about veterinary medicine, pet owners, and pets. Good for you! So, what's next? Armed with diplomas, licenses, old class notes, and optimism, you bravely go to work. Welcome to the world of veterinary medicine.

WHAT NEW GRADUATES LOOK LIKE

You may be wondering: What does a typical entry-level veterinarian look like? This was a question I first posed publicly at the annual AVMA convention in 1998 to a panel of veterinarians from corporate and private practice, academia, and industry. Of course, there was no one answer. But we can say that more than 70% of new graduates are female, white, and between the ages of 27 and 30. More than half carry a student loan debt of $70,000 or more. Less than 40% of you new graduates are able to meet your financial obligations with the money you make at your first jobs.

For the most part, you still seem to like animals and have pets of your own. Your childhood was likely spent in a fairly peaceful world in a middle- to upper middle-class family in an urban society. You are likely skillful at using computer applications as tools for information services that make your life easier.

Upon graduation from veterinary school, you will have at least eight years of college-level education, minimal hands-on experience in most veterinary disciplines, and little, if any, business knowledge or experience. This is possibly the first full-time job with which you'll support yourself.

You want to practice quality veterinary medicine, but not longer than forty hours a week. You're probably not really a "joiner" in established professional organizations. You may have a spouse with his or her own professional life, and you want a healthy lifestyle with time for family, church, hobbies, personal growth, and development. Your work ethic tends to be lifestyle first, work second. Often, your work ethic dismays the baby-boomer generation—your bosses.

Some 60% of new graduates enter small-animal practices as an associate. Along with clinical duties, you may be given supervisory responsibilities, especially in the areas of personnel management, finance (budgets and pricing), and marketing of the business (primarily client communication), for which you feel somewhat adequately trained. Yet these very same issues—client financial issues, management problems, and personnel management—are the ones you report as major sources of frustration on the job.

Personal financial issues are also troublesome—it's tough to try to make enough money to get by and repay student loan payments. Somewhere between 70% and 80% of you will have some sort of an employment contract as part of the service agreement. Health insurance, more than a week of vacation time, sick leave, a retirement or investment plan, paid journal subscriptions, and continuing education are high on the list of preferred benefits.

WHAT EMPLOYERS EXPECT

So that's you, but what about your boss? Older private practice owners really don't want you to rock the boat the moment you come on board. They would prefer that you learn about the existing way of doing things before trying to change it. Whining, complaining, or comparing everything in the practice to the way it was done in school does not endear you to your boss. Baby-boomer bosses will be quick to retaliate with detailed stories of making do with nothing in the worst of conditions, when the only therapeutics were penicillin or streptomycin, vaccines caused "blue eye," you had to tube a horse to deworm it, and parvo was the nastiest thing on earth.

In general, modern-day practice owners view the new associate as an investment and want associates to be productively engaged and involved 100% of the time they are on the clock. Although this is a business relationship, more progressive practices also empower and encourage new associates and want to help you increase your self-confidence and learn new skills. Human nature being what it is, this is not always an unselfish or benevolent position on the part of the employer. Practice owners hope that you, in turn, will share fresh ideas, perspectives, advances in medicine, and experiences from academia with the entire staff.

In not-so-infrequent situations, owners also hold their breath and hope that you will be capable enough, early on, to relieve the burgeoning workload of everyone in the practice, maintain a sense of humor, be a joy to work around, and, they hope, stay for more than a year.

We live in exciting, transitional times for veterinary medicine. It's a time of weeding out some of the old ways that may have outlived their usefulness, challenging the new directions that veterinary medicine is taking, and strengthening our commitment to make the world we live in a healthier place. I truly believe that it's also a time filled with significant opportunities for those who work hard and do their best. I encourage you to take an active role. Welcome to the family!

— Dr. Samuel Fassig

▶ **PART ONE** ◀

Taking Charge
of Your
Personal Life

CHAPTER ONE

Balancing Career, Family, and Life

Shannon Pigott, CVPM

Samuel M. Fassig, DVM, MA

Elizabeth I. Fassig, MA, PsyD

IN THIS CHAPTER, YOU'LL LEARN:

- **What gets in the way of life balance**
- **Key questions to ask yourself about your need for balance**
- **Why it's important to determine your core values**

One of the biggest hurdles to achieving personal satisfaction with life, family, and work is *balance*—a life that does not force you to focus on career above all else. It is important to laugh, have fun, face challenges, and go on an adventure every day—not just during vacation.

WHAT GETS IN THE WAY OF BALANCE

There are four primary factors that will influence your career and may impair your ability to find life balance:

- a growing public awareness of the human-animal bond and changing client expectations

- low professional salaries and exorbitant student debt

- the desire to work less and play more

- the desire to have a family

Growing Public Awareness and Changing Client Expectations

The general public's awareness of the role of companion animals is at an all-time high. The catch phrase "human-animal bond" is becoming commonplace as university teaching hospitals and small-animal practices throughout the world adopt and use the slogan to promote the role that pets play in people's lives.

Clients are signing on to the Internet to buy prescriptions and verify diagnostic information provided by their veterinarians. According to the *2000 AAHA Pet Owner Survey*, approximately 74% of pet owners surveyed indicated that they would go into debt to provide for their pets' well-being. Ninety-three percent had bought presents for their pets. Fifty-eight percent reported spending $351 to more than $1,000 on veterinary care for their pets during the preceding twelve months.

These statistics prove that pet owners want to provide the best possible care for their companion animals and suggest that the demand for veterinary services will increase in the coming years. Heightened demand for greater levels of medical care and client service will cause the profession to specialize. The growth of the number of referral-only and species-specific hospitals is evidence of this transformation. Competitive forces will cause hospitals to find distinct and different ways of providing veterinary services to capture and retain clients.

In terms of your career, it is critical to determine the type of practice in which you envision yourself working, the business and medical philosophies of the employer, and your role in the organization. If a high-volume, low-cost wellness practice offers you an attractive starting salary of $65,000 with a guaranteed $5,000 raise in one year, would that position truly serve you if you aspire to pursue an internal-medicine specialty? If a practice offers a reasonable starting salary but expects you to handle all inpatient treatments and surgeries without the opportunity to see new clients, how can you generate adequate income and gain enough experience to advance?

Even if you get the ideal job, clients will dictate when and how their pets are treated. For the most part, clients view veterinary medicine as a service industry. Clients want appointments on certain days and at particular times, and most practices attempt to accommodate those requests or risk losing the business to another hospital.

Consumers' awareness and knowledge of their pets' medical conditions is greater than ever before. Drug manufacturers now direct their marketing messages to the end consumer (pet owners) in print and television media, requiring the veterinarian to be prepared for clients' requests for name-brand products.

The trend is that every client will demand individualized products and services. The challenge is that all customers must be treated the "same" yet different, and they expect to develop relationships with their animal healthcare providers. Smart, affluent customers will demand the latest technological advances as well as Internet connections and constant access to animal healthcare providers.

By understanding and anticipating the growing expectations of clients, you will be better able to determine the quality of care you'll need to provide. How important is quality of care in your list of priorities for balancing your life?

Low Salaries and Exorbitant Student Debt

Are veterinarians' salaries too low or their debt too high? The difficulty in repaying student loans, according to *The Current and Future Market for Veterinarians and Veterinary Medical Services* (published by the American Veterinary Medical Association in 1999), is that the veterinarian's ability to repay student loans lags behind that of other professions. The bottom line is that veterinary salaries have not increased in proportion to the increases in education expenses. The crux of this problem is more complex than determining how you will be able to afford a home, a family, and school loans—the issue is how your life must change to meet financial demands. According to AAHA's *Compensation & Benefits*, Third Edition, the average associate with five or fewer years of experience makes $59,279.

> Even if you get the ideal job, clients will dictate when and how their pets are treated.

Most first-year and second-year veterinary students expect to earn a sufficient income upon graduation to repay school loans. How reasonable is the expectation that a $59,000 salary will satisfy living expenses and school loans?

To a large extent, your ability to generate income from products and services dictates your pay. Pay is determined by the number of hours worked per week, the number of patients treated, the average client transaction charge, your level of experience, as well as many other factors. Not everyone is motivated by money, but the reality is that money dictates the degree of control you have over many other areas of your life. The desire to work thirty hours per week may not be a reasonable expecta-

> Not everyone is motivated by money, but the reality is that money dictates the degree of control you have over many other areas of your life.

tion if you are obligated to repay $80,000 in school debt. Eighty thousand dollars financed at 6.25% for ten years equates to, in round numbers, a $900 monthly payment.

Focusing on income generation does not directly translate into a balanced life; rather, it gives you the flexibility to control and improve your life. Straight production-based compensation or a combination of production and base salary offers the best opportunity to increase your take-home pay. Although the ability to generate income is directly tied to the number of patients available to treat, most associates will earn a higher income in fewer hours with a production-based compensation package. Through production-based compensation, you can chart your own financial course while simultaneously increasing your value, in real dollars, to the practice owners. Furthermore, associates who can generate adequate revenue to meet the owner's income objective are often given the opportunity to buy in.

To be able to afford a modest home and reliable vehicle, provide for a family, and repay school debt, revenue production and the resulting paycheck must be one of your primary considerations. Without a reasonable salary, you cannot achieve life balance. Where does money rank in your list of priorities?

The Desire to Work Less and Play More

The work ethic of older veterinarians clashes with that of younger veterinarians. How many times have you heard, "The younger workforce just does not seem to have the same work ethic as previous generations?" The two generations are not vastly different in aspirations, but they do differ in their perception of how work should be done, what constitutes job loyalty, and how they approach work in general.

By necessity, the veterinary profession has made some attempt to transform rigid forty- to sixty-hour work weeks to accommodate the growing number of women in the profession. In 1998, the AVMA reported that female associates were twice as likely as their male counterparts to work fewer than forty hours per week. Fully 27% of female associates worked fewer than forty hours per week, compared with 14% of male associates. Current data from AAHA's *Compensation & Benefits* study shows there is still a significant difference between male associates' average of 44.8 hours worked per week and the females' average of 43. This transformation in the number of working hours per week by women testifies to the priority placed on balancing work with family. The common sentiment of younger workers, male and female, is to work less and play more. Playing more implies spending more time pursuing other life interests outside of work.

It is important to understand that veterinarians who have practiced for twenty or thirty years emphatically believe that commitment to a job requires being physically present in the practice forty to fifty-five hours per week. Working fewer hours equates to laziness and lack of ambition in the eyes of these veterinarians. Most veterinarians of this era cannot fathom how the majority of recent graduates decline emergency calls, especially when they are given a financial incentive.

Once you understand what the employer expects, you are better able to satisfy the employer's objectives while still meeting your own. If you wish to work thirty hours per week (and can afford to do so), but the employer requires a full-time, forty-hour-per-week veterinarian, you might suggest job sharing with another veterinarian and splitting emergency-call duty. If you negotiate a production-based compensation package, the employer does not risk a hefty paycheck without the revenue to justify it.

The ability to take time off and work fewer hours is a reasonable expectation, providing that the mission of the practice is met. How important are time off and working fewer hours per week to you?

5

The Desire to Have a Family

The majority of recent graduates are attempting to balance more life issues than previous generations. The growing number of female veterinarians in the workforce and an increasing desire on the part of males to have an active role in child rearing are forcing the life–balance issue. Veterinarians who graduated before 1980 were predominantly men focused on owning a practice and working in their area of specialization without consideration of childbearing or child nurturing. Most of these men graduated with the explicit objective of owning a practice after just a few years as an associate veterinarian. They had clear expectations of their careers, and the career was prioritized before family or personal interests.

Today, the number of graduates who want to own a practice within a few years of graduation are far fewer than previous generations, due to a variety of new hurdles, including excessive school debt and the number of graduating women who desire to bear and raise children before owning a practice. According to the National Commission on Veterinary Economic Issues (NCVEI), women presently make up about one-third of practicing veterinarians. By the year 2015, the number of female veterinarians will increase to two-thirds of the entire workforce. This growth is due to the increase in number of women who are graduating from colleges of veterinary medicine.

The desire to have a family creates challenges for the veterinary profession because of the sheer number of women coming into the workforce during the past decade. For the most part, women who work in veterinary hospitals are of childbearing age, are planning a family, and are eager to settle down. Many new graduates want to start a family shortly after graduation.

Even a subtle signal of interest in starting a family causes tremendous anxiety for a practice owner who has anxiously awaited the addition of an associate. In many cases, the position may have been vacant for a year or longer. By the time you have been hired, the owner expects to take a much deserved vacation. Contrary to Equal Opportunity employment laws, some owners go so far as to question an applicant about whether they are planning a family in the immediate or near future. (This is an illegal question that you are not obligated to answer.) In some cases, the decision to hire hinges on how soon an associate can take over the practice.

To balance the desire to have a family and develop a career, you must establish a plan of action. As Dr. Kevin Elliott (University of Georgia, 1998) shared, "My wife and I sat down together and established a five-year plan that included financial, family, and practice ownership goals. We decided to wait to start a family until five years after graduation so that my school loans could be paid off. We agreed that once we had children, I would continue to work as an associate so that I could spend as much time with the kids as possible while they were young. We thought that if I started a practice when the kids were young, I would miss out on all the wonderful developmental years. We plan to start up or buy into a practice once the children start school."

Having a well-thought-out plan is an important step in achieving life balance. How important is family to you?

CORE VALUES

Paramount to balancing your life with a career in veterinary medicine is self-exploration. What were your reasons for entering the profession? If your reason for entering the profession was a love of animals, how happy will you be working in a practice where analgesia is rarely administered to patients experiencing pain? If your reason for entering the profession was the desire to generate unlimited pay through revenue production, how satisfied will you be working for a set salary? If you wish to have children, how comfortable will you be working long hours and handling after-hours emergencies? By exploring your core values, you are

> Even a subtle signal of interest in starting a family causes tremendous anxiety for a practice owner who has anxiously awaited the addition of an associate.

better able to align yourself with practices that will satisfy your fundamental needs.

You create your own reality. Here is an example:

Once upon a time there lived a veterinarian named John Albert Buford. He knew from a young age that he wanted to become a veterinarian, and he carefully focused his academic studies to achieve his goal.

After graduation from veterinary school, John entered his career with drive, ambition, and commitment. He was like a sponge, taking in everything around him. He learned so many essential things that they didn't cover in veterinary school from his new boss—Ole Doc Reed.

In this busy mixed-animal clinic, nestled in the mountains of western Colorado, there was only one other veterinarian, Dr. Mary Crawford, a caring woman boarded in internal medicine. The three of them crystallized as a team. After four months on the job, another milestone event happened—John's wife, Diane, gave birth to twin daughters, Katie and Irene.

After only seven months of John being on the job, Dr. Reed had a heart attack and died. His widow came to John and asked if he wanted to purchase the business. After some creative financing, John was able to secure a loan from the local bank to purchase the clinic.

That was almost three and a half years ago. Today, John maintains a thriving practice. He brought into the business one full-time and a second part-time veterinarian to do supplemental flex-time with Dr. Crawford. In addition, he added two veterinary technicians and a bookkeeper to the staff. He plans to add a part-time practice manager in the fall. The client demographics continue to improve, and the outlook for the business is good.

Since he acquired the practice, John has spent more and more of his time working, immersed in managing the staff, handling finances, and doing an exorbitant amount of case work. A typical schedule consists of long hours—often seven days per week, fourteen hours per day, and the ever-interrupting night emergency.

The late hours mean missing family dinners nearly every evening. He is finding his time with his daughters is limited to kissing their foreheads when they are already asleep in bed. Time with Diane is nearly nonexistent. They are like two roommates sharing a home. Laughter, play, and fun for them as a couple have become exceptions instead of the rule.

One late evening at his desk, John, drink in hand, reflected on his work, his life, and his thoughts on the future. It was true that finances were improving, and there certainly wasn't a shortage of work to be done. Yet, he felt as if something were missing in his life. He didn't want to admit it, but John felt physically, mentally, and emotionally drained. It seemed that Diane was always on his case and there never was enough time. He seemed to be forgetting things and was frustrated by little things that never used to be a problem.

He had flashes of walking away from it all— Diane, the kids, the clinic—everything.

It wasn't that John had planned for life to turn out this way; it just seemed to sneak up on him. Suddenly, John felt he had become incredibly boring and narrowly focused. Where was the fun, enthusiastic, optimistic person he once was? He knew a lot of folks but had only a few good friends—and he was ignoring them. It was at this moment that a cloud of depression came over John.

"What am I doing wrong?" he questioned. John picked up the picture of Diane, Katie, and Irene that was on his desk. In the midst of all he was building— all this that looked like success—he felt like a failure.

John knew one thing for certain. He sensed that a train wreck was inevitable. He didn't want his life to continue this way. He wanted to feel alive, energetic, enthusiastic, and creative, with a passionate, fun view of the world. He wanted to feel good physically again, sleep restfully, and say goodbye to the daily headaches.

He wanted to be able to turn off the negative thoughts that ran through his head like a never-ending marathon, stop the excessive worrying, and figure out a way to relax. He wanted balance in his life. He knew he was at the brink of chronic depression and burnout.

> Balancing your life with your career does not begin after accepting a job offer; it begins before the first interview.

Balancing your life with your career does not begin after accepting a job offer; *it begins before the first interview.* To enjoy a balanced life, you must gravitate to a working environment that fosters the same values you have. Sadly, too many graduates secure the highest paying job without consideration of their core values. What are your core values?

HUMAN NEEDS AND BELIEFS

Understanding Your Needs

It is important to acknowledge what you need in order to achieve a sense of balance and control over your life. Much of human behavior can be explained in terms of trying to satisfy one or more individual needs, sometimes at the expense of everything else. These pursuits can disrupt all your other goals, visions, plans, and good intentions.

Based on comments from Hyrum Smith in *The 10 Natural Laws of Successful Time and Life Management*, these needs include:

- **The need to live**—it is an incredibly strong, natural instinct—so powerful that if you feel yourself in danger, you will do many things that you would otherwise never even consider. You want to feel safe and secure. When you do, your desire to live manifests itself in your positive, productive job performance, in your efforts to maintain good health, and even in your ability to pay attention to your finances by sticking to your budget, saving money, and making sound investments.

- **The need to love and be loved**—loneliness, isolation, and a sense of abandonment are devastating. You go to great lengths to win love and have a sense of belonging. You put up with behaviors that you don't like. You make incredible sacrifices as a husband, wife, or friend because of your desire for love.

- **The need to feel important**—from the time you first hollered, "Mom, watch me!" you expressed the need to have another person pay attention to you. You want other people to value and notice you, and if you cannot win their love, you at least want to win their respect. As an adult, there are times you want to shout, "Look at me! I really did well! I am important!" Because this kind of behavior would most likely be considered at the least egotistical, you often resort to less genuine, more stressful means of attracting others' attention—like claiming all the credit for a group project or someone else's work.

- **The need to experience variety**—it is the basic reason you wear different clothing every day, eat an assortment of foods, watch movies, surf the web, listen to new music, take vacations, and go to sporting events. You do these things just to change your sensory inputs. Sometimes the need for variety is so compelling, you take risks and jeopardize your safety at the expense of other needs, just for the thrill.

Recognizable in these four categories of need is the demand to fulfill your emotional, physical, spiritual, social, and security needs.

Understanding Your Beliefs

In addition to your needs, your beliefs—whether based on scientific fact or your own untested assumptions—drive your actions. They also reflect your personal values. How do you look at each of these issues? Are your beliefs the same as everyone in your family, friends on the bowling team, or the political party your boss belongs to?

- Military spending and buildup

- The school system—go back to basics or explore new educational methods?

- Wages and benefits—do you get paid what you are worth?

- Politics and the political system—does it work?

- Religion

- Music

- Self-esteem—how is your worth as a person determined?

Everyone has specific beliefs that influence behavior. Scientists test their beliefs and continually challenge them based on new information. You, on the other hand, often do not test your personal assumptions and continue to act and conduct your life on these assumptions as if they are true and written in stone. In addition, sometimes you have to make a choice about how you act, even if it conflicts with your beliefs.

For example, at work, the organization may insist on a high degree of conformity among employees. There is a right way and a wrong way, and the right way to do something is how the boss says to do it. Or it has always been done that way. For subordinates, it is accepted that the boss's way is *the* way. However, your own belief system says that individuality and creativity are very important. For you, finding a more efficient way of accomplishing something is of a high priority. In this example, if you choose to conform, you may find yourself highly frustrated. If you choose to express your individuality at work, you may be branded a maverick and not a team player, and you may be overlooked for promotions and raises because you are not a "good corporate citizen."

There are other options—to quit outright and find a working environment that has values similar to yours, or sabotage your work to the point you are fired and then be forced to go out and find a working environment with people that share your values. What's most important is to find those shared values *before* you accept the job.

GETTING TO BALANCE

If you are a beginner at snowboarding, you will fall. You get up and try again. With each cycle of up, fall, up, fall, you learn a bit more about how to manage everything within your control. The more you learn, the less angry and frustrated you are, and the greater your joy in your accomplishment becomes. As you learn to get your balance, you learn more "how to" and can move on to bigger thrills, like snowboarding down the hill. As you progress, so will your awareness of the environment (e.g., weather, snow conditions, objects in your path) that you cannot control. If you do not adjust to them, they may have a negative impact on your experience.

Whether it's your first job as a veterinarian or your first time snowboarding, you may feel as if you have no control. In spite of that, once you understand that you can control certain elements of the process, living through the experience becomes an entirely different process. Ultimately, you feel a sense of "blending in" or "being in harmony" with the universe around you.

Don't make work a four-letter word. As you will see, it is important to strive for balance in your life, making time for family, friends, hobbies, and fun. The chapters on stress and time management will provide some insights into developing good habits in order to manage events in your life, find perspective, visualize what is important for you, and avoid burnout in your career and at home.

REFERENCES

American Animal Hospital Association. 2000. AAHA Pet Owner Survey.

Brakke, R. 2002. Brakke Management and Behavior Study. Brakke Consulting Inc.

Brown, J. and Silverman, J. "The Current and Future Market for Veterinarians and Veterinary Medical Services in the United States." *Journal of the American Veterinary Medical Association*, 215. No. 2: 161–183.

Johnson, S. and Blanchard, K. *One Minute Manager*. Berkley Pub Group, 1983.

McGraw, P. *Relationship Rescue: A Seven-Step Strategy for Reconnecting With Your Partner*. Hyperion, 2000.

McGraw, P. *Life Strategies: Doing What Works, Doing What Matters*. Hyperion, 2000.

Smith, H. *The 10 Natural Laws Of Successful Time And Life Management*. Warner Books, 1995.

Tannenbaum, J. *Veterinary Ethics*. Mosby Yearbook, 1995.

Wilson, J. DVM, JD. *Law and Ethics of the Veterinary Profession*. Priority Press, Ltd., 1990.

RESOURCES

Books

Beyond Anger—A Guide for Men by T. Harbin.
Do What You Are by P. Tieger and B. Tieger.
Home Coming—Reclaiming and Championing Your Inner Child by J. Bradshaw.
Win Your Life in 90 Days by S. Kelly.

Websites

Brakke Consulting
www.brakkeconsulting.com
A management consulting firm serving the worldwide animal health and nutrition, pet product, and specialty chemical industries and the veterinary profession.

Dr. Phil
www.drphil.com
An expert in human behavior, Dr. Phil McGraw provides strategic life guidance on many topics.

► CHAPTER TWO ◄

Planning for Your Financial Future

Samuel M. Fassig, DVM, MA

IN THIS CHAPTER, YOU'LL LEARN:

- **How to calculate your net worth**
- **How to develop a budget**
- **Where your money goes**
- **About the different types of insurance**
- **The importance of investing early**

THE ROLE OF FINANCES IN YOUR LIFE PLAN

According to a survey by Intuit, Inc., for each American who thinks about sex, there are three others who think about money. Increasingly, people are focused on more than paying the monthly bills. They also care about their long-term financial goals and objectives.

Personal financial planning is the process of organizing your financial goals into a workable plan so that you can live the life you want, with financial security.

Whether you begin practice as an associate and plan to stay in a multi-person practice or have aspirations to purchase a practice of your own, prioritizing your financial goals is a critical step in mapping your future.

It's tough enough to apply everything you've learned to everyday veterinary practice without worrying about how to file your tax return, purchase insurance, or invest your retirement money. Find a good accountant, attorney, and financial advisor, and pick their brains for advice. Be sure you fully understand what they are doing for you, and learn to interpret and use basic accounting, legal, and financial tools yourself.

The Choices You Make

Contrary to popular belief, most of America's wealthy did not inherit their fortunes but made them through hard work. The characteristics that make one person a millionaire and another a pauper have more to do with their spending and saving habits than with their level of income. Thomas Stanley, author of *The Millionaire Next Door*, says that the key is to *save more and spend less*. Answer these questions:

A. You receive an unexpected inheritance. Do you:

1. Remodel your bathroom and kitchen?

2. Pay off your credit cards and student loans?

3. Save some and go on a vacation with the rest?

B. Your five-year-old Saturn sedan is a little banged up but overall is in great shape. Your friends drive snazzy, high-end SUVs, and your spouse has his eye on a sports car. You can afford the payments because of the family's two incomes, although it might mean putting off adding to your retirement account for a little while. Do you:

1. Trade in your wheels and lease a new Jaguar or Porsche?

2. Sell your old car and buy a used Mercedes?

3. Keep your old car and tuck the money into your retirement investment account?

These are pretty easy questions, and since you were sharp enough to graduate from veterinary school, you most likely see right through them. But, think for a moment about how you spend your money. Do you look at your pay stub and wonder, "Where did it go?" Or do you actively budget your funds, set financial goals, and plan for the future?

Several recent studies commissioned by a major brokerage firm concluded that today's most important financial goals are saving for retirement, paying medical bills, and saving for your children's education. You might want to throw "paying off student loans" into that mix, but the only way to do it is one step at a time.

NET WORTH

Your net worth is one of the tools that financial lenders use when evaluating your creditworthiness. Net worth equals your total assets minus your total liabilities. The higher your net worth, the more likely you'll be to get the loan you apply for. Use Worksheet 2-1, to track net worth over time and measure progress toward your financial goals. To determine your net worth, use Worksheet 2-1 on page 13. This is also pro-

vided as an interactive worksheet on the companion CD.

CREDIT REPORTS

A strong, accurate credit report is one of your most important financial assets. It is a clear picture of your indebtedness, and it can reveal problems or discrepancies that may prevent you from gaining access to further credit and reaching your financial and life goals. Getting a problem repaired now is much easier than attempting to do it after you have applied for a mortgage or car loan. The key words "credit report" will get you to sites online that provide credit reports either at no or low cost. As always, be careful what information you give out to unsecured sites.

BUDGETS

Spend less, save more—this may sound simplistic, but simple concepts are often the basis for effective life changes. Budgets are financial plans that help you make the best use of your money.

Getting control of your finances means more than simply controlling your money. It means understanding how you think about money and how you spend it, as well as being able to identify long- and short-term goals. Getting control of your finances may lead to a more satisfying family life by reducing stress. It will also help prepare you for the future as the family matures.

Keeping a budget consists of three major steps:

- Estimating income

- Estimating expenses

- Keeping financial records

Estimating Income

If you are paid a base salary plus a percentage of production, the exact amount may be difficult to determine; therefore, an estimate will have to suffice. As you gain experience, the amount you estimate will become more accurate.

WORKSHEET 2-1
Your Net Worth

This worksheet is also available on the companion CD.

Assets

List the balances in your accounts and the market value of your assets.

Bank accounts (savings, checking)	$_____
Certificates of deposit, money-market funds, brokerage accounts	$_____
401(k)s, mutual funds, other retirement accounts	$_____
Insurance cash value	$_____
Vehicles	$_____
Home	$_____
Personal property (furniture, antiques, jewelry, etc.)	$_____
Other assets	$_____
	$_____
	$_____
	$_____

Total Assets $_____ **A**

Liabilities

List the unpaid balances of the following types of loans, along with any other debt.

Mortgage	$_____
Vehicle loans	$_____
Credit cards	$_____
Student loans	$_____
Money owed to friends and family	$_____
Other debt	$_____
	$_____
	$_____
	$_____
	$_____

Total Liabilities $_____ **B**

Net Worth = Total Assets - Total Liabilities (A - B) $_____ **C**

Estimating Expenses

Certain major expenses remain the same, month after month. For expenses like rent, a house payment, a second-mortgage payment, insurance premiums, monthly installments, and other fixed-cost items, set aside the same amount of money each month. Other monthly expenses, although necessary, are somewhat under your control. These include food, entertainment, utilities, clothing, recreation, transportation, and leisure items.

When estimating expenses, consider your wants and needs and establish your priorities. You may want to include savings and investments as well as an emergency fund for unexpected expenses in your personal family budget.

Keeping Financial Records

Most people who follow a budget keep a list of monthly expenses and prepare a yearly summary. These records of actual spending habits help you plan future budgets. They show you where you need to make adjustments.

If you ever are in a practice ownership position, you will need to apply the same principles in order to create a successful small business. On their own, budgets will *not* solve all your financial problems, force you to use them, eliminate all decision making regarding money, or balance by themselves.

When using a budget:

- Keep it visible and available for use.

- Set achievable goals, estimates, and priorities.

- Establish a set time and day to review budgeted versus actual spending (*preferably in the middle of the bill-paying cycle or when there may be less tension*).

- Make changes and alter the plan as circumstances warrant.

- Keep a file copy each year with your tax-return records as a reference.

- Don't count on windfalls to bail you out.

- Save a percentage of every paycheck for yourself. Aim to spend no more than 90% of your income, leaving 10% for the emergency fund or big expenses.

- Watch out for cash leakage, where withdrawals from the cash machine seem to evaporate without explanation. Keep a record of cash expenses.

- Beware of luxuries dressed as necessities. If your income does not cover your costs, and you are making a fair wage for your job, then some of your spending is probably going for luxuries that you think fill a real need.

Worksheet 2-2 on pages 15–19 gives you a format for developing a family budget and understanding your monthly income and expenses. This worksheet is also provided as an editable spreadsheet on the CD that accompanies this book.

Enter your current income and monthly expenses to determine how much more you need to earn and/or how much less you need to spend. Use the proposed monthly payment column to enter an alternate or proposed budget. This can be easily completed in the electronic spreadsheet version of this worksheet where the math is done for you. Also, that version allows you to see several budget proposals side by side.

The idea of making a budget may cause you to shudder for fear it will be too restrictive. You may assume it will take away spending freedom and reduce the amount of pleasure you take in your life. In reality, an effective budget does the opposite. By keeping track of expenses, you can concentrate on the items that bring you the highest reward, both financially and personally. An effective budget puts you in control.

> By keeping track of expenses, you can concentrate on the items that bring you the highest reward, both financially and personally.

Target Goals for an Ideal Budget Allocation

- **Housing and debt**—Mortgage or rent, credit cards, auto loans, personal loans, school loans, child support, and alimony combined should

WORKSHEET 2-2
Your Family Budget

This worksheet is also available on the companion CD.

For the Month of: _____   Year: _____

Prepared by: _____   Date Prepared: _____

	CURRENT Current Monthly Payment	**OPTION A** Proposed Monthly Payment	**OPTION B** Proposed Monthly Payment	**OPTION C** Proposed Monthly Payment
A. TOTAL INCOME				
List income before taxes and other deductions.				
Yours	_____	_____	_____	_____
Spouse	_____	_____	_____	_____
Other	_____	_____	_____	_____
	_____	_____	_____	_____
EXPENSES/PAYMENTS				
HOUSING				
Mortgage/Rent	_____	_____	_____	_____
Second Mortgage	_____	_____	_____	_____
Electric	_____	_____	_____	_____
Phone	_____	_____	_____	_____
Water/Sewer	_____	_____	_____	_____
Gas/Oil	_____	_____	_____	_____
Trash Removal	_____	_____	_____	_____
Supplies	_____	_____	_____	_____
Maintenance/Repair	_____	_____	_____	_____
Subtotal Housing	_____	_____	_____	_____
AUTOMOBILES				
Payment 1	_____	_____	_____	_____
Payment 2	_____	_____	_____	_____
Gas/Oil	_____	_____	_____	_____
Maintenance	_____	_____	_____	_____
Licensing	_____	_____	_____	_____
Subtotal Automobiles	_____	_____	_____	_____

WORKSHEET 2-2 (continued)
Your Family Budget

Expenses/Payments	CURRENT Current Monthly Payment	OPTION A Proposed Monthly Payment	OPTION B Proposed Monthly Payment	OPTION C Proposed Monthly Payment
INSURANCE				
Homeowners'	_____	_____	_____	_____
Auto	_____	_____	_____	_____
Life	_____	_____	_____	_____
Health/Dental/Vision	_____	_____	_____	_____
Disability	_____	_____	_____	_____
Subtotal Insurance	_____	_____	_____	_____
FOOD				
Groceries	_____	_____	_____	_____
Meals Outside the Home	_____	_____	_____	_____
Snacks/Coffee	_____	_____	_____	_____
Subtotal Food	_____	_____	_____	_____
PROFESSIONAL FEES				
Physician	_____	_____	_____	_____
Dentist	_____	_____	_____	_____
Eye care	_____	_____	_____	_____
Veterinarian	_____	_____	_____	_____
Attorney	_____	_____	_____	_____
Hair Stylist	_____	_____	_____	_____
Subtotal Professional Fees	_____	_____	_____	_____
ENTERTAINMENT AND TRAVEL				
Movies/Videos	_____	_____	_____	_____
Sporting Events	_____	_____	_____	_____
Concerts	_____	_____	_____	_____
Travel	_____	_____	_____	_____
Cable/Satellite	_____	_____	_____	_____
Subtotal Entertainment and Travel	_____	_____	_____	_____

WORKSHEET 2-2 (continued)
Your Family Budget

Expenses/ Payments	CURRENT Current Monthly Payment	OPTION A Proposed Monthly Payment	OPTION B Proposed Monthly Payment	OPTION C Proposed Monthly Payment
CLOTHING				
New Clothes	_____	_____	_____	_____
Cleaning/Repair	_____	_____	_____	_____
Subtotal Clothing	_____	_____	_____	_____
LOANS				
Personal Loans	_____	_____	_____	_____
Student Loans	_____	_____	_____	_____
Credit Card	_____	_____	_____	_____
Credit Card	_____	_____	_____	_____
Credit Card	_____	_____	_____	_____
Credit Card	_____	_____	_____	_____
Payments on a Lien or Judgement	_____	_____	_____	_____
Subtotal Loans	_____	_____	_____	_____
CONTRIBUTIONS				
Charity	_____	_____	_____	_____
Church/Synagogue	_____	_____	_____	_____
Subtotal Contributions	_____	_____	_____	_____
TAXES				
Federal Income Tax	_____	_____	_____	_____
State Income Tax	_____	_____	_____	_____
Local Income Tax	_____	_____	_____	_____
FICA Taxes (Social Security and Medicare)	_____	_____	_____	_____
Subtotal Taxes	_____	_____	_____	_____

17

WORKSHEET 2-2 (continued)
Your Family Budget

Expenses/ Payments	CURRENT Current Monthly Payment	OPTION A Proposed Monthly Payment	OPTION B Proposed Monthly Payment	OPTION C Proposed Monthly Payment
SAVINGS AND INVESTMENTS				
Toward Short-Term Goal	_____	_____	_____	_____
Toward Long-Term Goal	_____	_____	_____	_____
Contribution to Retirement Plans	_____	_____	_____	_____
Subtotal Savings	_____	_____	_____	_____
JOB-RELATED EXPENSES				
Organizational Dues	_____	_____	_____	_____
Licensing Fees	_____	_____	_____	_____
Professional Liability Insurance	_____	_____	_____	_____
Professional Clothing	_____	_____	_____	_____
Books/Journals	_____	_____	_____	_____
Subtotal Job-Related Expenses	_____	_____	_____	_____
MISCELLANEOUS				
Health Club	_____	_____	_____	_____
Postage	_____	_____	_____	_____
Child Care	_____	_____	_____	_____
Alimony/ Child Support	_____	_____	_____	_____
Other Items	_____	_____	_____	_____
	_____	_____	_____	_____
	_____	_____	_____	_____
	_____	_____	_____	_____
	_____	_____	_____	_____
	_____	_____	_____	_____
	_____	_____	_____	_____
Subtotal Miscellaneous	_____	_____	_____	_____

WORKSHEET 2-2 (continued)
Your Family Budget

Expenses/ Payments	**CURRENT** Current Monthly Payment	**OPTION A** Proposed Monthly Payment	**OPTION B** Proposed Monthly Payment	**OPTION C** Proposed Monthly Payment

List the subtotals from previous pages here to make them easier to add and to see their relative sizes.

	CURRENT	OPTION A	OPTION B	OPTION C
Subtotal Housing	_____	_____	_____	_____
Subtotal Automobiles	_____	_____	_____	_____
Subtotal Insurance	_____	_____	_____	_____
Subtotal Food	_____	_____	_____	_____
Subtotal Professional Fees	_____	_____	_____	_____
Subtotal Entertainment and Travel	_____	_____	_____	_____
Subtotal Clothing	_____	_____	_____	_____
Subtotal Loans	_____	_____	_____	_____
Subtotal Contributions	_____	_____	_____	_____
Subtotal Taxes	_____	_____	_____	_____
Subtotal Savings and Investments	_____	_____	_____	_____
Subtotal Job-Related Expenses	_____	_____	_____	_____
Subtotal Miscellaneous	_____	_____	_____	_____
B. TOTAL EXPENSES	_____	_____	_____	_____
C. NET INCOME OR NET LOSS (A - B)	_____	_____	_____	_____

be no more than **30% of your gross monthly income.**

- **Taxes**—Federal income, state income, local property, FICA withholding, and Medicare withholding combined will be about **25% of your gross monthly income.**

- **Savings and investments**—401(k), IRA, mutual funds, stocks and bonds, college savings, and other savings combined should be at least **15% of your gross monthly income.**

- **Insurance**—Life, health, disability, professional liability, auto, homeowners', umbrella liability, and other insurance combined will be about **4% of your gross monthly income.**

- **Transportation**—Gas and oil, car maintenance and repair, public transportation, and parking combined shouldn't be more than **2% of your gross monthly income.**

- **Household expenses**—Food, clothing, utilities, cable TV and Internet, home maintenance and repair, garbage, pest control, personal care, doctor, dentist, prescription drugs, entertainment, hobbies, magazines, club dues, day care, private school tuition, etc. combined should be about **24% of your total income.**

Stretching the Family Budget

There are multiple websites, articles, and self-help books that have strategies for stretching the family budget and saving money on those items you really need. Listed here are a few ideas to help you control and enhance your budget.

- **Home Mortgage**—Do you have the best interest rate? The difference between a $100,000 mortgage at 9.75% and at 7.25% is $142.74 per month, or $1,712.88 per year. Compare products, rates, and restrictions, then choose the best one for you. Over eight years you could save as much as $13,703.04. If *only one* house payment of $1,712.88 were invested at about 5% interest, the amount saved would double in about fourteen years. Think what an investment portfolio you would have created if each year you had

invested that amount. Your kids' college fund would be off and running.

- **Home repairs**—Do it yourself whenever possible. Get at least three to four competing bids from prescreened (e.g., Better Business Bureau members) contractors before having the work done on your property if you are not experienced enough to do it yourself.

- **Cars**—Cars are a big expense for most families. Do you own too much vehicle for your needs? Do you have equity in a car, SUV, or truck you no longer use frequently? Could you downsize and save money, not only on payments, but also on maintenance, insurance, and operating expenses? Can you take advantage of an auto-club discount to help with discounts on repairs and preventive services that you do not usually do yourself?

- **Banking and financial services**—Do you just pay whatever the bank charges? Shop around for the best rates on monthly fees, check costs, interest rates, ATM fees, and other services. These little fees can add up to $15 to $20 per month or $180 to $240 per year.

- **Credit cards**—Use cash whenever possible. Get rid of the high-interest cards. Pay them off or transfer balances and close the accounts.

- **Insurance**—Shop around for a fair price and excellent service. Raise your deductibles. If you raised the deductible on your homeowners' policy, for example, from $250 to $500, you could save up to 12% on the premium. Beefing up home security with heat and smoke detectors, burglar alarms, and dead bolts can generate discounts of another 5%.

- **Food expenses**—We all have to eat. Yet if you can save just $20 per week on food, it adds up to just over $1,000 in savings in one year.

    Try to plan food shopping in advance. Make a list, consider larger quantities (price compare per unit), and cut down on convenience food purchases (almost always more expensive). Once you are in the habit, you can plan two weeks of meals and make a shopping list in less than half an hour.

If you use national brand products, consider store brands or generics. Use the sales to stock up on items you use frequently and regularly.

Shop the grocery store that is the cheapest overall. Surveys show there is sometimes as much as a 10% to 15% difference on identical grocery orders at two different stores in the same area. If you spend $500 a month on groceries, that can translate into $600 to $900 a year in savings. You may also want to look at items you buy regularly. Select stores in your area that always carry that category of product at a lower cost.

> While it is understandable that any young professional just out of school finds it hard to think about the future, planning for the future may be one of the most important budgetary issues you face.

- **Clothing**—Although the costs of many consumer items (like computers and electronics) have decreased in the past few years, the cost of clothing continues to spiral upward while quality decreases. Buy separates that can be mixed and matched to make numerous combinations. The goal is to create a versatile wardrobe with minimal expense. Perhaps your employer can be persuaded to furnish or contribute to the purchase of scrubs, lab coats, and shoes used on the job.

   Buy clothes a season ahead (next year's winter clothes at this year's closeout prices). If you are hard on clothes, buy quality. Look for quality in discount stores. Shoes that hold up are often cheaper in the long run than several pairs of inexpensive ones. If you are on your feet all day, it is important for your health, well-being, and mental attitude to make sure your feet are protected and comfortable.

   Try to stay away from trendy fashions. Stick with the basics. Using the Internet can help you comparison shop on most items, even if you purchase through a buying club. In addition, Internet ordering often reduces the sales taxes you have to pay on an item, but beware of shipping costs.

- **Luxury items**—As your annual income increases due to raises, promotions, and smart investing, try not to spend money on luxuries

until you know your increases in income are outpacing inflation.

PLANNING FOR THE FUTURE: THE FAMILY LIFE CYCLE

While it is understandable that any young professional just out of school finds it hard to think about the future, planning for the future may be one of the most important budgetary issues you face. Taking a look at the typical family life cycle helps you see how you can structure your finances to meet your family's needs as it evolves through each stage (see Figure 2-1). You may be single now or already married, which may affect the position of one or two stages, but this cycle applies to most people.

Cost of Raising Kids

Having a child and seeing the world through the eyes of a child as he or she grows is a wonderful and joyous experience. It is also a great responsibility that requires you to be loving enough to plan for your children's needs. This can become a major focal point of your family financial plan.

The U.S. Department of Agriculture, in its annual Consumer Expenditure Survey on the cost of raising children to age seventeen, estimated the costs for raising a child in the United States in 2001. Table 2-1 shows the results. The figures in Table 2-1 do not take into account expensive medical bills, special accommodations, pricey private schools, advanced sports training, or any college prep or college expenses. (College expenses, by the way, are estimated at $20,000 to $150,000 for a basic four-year education.)

According to this survey, the expense breaks down to more than $12,500 per year from birth to two years of age for families in the $61,900 and over income bracket. As the child ages, the cost to raise the child increases. For the years fifteen to

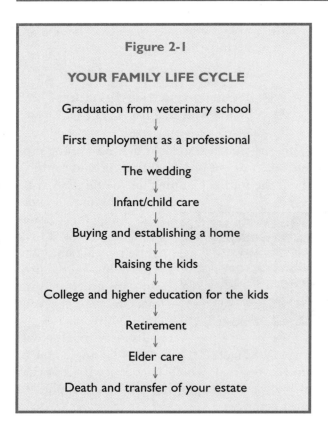

Figure 2-1

YOUR FAMILY LIFE CYCLE

Graduation from veterinary school
↓
First employment as a professional
↓
The wedding
↓
Infant/child care
↓
Buying and establishing a home
↓
Raising the kids
↓
College and higher education for the kids
↓
Retirement
↓
Elder care
↓
Death and transfer of your estate

not many couples decide to have children on the basis of economics.

If both parents are working, the biggest question is whether one of them will stay at home with the baby. This, of course, is the alternative to day care or some sort of nanny arrangement. The stay-at-home decision involves more than money and warrants much discussion and investigation. It is a choice that can affect career plans, the pace of family life, the baby's health, the harmony of the home, and the emotional well-being of both parents.

Choosing whether or not to have a stay-at-home parent is not an easy decision, although many parents are surprised to find out how little money is actually earned by the second breadwinner after expenses and taxes are deducted. Someone earning $20,000 per year ($9.61 per hour) could find their take-home pay reduced by as much as 75% when taxes and additional expenses are factored into the equation.

Once the child enters the picture, the family finances and goals will need to be readdressed and priorities rearranged. Additional expenses, such as medical costs, must be addressed, especially if you have no insurance coverage and there are concerns about depleting the savings account to pay for prenatal and labor and delivery costs. Other issues, such as having a valid will for each parent, appropriate life and disability insurance, and a plan for raising a child in a one-parent home in case one parent dies, also need to be addressed.

seventeen, it reaches $13,800 per year. The more significant costs in raising a child are listed in Table 2-2.

Today, raising a child is a quarter-of-a-million-dollar investment or more. That figure assumes your child does not wreck the minivan, go to college, or have special needs. The good news is that

Table 2-1
COSTS OF RAISING A CHILD IN THE UNITED STATES IN 2001

Family Income Level	Cost to Raise a Child Through Age Seventeen
$61,900 per year or more	$234,000+
$38,600–$61,900 per year or more	$160,140
Less than $38,600 per year	$117,390

Table 2-2
COSTS OF RAISING A CHILD (BY TYPE OF EXPENSE)

Expense Category	Percent of Total Cost	Cost Through Age Seventeen
Housing	33%–37%	$38,550–$86,610
Food	15%–19%	$23,340–$34,920
Transportation	13%–14%	$16,470–$30,870
Clothing	6%–8%	$9,210–$13,980
Health Care	5%–7%	$8,640–$12,840
Child Care/Education	7%–11%	$9,060–$25,200
Miscellaneous	10%–13%	$12,120–$29,430
TOTAL		**$117,390–$233,850**

INSURANCE

After years of study you are now ready to face the challenges of practicing your profession in a highly competitive and changeable business world, with its inherent uncertainty and risk. Fortunately, you do not have to assume all those risks alone. The unpredictable and uncontrollable events that cause financial hardships can be offset, at least in part, with a well-constructed insurance program. Purchasing insurance does not have to be a cure for insomnia or a cause for bankruptcy.

While you can buy insurance to mitigate just about every possible risk, only a few kinds of insurance make sense. Insurance is a form of security against events that could prove financially devastating. According to Leslie A. Woods, CPCU, ALCM, ARM, an insurance sales director with thirty years of experience, "Proper insurance protection includes coverage for the current and future value of both your business and personal assets."

Insurance Industry Terms

You'll be able to understand your insurance options much more easily if you learn a few industry terms.

- **Premium**—The premium is what you must pay for insurance protection. You can pay premiums monthly, quarterly, or once a year; this may vary by company and coverage. Monthly payment plans often have a finance charge associated with them.

- **Waiver of Premium**—Some policies allow insurance coverage to continue without premium payments in the event an insured person becomes disabled before a certain age. The waiver-of-premium provision is usually associated with life, health, and disability policies.

- **Deductible**—A deductible is a dollar amount—part of the loss—that you pay or absorb yourself. The insurance company pays the amount of the loss exceeding the deductible up to the limit of liability. In general, the larger the deductible you choose, the lower your premium.

- **Coinsurance**—In a health insurance policy, coinsurance refers to the percentage of a covered loss you must absorb after satisfying any up-front per-person or per-family deductibles.

- **Veterinarian Professional Liability**—This is a specific type of liability coverage that is normally excluded from standard liability policies. Professional liability can be defined as all money that the insured shall become legally obligated to pay as damages because of injury caused by a medical incident. A medical incident is any act or omission in the furnishing of professional veterinarian services.

Types of Coverages Available

There are several basic types of insurance, including life, health, disability, malpractice, and personal liability. Information on insurance-company ratings is available at the library or you can call a rating service for more information. Standard & Poor's will provide a free rating over the phone (212/208-1527). A.M. Best charges $2.50 per minute (900/420-0400).

> There are several basic types of insurance, including life, health, disability, malpractice, and personal liability.

Here are tips to help you avoid some common insurance mistakes:

- Choose the type of coverage you need, then select a policy.

- Check out the company before you sign up. Ask colleagues about their experiences with the company.

- Use a reputable agent. There are two types of agents—those who sell one company's products (captive agents), and those who sell several policies from several companies (independent agents). To check an agent's credentials and professional record, call your state insurance commission. Find out how the agents are compensated, and determine if they will be there for you if you need them.

- Remember that insurance is sold, not bought. Agents, especially those selling life insurance, have a vested interest in pushing high-commission (and high-profit) whole-life policies.

- Don't buy insurance that you don't need. This includes life insurance for your children. (Most children will be able to get insurance later; it is not a good way to save for college; and your family, while grief stricken if a child dies, can probably function financially without him or her.) Credit-protection life insurance (to pay your bills and credit card balance if you die) is overpriced and a waste of money. If you become disabled, it will only make the minimum monthly payment.

- Rental-car insurance may not be a bargain either. Some credit cards provide rental-car protection; you may also be covered under your auto policy. Be sure to know what coverage options are available to you long before you go to the car-rental agency. If you are not covered under a credit-card policy or under your own auto policy, buy the rental-car insurance.

- Keep your investing and insurance strictly separate. There are better places to invest for the future than in high-commission, whole-life insurance policies.

- Buy life insurance when you are young and healthy. Older people and those not in the best of health pay considerably higher rates. You may not need much life insurance until you have dependents. However, buying early may allow you to increase the coverage amount without an additional physical examination. And yes, the insurance physical may include blood tests for drug screens and HIV, whether you are informed of it or not. So ask.

- Be truthful on your life-insurance application. Be assured that if a large claim is made, the insurance company will investigate before making payment. For example, if your neighbors and coworkers know you are a smoker at the time you are applying, do not indicate on the application form that you are a nonsmoker.

- Use the Internet to shop for life insurance. It will cut out the pushy salespeople, and you can get a number of rate quotes and products to compare.

LIFE INSURANCE

In estate planning, it is important to provide enough assets to pay off your liabilities, to cover the cost of your funeral, and to help your loved ones, including money for child care and the surviving partner's short-term expenses. In general, life-insurance products are not good investment vehicles, but rather a tool for debt annihilation and keeping the survivors afloat.

24

How much life insurance do you need? There is no one answer. Some financial planners say five to seven times your annual income is sufficient, while others argue you need twice as much. That would mean a person making $50,000 a year should have a policy for $250,000 to $350,000 or more.

While it may be difficult to think about life insurance when you are just starting out, now is the best time. When you are young, the cost of life insurance is lower. In addition, future changes in your health status may make it difficult or impossible for you to get coverage. The AVMA Group Health and Life Insurance Trust, as well as other professional organizations, offer insurance packages as member services. Often these are very competitive products due to group rates offered to organizations. Your employer may offer group life, accident, and health coverage as part of your benefit package, or you may choose to purchase individual or family coverage on your own.

Term Life Insurance. For a specified period of time, or the "term," you will be afforded with coverage should you die. There may be exceptions that are not covered, such as suicide, war, and self-inflicted injuries while insane. As your age increases, so do premiums. Many companies offer term insurance that can be transferred to other insurance products. Remember, though— each renewal date provides the company with the opportunity to not renew your coverage based on medical information they may have obtained. There is no cash value on the policy and no death benefit once the specified period of time has elapsed. Although there may be a short grace period, it is especially important to pay these premiums on time. If they become overdue, you may have to reapply and have another physical examination.

Whole-Life Insurance. For a specified period of time, you will pay premiums at rates established for your age at the time you buy the insurance. With some products, after a certain number of years, your payments or contributions may stop. Again, premium rates are lower the younger you are. Once you have been accepted, it is difficult for the insurance carrier to drop you due to illness.

Monies from premiums, which are considerably higher than those for term life insurance, are invested by the insurance company. The company, depending on its structure, pays you a dividend or reinvests a portion of the returns on that investment into your policy, giving it an additional cash value beyond the death benefit. Therefore, when you die after twenty years of holding a $100,000 policy, it would pay your spouse the $100,000 death benefit and may have a cash value of an additional $28,000. The check would be for $128,000. It is possible to borrow money against whole-life policies based on their cash-value features.

HEALTH INSURANCE

Are you young and healthy? Why spend the money on health insurance when there are so many other things you need? Good health is great, but good health insurance is almost better. Unfortunately, affordable health insurance is hard to come by, and not having a minimum level of coverage can be financially devastating. Any policy you select should cover 80% of your doctor and hospital bills after your deductible is paid. To reduce your premiums, raise your deductible.

Your policy should have a maximum lifetime benefit of at least $250,000 and should cover all diseases. Try for at least one or two million as a lifetime benefit if you can afford it. Healthcare costs are not forecast to decrease anytime soon. If you have a serious preexisting condition, insurance may be more difficult to secure. In many states, Blue Cross and Blue Shield insurers offer quality coverage for a competitive price and may package individual coverage for self-employed persons as a group of one. Their health maintenance organizations (HMO) and individual insurers offer open enrollment periods several times per year. Health insurance may be available from professional associations, including the AVMA and state veterinary medical associations.

Accessing Medical Benefits. Take time to understand what is included in your health plan. Become familiar with the costs, the process to make claims, and the manner of contacting the administrator before you need to file a claim. Benefits and deductibles vary with programs and providers, as does the need for preapprovals for services.

25

To help understand types of coverages available under group plans, here are a few definitions:

- **HMO**—An HMO plan requires that all care be received within the carrier's network list of providers. Generally, a PCP (primary-care physician) is responsible for coordinating and referring all the patient's healthcare needs. Basically, you are assigned (in some cases you can pick from a list) a doctor you must see first in order to receive any care.

- **POS**—The POS is a point-of-service plan. The in-network benefits operate just like an HMO (you must use a PCP), but an out-of-network benefit is also available. The out-of-network benefits for both plans are provided at a higher out-of-pocket expense. Out-of-network may still require the physician to be on an approved list. Call your program administrator to find out the rules before you need to use the services.

- **PPO**—The PPO plan is a preferred-provider-organization plan that allows you more latitude in accessing care. In this plan, you can use any network physician, including a specialist, directly, without a primary-care physician referral, or you can go out of network and use any physician. A PPO plan is generally the most costly and typically uses coinsurance (10% to 40%) rather than copays. Again, study the program guides and become familiar with the administrator access as listed on your PPO insurance card.

DISABILITY INSURANCE

Most people have some life insurance, even if it is a free benefit of a checking account at a bank. Unfortunately, though, many practitioners do not carry disability insurance—an unforgivable error. While death is a catastrophe for your loved ones, disability can be an even larger financial problem. If you are not able to work due to injury or a medical condition, you still must have a source of income to pay monthly living expenses. The right type of disability insurance can help you secure that income.

> Many practitioners do not carry disability insurance—an unforgivable error. While death is a catastrophe for your loved ones, disability can be an even larger financial problem.

Disability coverage comes in short-term and long-term packages. Ideally, it is best to be covered for both. Before selecting a policy on your own, check to see if your employer has one. Workers' compensation will cover you for accidents that occur on the job only. If you break your leg while skiing, have a car accident while out of town, or have a stroke on the golf course, you're out of luck unless you have disability insurance.

Disability income protection provides a monthly benefit to the insured who is unable to perform the substantial and material duties of his or her job due to accidental injury or illness. Approximately one in three people suffer an accident or illness that deprives them of employment for an average of ninety days. For most disability policies, there is a waiting period of thirty to ninety days before coverage becomes effective. The benefit period (the length of time the insurance company will pay) can vary by the policy. The longer you wait to draw benefits after an illness or accident, and the shorter the benefit period, the lower the premium.

If your employer has a disability policy, find out when your coverage begins, your benefit amount, the amount of time before benefits start, the cost (if any) to you, and how the policy defines "disabled." The less broad the definition of what being a veterinarian means, the more it is in your favor. For example, if the policy says you cannot work as a veterinarian (meaning anything related to veterinary medicine), it is more restrictive about paying benefits (more inclusive about ceasing payments if you accept some other type of work). A more specific definition of your work would be "a small-animal practitioner in private practice," or the exact work you were doing when you were injured.

If long-term disability payments begin because you cannot work in a clinic setting as defined by your coverage, you may still be eligible for disability payments while having other employment, such as a technical service job for a veterinary distributor in which you use the phone and still provide advice as a veterinarian but do not perform patient care. If the definition of disability indicates in more general terms that you could not work as a veterinarian, working for the distributor might disqualify you from receiving disability payments. Seek written clarity from the provider as to how disability is defined and under what situations benefits will continue to be paid.

Employer-paid disability insurance will usually help supplement your income if you become disabled, but benefits are often short-lived. Remember, too, that benefits paid from employer-provided policies are taxable.

Whether or not your employer provides disability insurance, this type of coverage should be a priority. To figure out how much you need, do a quick financial inventory. Take a look at your net-worth statement on page 13 and calculate how long your savings would last if you had to invade it in an emergency. Don't panic—this is what insurance is *for*. Premiums increase with age, risky hobbies, or self-employment. Several companies provide this type of insurance; therefore, talk to a few agents before signing up.

When you are considering the amount of benefit, think in terms of replacing *part* of your income—not all of it. Unlike your regular income or benefits from employer-sponsored disability plans, benefits paid to you from a policy that you pay for *yourself* are *not* taxable. Consider a maximum benefit of 65% to 70% of your current income. To lower the premium, go back to your net worth and figure out how much you'd need to pay your bills and put groceries on the table, then work backward from there. Some people take into account potential Social Security benefits, but it can be difficult to qualify for these payments; therefore, include them in your calculations at your own discretion.

ACCIDENTAL DEATH AND DISMEMBERMENT (AD&D) INSURANCE

The basic tools of a veterinarian are his or her hands, and an AD&D policy offers financial compensation for the accidental loss of life or dismemberment. A special policy endorsed by the AVMA covers the *loss of use of hands,* even if actual dismemberment does not occur. Be sure to clarify exactly what is covered.

MALPRACTICE INSURANCE (PROFESSIONAL NEGLIGENCE, VETERINARIAN PROFESSIONAL LIABILITY)

In today's litigious society, you are expected to be perfect or risk paying the price. To keep a disgruntled client from taking a bite out of your income, you need adequate coverage. The Professional Liability Insurance Trust (PLIT), a membership service of the AVMA, is the primary source of personal malpractice insurance for an associate. Even if your employer carries a policy for you, make sure that you are covered by the policy (get it in writing). Also, you may not be covered outside the practice if you are moonlighting, doing relief work, or consulting. If you purchase the policy as an individual, the AVMA product policy will cover you wherever you go and your relationship and history with the insurer will be consistent and long term; this may help keep your premiums lower if you need to file a claim.

If allegations of professional negligence are levied, the AVMA PLIT will respond in your defense. The coverage provided through the AVMA PLIT is comprehensive; the insurance carrier will not settle unless negligence is involved and the veterinarian in question gives his or her consent. A board of eight trustees, all of whom are veterinarians, directs this program. A network of attorneys who specialize in malpractice defense is used, pointing carriers to the best expert witnesses when needed. For more information, call 800/228-7548.

AUTO INSURANCE

We all need auto insurance. Here are a few things to think about:

* As far as the insurance company goes, you represent a set of risks. An insurance company bases its premium decisions (the decision to insure you) on your "risk factors," some of which have nothing to do with driving a car—including your occupation, how you live, and your credit rating.

* Different companies charge different prices for what seems to be the same product.

* Research the insurer's record for claims service and financial stability. If they take forever to settle a claim or there are many Better Business

Bureau complaints, the policy may not be a bargain.

- Most states require only a minimum of liability insurance. Consider insuring yourself for more than the minimum.

- Ask for discounts. If you have your homeowners' or renters' policy with the same company, if you have multiple cars, if you own more vehicles than you have drivers, if you have highly rated safety equipment installed in the vehicles, and if you have a clean driving record, you might be entitled to discounts. Insurance companies reward behavior that reduces risks, including driving vehicles that have lower theft and better accident performance ratings.

- Demand that parts by the original equipment manufacturers be used for replacement. Insurance companies often save money by using inferior after-market or reconditioned parts.

- If your employer requires you to use your vehicle for work, be sure the employer has nonownership liability coverage that will protect you. Ask to see his or her policy, or get the policy in writing from the agent. If you have not reported to your carrier that you are required to use your vehicle for business, claims may be disallowed.

HOMEOWNERS' AND RENTERS' INSURANCE

As a professional, you are a lucrative potential target for liability and injury claims that happen to others on your property or in your residence. Chances are you will not be able to close on a home loan until a homeowners' insurance policy is in place. If you are renting, get low-cost renters' insurance. This protects you against a lawsuit from the property owner if anything you or a family member does causes damage to the property. It will also provide replacement protection for your belongings.

UMBRELLA LIABILITY COVERAGE

Depending on your other insurance carriers, you might also consider a personal liability umbrella policy as part of your homeowners' or renters' portfolio to protect you from actions against you that arise from situations on your personal property,

or when you or a family member does something on someone else's property.

This type of liability insurance provides $1 million of coverage or more, over and above all your existing liability coverage. If you coordinate this with your renters', homeowners', and auto insurance, it can sometimes actually reduce those premiums, almost paying for itself in the process. A good insurance agent can explain how it works.

Here is an example:

It's Sunday afternoon and you are out in the yard putting in a new walkway. The area is dug up and your tools are lying on the ground. A young neighbor, Nancy, who knows you are a veterinarian and is a client at the hospital where you work, rushes over with her two-year-old Jack Russell terrier, Champ. Champ has just been bitten by a raccoon that was "acting strange." There are small wounds on Champ's face, but you do not think they are life-threatening. You apply first aid to the dog's muzzle and neck to stop the bleeding and treat the wounds right there on the lawn with some iodine scrub from the house.

You say to Nancy that because Champ is vaccinated, he should be okay. However, in the process of holding the dog, Nancy is bitten by Champ, stumbles, and trips over your tools. She falls rather unceremoniously to the ground and grabs her wrist. In the confusion, you did not tell her to have the animal rechecked in a few days. At the time, you feel bad that Nancy is injured, but she insists she is okay and leaves with Champ, walking away with a slight limp. You are busy at the clinic and forget about the incident, and you don't hear from Nancy for weeks. You assume everything worked out okay.

Unbeknownst to you, the county quarantined the dog, the bite wound on the animal abscessed, and Nancy fractured a bone in her wrist and severely sprained her ankle, forcing her to be on crutches for weeks. She also underwent a series of rabies prophylaxis injections because the raccoon that attacked her dog could not be found and the county public-health department urged her to have the medical treatment. She did not have medical insurance—only workers' compensation—which would not cover the incident.

A single parent, Nancy is a computer programmer and will be out of work for many months. She will require rehabilitation services for her wrist and ankle and has to hire someone to help her with her children and to drive her around.

She sues you for professional negligence (regarding the handling of her dog and the raccoon-bite wound), the treatment costs at the animal clinic down the street (for Champ's care), and separately for her medical expenses, lost wages, and in-home assistance due to tripping on the "hazards" (the tools) you had in your yard.

Looking back, the easiest thing would have been for you to show concern and either refer Nancy to an emergency clinic for the dog right then or have her transport the animal to your facility, where you could have treated the dog under optimum conditions, advised Nancy of the rabies precautions, and set up an appointment to recheck the dog either in quarantine or afterward. Your actions—cleansing the wound and treating the animal on the lawn, even without charging a fee—may or may not qualify you for a Good Samaritan scenario for the dog, especially because there was already a client-patient-veterinarian relationship. The wound was not life-threatening, and you failed to discuss owner safety regarding a potential rabies exposure (professional liability).

This case could be complex because you have several types of liability. Chances are the personal liability (injury to the owner) is beyond the scope of your employer's liability for the clinic, because it all took place on your property. The damages may also exceed the limits on your homeowners' policy, or your insurance carrier might try to say you were running a business out of your house for which you were not insured. It is questionable if your own malpractice insurance would completely cover all of your liability in this case, because it would apply only to the dog. Also, services were not performed at the clinic, and you do not usually make house calls.

Unfortunately, the scenario is not that far-fetched. Be sure you are comfortable with your liability coverage—you never know when a seemingly harmless scenario will turn into a liability nightmare.

> You do not have to be entirely debt-free before you invest in retirement funding. This is because you have what is called "compound interest" working for you.

INVESTMENTS AS PART OF THE PLAN

Dr. John S. Mitchell, an equine veterinarian, retired at the age of forty-eight, healthy and reportedly very happy. This was in large part due to his retirement plan. In an article that appeared in Intervet's *Partners In Practice* (October 2001), he wrote: "It's been said that if you want a large shade tree in your yard, the best day to plant it was 20 years ago, and the second best day is today." His message is that we are responsible for taking control of and managing our own retirement dollars.

The number of small-business retirement plans has grown markedly in the last fifteen years. Practitioners can choose among IRAs, Simplified Employee Pension (SEP) plans, SIMPLE accounts, or traditional money-purchase and profit-sharing plans. The American Animal Hospital Association sponsors a retirement program as well.

Investment Strategy

Developing a strategy is important. Pay off credit-card debt first. Then focus on these three areas:

- Retirement funding
- Elimination of student debt
- Mortgage-debt repayment

You do not have to be entirely debt-free before you invest in retirement funding. This is because you have what is called "compound interest" working for you. The power of compounding allows your money to earn interest and be reinvested with whatever principal was present at the beginning, even without additional contributions of principal from you. This accelerates the rate at which your money accumulates. Say, for example, you invest $2,000 in a Roth Individual Retirement Account (IRA) when you are twenty-five years old. If its average return is 9%, you will have amassed about $64,000, tax-free, by age sixty-five.

29

After paying for all the necessities of life, who has the money, time, or energy for investing? Volatile markets may be great for day traders, but as a new associate, the demands on your time will likely prevent checking the portfolio ten times a day.

You can still make the most of your money the easy way by dollar-cost averaging. Consider making a consistent monthly payment to yourself for deposit in your retirement fund, before you pay your other bills. Start small, saving as much as you can afford. If you are less than forty years of age, plan to set aside at least 10% of your income each year. If you are older and have not started investing, you may need to set aside a much higher percentage. Proprietary computer programs such as Quicken Deluxe® and Microsoft® Money are affordable and easy to use and will help you organize your budget, checkbook, investments, insurance, taxes, and retirement planning. Both have Internet connections to update stock prices and provide access to your bank summaries.

Haven't got a cent to spare? Well, you can give up that morning cappuccino and save $2.50 per day, five days a week, fifty weeks a year for a savings of $375 per year. Take your lunch to work four times a week and save another $5 per day, which will be $20 per week, or $1,000 per year. We won't even discuss cigarettes! Invest money automatically by having it drafted from your checking account *before* you have the chance to spend it. In no time, you'll find that you've saved money—and you just might be healthier, too.

The Tax Man

Before taking on an investment project, consider the tax consequences of your actions and get professional advice. If the practice has a retirement plan, consider making contributions. Many plans match employee contributions; therefore, *not* participating is like throwing money away. If your practice doesn't have a plan, that's no reason why *you* cannot have one. Consider a traditional IRA or a Roth IRA. Contributions to the former are currently tax deductible and grow tax-deferred. Distributions after age 59½ are taxed at the same level as taxable income. Roth IRAs provide no current tax savings, but funds grow tax-free. Distributions are also tax-free. Before you invest,

get more information on these options from your financial and tax advisors.

Diversification

"Diversification" seems to be the buzzword of the new century. However, ten different mutual funds or twenty different stocks do not really comprise a diversified portfolio. Good advice can be obtained from a reputable broker with whom you have developed a relationship. Just be sure that any recommendations fit in with your overall objectives and will help you reach your financial goals.

Just as a reminder, *always consult your tax and legal advisors before investing in financial products.* Select an advisor whose personality is compatible with yours, who is honest, and who is a good communicator, and who will keep your best interests at heart. Keep in mind the disclaimer: Take time to read the prospectus before you invest or send money. Remember, though, that past performance is no guarantee of future results when it comes to evaluating financial products. Explained below are a few of the major types of investment vehicles.

INSURED SAVINGS AND MONEY-MARKET ACCOUNTS

Insured savings accounts and money-market accounts are the most secure because the investment is insured up to $100,000 by the Federal Deposit Insurance Corporation (FDIC). In addition, these accounts offer flexibility in that you can deposit and withdraw money on a personal schedule. However, the rate of return on investment (i.e., the interest paid) is relatively low. Certificate of Deposit (CD) accounts offer a slightly higher yield but are locked in for periods of time (six months to ten years) during which you cannot remove your money without paying a penalty.

STOCKS

Stock ownership by private individuals is still one of the best investments in history. The average annual return has been 11%, which is a better *long-term* investment vehicle than most. Experts are predicting, though, that the average return for the next ten to twenty years will be lower than average, at about 4% to 9%.

MUTUAL FUNDS

Mutual funds are collections of different funds (stocks, bonds, securities) that are managed by a professional fund manager in which individuals buy in at current prices. Each fund has an orientation and mix of investments and is categorized by the amount of risk associated with the investment. The more risk, the more potential for higher profits as the value and price rise. With more risk, however, there is a greater chance of loss if share prices fall. Because these funds are a mainstay of 401(k) and other retirement programs, it is important for you to educate yourself about them. Magazines like *Mutual Funds Magazine* or *Money* can help you get oriented; plus, there are numerous websites and, of course, a menagerie of brokers just waiting to help you invest your money.

REAL ESTATE

Real-estate investing may also be an excellent avenue for some individuals. When it comes to investing in real estate, buying and managing real estate is much different than buying your personal home, often with higher down payments and loan-qualification standards. Again, do your homework, get educated, and seek the advice of a trustworthy professional who will have *your* interests as the primary focus.

Investment Goal Planning

Whether you are saving for your children to attend college, for a second home, or for a dream vacation, the basic question is, "How much do I need to tuck away every month to make it happen?"

The examples in Tables 2-3 and 2-4 are based on an investment goal of $250,000 (today's price of what you want). Example one (Table 2-3) is based on twenty years to reach your goal; example two (Table 2-4) is based on thirty years. There are two assumptions. During the period of each example, the inflation rate will be 4% and the rate of return on investment will be 9%. Since no one knows for sure what these rates will ultimately be, these are best-guess models. The calculations were made using the interactive Internet site *www.msnbc.com/moules/commerce/newtoolkit/invest/goal.asp.*

In the ten years' difference in time reflected in the two examples from Tables 2-3 and 2-4, your monthly payment (investment from cash wages) was $377.26 less per month over the thirty-year period. Your total out-of-pocket expense was $37,394.23 *less* if you had the extra ten years in which to make the investment. However, over the ten years, the cost of the goal with inflation increased some $263,068.59. Still, you met that goal with less out-of-pocket cash.

Using the same assumptions as in examples one and two, but for forty years, the numbers would be:

- Monthly payment: $256.39

- Cost of your goal in future dollars: $1,200,255

- Total out-of-pocket cash wages invested: $123,068

Again, you can see the trend. The longer you have to save, the less money per month it will take to reach your goal, adjusted for inflation. The lesson is to invest what you can as early as you can—regularly.

The rule of 72 and the rule of 115 will tell you how long it will take you to double or triple your investment (see Table 2-5). Using Table 2-5, at a 1% rate of return, an investment will double in approximately 72 years and triple in 115 years. At a 10% rate of return, an investment will double in approximately 7.2 years and triple in 11.5 years.

These rules can also tell you how long before a given item will double or triple in price at an estimated average rate of inflation. For example: At an estimated average inflation rate of 8%, a loaf of bread will double in price every nine years.

> **Whether you are saving for your children to attend college, for a second home, or for a dream vacation, the basic question is, "How much do I need to tuck away every month to make it happen?"**

DETERMINING YOUR BEST INVESTMENTS

What is your best investment? First, find a trustworthy consultant with whom you can work. Do your own homework as well. You may hear that

Table 2-3
DOLLARS NEEDED TO REACH CURRENT-DOLLAR GOAL OF $250,000 IN TWENTY YEARS

Year Ending	Dollars You Invested	Dollars You Accumulated	Your Goal's Cost With Inflation
2001	$9,842.40	$10,258.35	$260,000.00
2002	$19,684.80	$21,478.10	$270,400.00
2003	$29,526.12	$33,752.22	$281,216.00
2004	$39,368.16	$47,176.76	$292,464.64
2005	$49,210.20	$61,860.62	$304,163.23
2006	$59,052.24	$77,921.92	$316,329.75
2007	$68,894.28	$95,489.88	$328,982.94
2008	$78,736.32	$114,705.83	$342,142.26
2009	$88,578.36	$135,724.38	$355,827.95
2010	$98,420.40	$158,714.61	$370,061.70
2011	$108,262.44	$183,861.48	$384,863.51
2012	$118,104.48	$211,367.30	$400,258.50
2013	$127,946.52	$241,453.36	$416,268.38
2014	$137,788.56	$274,361.70	$432,919.11
2015	$147,630.60	$310,357.70	$450,235.88
2016	$157,472.64	$349,729.50	$468,245.31
2017	$167,314.68	$392,794.39	$486,975.12
2018	$177,156.72	$439,899.56	$506,454.13
2019	$186,998.76	$491,423.52	$526,712.29
2020	$196,840.80	$547,780.79	$547,780.79

In this example, we assumed a goal of $250,000, 4% inflation, and a 9% rate of return. In twenty years, the cost of your goal in future dollars will be $547,780.79. You would have to save $820.17 a month to get there. You would have invested $196,840.80 of your cash wages.

real estate, such as your house, is your best investment. Is it? Real estate has performed well over time. In 1950, the median-priced home in the United States sold for $12,600. Today that house, based on U.S. Census Bureau estimates, would be worth $141,400. However, if in 1950 you had invested that $12,600 in stocks and reinvested all dividends, it would have grown to $4.3 million. Remember—past performance of stocks, funds, and the real-estate market does not guarantee future results.

Gather as much information as you can, make a plan, be disciplined, pay down your debts, save, and invest. As Suze Orman, author of *The 9 Steps to Financial Freedom*, would say, "Have the courage to be rich and create a life of material and spiritual abundance."

FINANCIAL RESOLUTIONS FOR THE NEW ASSOCIATE

- Pay yourself first every month. Your savings should be the first bill you pay. Live within your means and create only "good debt."

- Put your financial papers in order. Organize and review them on a regular basis. Make your will or update it. Make sure your spouse knows where these papers are located. Discuss finances with your spouse regularly and develop a financial plan.

- Read one or two financial publications such as *Money* (*www.money.com*), *Kiplinger's Personal Finance Magazine*, or *Fortune*. Visit "CNN Money" on the web. Read the articles.

Table 2-4
**DOLLARS NEEDED TO REACH CURRENT-DOLLAR GOAL
OF $250,000 IN THIRTY YEARS**

Year Ending	Dollars You Invested	Dollars You Accumulated	Your Goal's Cost With Inflation
2001	$5,314.89	$5,539.70	$260,000.00
2002	$10,629.77	$11,599.60	$270,400.00
2003	$15,944.66	$18,226.83	$281,216.00
2004	$21,259.54	$25,476.33	$292,464.64
2005	$26,574.43	$33,405.89	$304,163.23
2006	$31,889.31	$42,079.29	$316,329.75
2007	$37,204.20	$51,566.32	$328,982.94
2008	$42,519.90	$61,943.29	$342,142.26
2009	$47,833.97	$73,293.70	$355,827.95
2010	$53,148.86	$85,708.86	$370,061.70
2011	$58,463.74	$99,288.64	$384,863.51
2012	$63,778.63	$114,142.30	$400,258.50
2013	$69,093.52	$130,389.33	$416,268.38
2014	$74,408.40	$148,160.45	$432,919.11
2015	$79,723.29	$167,598.62	$450,235.88
2016	$85,038.17	$188,860.23	$468,245.31
2017	$90,353.60	$212,116.32	$486,975.12
2018	$95,667.94	$237,553.99	$506,454.13
2019	$100,982.83	$265,377.89	$526,712.29
2020	$106,297.72	$295,811.87	$547,780.79
2021	$111,612.60	$329,100.76	$569,692.20
2022	$116,927.49	$365,512.38	$592,479.70
2023	$122,242.37	$405,339.67	$616,178.89
2024	$127,557.26	$448,903.20	$640,826.40
2025	$132,872.14	$496,552.92	$666,459.80
2026	$138,187.30	$548,672.71	$693,117.45
2027	$143,501.92	$605,681.69	$720,842.14
2028	$148,816.80	$668,038.51	$749,675.83
2029	$154,131.69	$736,244.83	$779,662.86
2030	$159,446.57	$810,849.38	$810,849.38

In this example, we assumed a goal of $250,000, 4% inflation, and a 9% rate of return. In thirty years, the cost of your goal in future dollars will be $810,849.38. You would have to save $442.91 a month to get there. You would have invested $159,446.57 of your cash wages.

- Be an informed investor. Do not speculate blindly.

- Create a financial library and notebook. Keep articles for review and file them for easy reference.

- Spend fifteen to twenty minutes, several times a week, reading about or listening to things that pertain to financial matters.

- Only invest in things you understand and have taken the time to become knowledgeable about.

- Ask questions of others who may be informed. Find out their sources of financial information and explore them for yourself.

- Examine your plan on a regular basis. Often the best time to review your progress is at the end of

Table 2-5
RATES OF RETURN USING THE RULES OF 72 AND 115

Rate of Return	Years to Double	Years to Triple
1%	72	115
2%	36	57.5
3%	24	38.3
4%	18	28.8
5%	14.4	23
6%	12	19.2
7%	10.3	16.4
8%	9	14.4
9%	8	12.8
10%	7.2	1.5
11%	6.5	10.5
12%	6	9.6
13%	5.5	8.8
14%	5.1	8.2
15%	4.8	7.7
16%	4.5	7.2
17%	4.2	6.8
18%	4	6.4
19%	3.8	6.1
20%	3.6	5.8
21%	3.4	5.5
22%	3.3	5.2

the calendar year at tax time. Keep a written record of your plan with your tax documents for your own personal reference.

- Reward yourself. Build in rewards as you reach your targets—perhaps a trip to the islands with your significant other when you reach your goal of keeping within your budget and having a new $5,000 CD in the bank for each of the last three years.

REFERENCES

Edelman, R. *Discover the Wealth Within You: A Financial Plan for Creating a Rich and Fulfilling Life.* Harper-Collins Publishers, 2002.

Gardner, D. and Gardner, T. *The Motley Fool's What to Do With Your Money Now: Ten Steps to Staying Up in a Down Market.* Simon & Schuster, 2002.

Gitman, L. and Joehnk, M. *Personal Financial Planning with Financial Planning Software and Worksheets.* Lawrence South-Western College Publishing, 2001.

Hallman, G. and Rosenbloom, J. *Personal Financial Planning.* McGraw-Hill Professional, 2000.

Hansen, M. and Allen, R. *The One-Minute Millionaire: The Enlightened Way to Wealth.* Crown Publishing Group, 2002.

Kobliner, B. *Get a Financial Life: Personal Finance in Your Twenties and Thirties.* Simon & Schuster Adult Publishing Group, 2000.

McCurnin, D. *Veterinary Practice Management.* Lippincott Williams & Wilkins, 1991.

Monheiser List, L., *Personal Financial Planning for Veterinarians,* AAHA Press, 1998.

Orman, S. *The Courage to Be Rich.* Running Press Book Publishers, 2001.

Orman, S. *Suze Orman's Financial Guidebook: Put the 9 Steps to Work.* Crown Publishing Group, 2002.

Orman, S. *The 9 Steps to Financial Freedom; You've Earned It, Don't Lose It.* Running Press Book Publishers, 2001.

Prechter, R. *Conquer the Crash: You Can Survive and Prosper in a Deflationary Depression.* Wiley, John & Sons, Incorporated, 2002.

RESOURCES

Books

Personal Financial Planning for Veterinarians by L. Monheiser List. Available through AAHA Press.

Magazines

Kiplinger's Personal Finance Magazine
Money
Smart Money
Worth

Websites

Benefits & Incentives Group, Inc.
www.bigroupinc.com
BIG, Inc. is a full-service consulting and brokerage firm that specializes in employee/group benefits.

U.S. Department of Labor Consumer Expenditure Survey
www.bls.gov/cex/home.htm
The Consumer Expenditure Survey provides information on the buying habits of American consumers.

CHAPTER THREE

Understanding Debt and Debt Management

Lorraine Monheiser List, CPA, MEd

IN THIS CHAPTER, YOU'LL LEARN:

- How to calculate your debt-to-income ratio
- The six basic rules of debt management
- How to know when you have too much debt
- The ins and outs of student loans

Now that you're out of school and embarking on your veterinary career, one of your main concerns is likely repaying your student loans. According to the KPMG Megastudy of 1998, the new graduate in 1995 had accumulated a median of $39,483 in student-loan debt while in school; that figure will only increase as tuition continues its upward spiral. At the same time, starting salaries for new graduates are rising, but not at the same rate as the average graduate's student debt. That means each year's graduating class will likely be repaying more debt on proportionately less income than the previous class.

And it isn't just student loan debt that can cause you to lose sleep at night. You also need to think about rent (or mortgage payments), taxes, insurance, and credit card debt.

Is this debt burden unique to veterinarians? Student loans certainly are not, since many professionals must incur significant debt in order to get the training they need. In fact, the debt burden for physicians and dentists is actually higher than for veterinarians, according to the KPMG study.

However, the study also noted that the veterinary profession is unique in that real salaries (salaries adjusted for inflation) have not risen as fast as for other professions. In fact, veterinarians pay a higher portion of their income to decrease their student debt than any other professionals. Here we discuss how to manage your debt and credit wisely.

BASIC RULES OF DEBT MANAGEMENT

Debt Management Rule #1

Regardless of the reason you're borrowing, don't borrow more than you really need. You're just going to have to pay it back later, plus interest.

Ideally, someone should have counseled you to borrow the minimum amount you needed, because you now would have less to pay back. The reality, however, is that student loans are readily available, and they seem like "free money" at a time when you're feeling very strapped for cash. Consequently, many students borrow money not just for tuition, books, and basic living expenses, but also for spending money, entertainment, new clothes, travel, and eating out. Most students don't give a lot of thought to whether they could get by with smaller loans. Chances are good that no one pointed out to you that by increasing your debt load, you were effectively prespending a significant portion of your first few years' salary.

Student loans have special features that can help you as you repay this debt. First, they have certain deferment provisions for situations like military or Peace Corps service, and repayment is also deferred if you continue your education. When this deferment ends, student loans generally have low monthly payments, fairly low interest rates, and grace periods ranging from fifteen days to several months, depending on the kind of loan and the circumstances. Also, there is no prepayment penalty should you win the lottery and decide to pay them off in a lump sum. Another advantage of student loans is that part of the interest may be deductible on your income tax return. The rules are fairly complex, so consult your tax advisor.

So why does all this matter now? It matters because whatever the level of debt you incurred while in school, payback time is here. And that monthly payment is a major expenditure in your household budget. At a time when you're getting your first paychecks, hoping to upgrade your car, moving to a new location, setting up a household, and marrying or starting a family, you have lots of ways to spend that paycheck. Unless you're careful, you could end up spending far more than you make. You may go further into debt by increasing the balance on your credit cards. You are probably being inundated with credit card offers, and it's tempting to accept a few. But that's a game you can play for only a short while, as it always comes back to haunt you eventually when you find you can't make the minimum payments on your array of credit cards or you can't get a loan for some other purpose—e.g., to buy your first house.

> If your salary won't pay for your lifestyle, then increase your salary or lower your living expenses—don't borrow more money!

Debt Management Rule #2

Borrow money for long-term assets (like your education or your home), not for day-to-day living expenses.

Your living expenses, including payments on the debt you already have, must come from your salary. If your salary won't pay for your lifestyle, then increase your salary or lower your living expenses—don't borrow more money!

Now about the debt you already have... If you borrowed $50,000 and repay it at 8% interest over ten years, the monthly payment is just over $600. However, to have that amount available each month to send to the lender, you must earn more so that you will have $600 left after paying income and FICA taxes. How much more depends on your personal income tax situation. Your share of FICA taxes is 7.65% of your salary, and the lowest income tax rate on an associate's salary is around 15% (ignoring state income taxes); therefore, almost a quarter of your income is spent before you even see it. Your challenge is to have enough money, after taxes, to cover your living expenses, to repay your debt, and to save for the future. How do you do that?

Debt Management Rule #3

Get a handle on your personal finances by taking advantage of software packages like Quicken® and Microsoft® Money. This is especially critical with credit card debt.

Knowing where you spend your money is essential to managing it well. Money-management computer programs are inexpensive and user-friendly, allowing you to track your income and outgoing expenses easily. You could manage your finances manually, but realistically, you won't—you'll never find enough time.

In order to know how much discretionary income you have available to spend, you need to know how much of your income is already consumed by your ongoing expenses, like rent, food, debt payments, taxes, and insurance. These

---

Figure 3-1

TIPS FOR CONTROLLING CREDIT CARD DEBT

- Use only one card (or one card for personal use and one for business expenses if you must separate them for tax or other purposes).
- Avoid credit cards that can be used at only one store. They usually have very high interest rates, and they keep you from shopping around for the best prices.
- Destroy all your other credit cards.
- If necessary, freeze your one card in a block of ice in the freezer so that you will use it only when absolutely necessary.
- Define specifically what you can charge; for example, your personal card is to be used only for gasoline purchases, and your business card (if applicable) is to be used only for professional continuing education, membership dues, computer supplies, and hotels when you are on a business trip.
- Pay off all charges each month, if possible.
- If you cannot pay off all charges each month, pay off high-interest debt first while making at least the minimum payments on your other bills.
- Transfer balances to cards with low introductory interest rates, as long as you have the discipline to either pay off the balance before the interest rate escalates or transfer the remaining balance to another card with a low rate.
- If you are part of a couple, make bill paying a family event so that you both know your financial situation. That way, it will be easier to stay on budget. Foster communication about your finances, ensuring wise expenditures and payment of credit card debt on a timely basis.

programs can generate reports that give that information quickly and easily. They also help you understand the true cost of borrowing money, because they calculate the principal and interest included in every payment you make on your loans and credit cards. They allow you to know exactly how much you owe your creditors at any point in time, and they help you determine whether you can afford to repay a new loan.

CREDIT CARD DEBT

The financial industry has made it extremely easy for you to spend more than you make by giving you the ability to charge nearly any expenditure on a credit card and then make only the minimum monthly payment on the outstanding balance. If you've looked closely at your credit card statement, you've probably observed that the minimum payment is only slightly more than the interest on the outstanding balance. With each payment, you are paying for the use of the money (interest), but you're not repaying much of the loan (principal). The credit card issuers have set it up this way,

because they're in the business of collecting interest from the use of their money. If you charge a $50 dinner on your credit card and routinely pay only the minimum balance, that dinner could easily end up costing you twice as much.

You must curb your current spending, pay more than the monthly minimum payment on your credit cards, and discipline yourself to pay the full amount of any new charges when the bill arrives. Just remember—it's not personally rewarding to make a credit card payment and not even remember what you're paying for.

It's hard to get out of the credit card trap, so try not to get caught in it in the first place. Credit counselors suggest tricks like cutting up all but one of your credit cards and freezing the remaining card in a block of ice in your freezer. That way, if you really need to use it, you can thaw the ice and retrieve the card. However, by not having the card in your wallet, you are more likely to curb your spending and pay cash or write a check for only what you really need to buy. If you don't actually have the money, you won't buy it. See the

"Tips for Controlling Credit Card Debt" listed in Figure 3-1 on the previous page for more helpful information.

Debt Management Rule #4

When you borrow money, try to pay it back as quickly as you can to minimize the interest you must pay.

A corollary to this rule is to avoid loans with prepayment penalties so that you can retain the option to pay off the loan sooner than the stated term. For example, let's say you borrow $150,000 to purchase a home. The interest rate is fixed at 7.5%, and the term of the loan is thirty years. The monthly payment (principal and interest only) is $1,048.82. The total interest paid over the life of the loan is $227,575.20, which, when added to the original $150,000 loan, means that you will pay a total of $377,575.20 over thirty years to buy your home.

Now let's say that the term of the loan is fifteen years. The monthly payment (principal and interest only) is $1,390.52—only $341.70 more per month than for a thirty-year loan. However, the total interest paid over the life of this loan is only $100,293.60. Therefore, the total payments are $250,293.60, and you own the home outright after only fifteen years. Furthermore, you could take out a thirty-year loan (to make it easier to qualify at the lower payment), but pay extra principal each month so that the actual payments are equal to those for a fifteen-year loan. By doing this, you get the benefit of the interest savings, and you'll own your home after fifteen years, not thirty.

Borrowers often point out that paying more interest isn't as bad as long as it is tax deductible. To a point, that is true. If you must borrow money, it's nice to arrange it so that the interest is deductible in computing your income tax. For example, interest paid to purchase your residence often falls in that category. But the fallacy is that even if you are at the highest federal income tax rate (and you're probably not), your tax deduction causes the government to subsidize less than 40% of the interest you pay. Stated differently, for every dollar of tax-deductible interest you pay, more than sixty cents must still come out of your pocket. Therefore, it's better to pay less total interest, even if the interest is fully tax deductible.

Debt Management Rule #5

Know how much debt you can handle and recognize the symptoms of having too much debt.

So is all debt bad? No. When you make a major purchase, such as a new home, you likely will need to borrow a large part of the purchase price (as discussed in Debt Management Rule #4). However, this does not violate Debt Management Rule #2 because you are borrowing long-term to purchase a long-term asset—your residence. For most people, their home represents their single largest asset and the one that gives them the most security over the years. Other large purchases such as buying or starting a practice will likely require you to incur additional debt as well. Just be sure that the quality of the investment justifies the cost of the loan. (See Table 3-1 on page 41 for guidelines concerning good debt versus bad debt.)

Experts agree that *your total monthly long-term debt payments, including mortgage (or rent) and credit card payments, should not exceed 36% of your gross monthly income.* Mortgage bankers use this as one major criterion for determining your creditworthiness as a potential borrower. Therefore, this is a good rule of thumb to follow. You will also know you have too much debt when you experience the following:

- **Your discretionary income falls.** Discretionary income is the money you have left over after paying your monthly bills and contributing to any investment plans you might have. Does this amount drop because you occasionally have to dip into savings to cover shortfalls in your checking account or borrow against your retirement?

- **You make only minimum payments on your debt.** If you make only minimal payments on a debt of $3,000 at 13.5% interest, it would take twenty-six years to fully repay the loan, and it would cost you a total of $7,860.

- **You repeatedly maximize credit limits on your credit cards.** This happens as you finally pay off the long-standing balances of your credit cards, only to find you have reached your credit limit again shortly after doing so. It is not wise to charge your way back into debt once you become debt free.

- **You have no dedicated emergency fund or savings cushion.** You should have a cash reserve of three to six months of expenses (perhaps more if you are worried about being laid off). An emergency fund is intended to bail you out if you face some costly, unexpected situation. Payment of debt should not prevent you from maintaining such a fund.

- **Your sleep is disturbed and you worry about your debt at night.** If you are worried about your debt to the point you are up at night feeling anguished, it is a symptom that you might be too deep in debt.

- **You are using credit cards for items you used to buy with cash.** Try to get rid of those credit cards so that you will buy only what you can pay for with cash.

- **Your ability to make payments right away would be jeopardized if you lost your job.** If you are living hand-to-mouth, spending your next check before it gets here, you may be in serious trouble.

- **Your debt-to-income ratio is out of balance.** The debt-to-income ratio is a borrower's monthly payments divided by his or her gross (before taxes) monthly income. It is a quick way to see where you stand and is one of the first tools a lender might use to evaluate your creditworthiness. The amount you owe is only relevant when measured against your income and ability to repay. The more you make, the more debt you can afford to take on, unfortunately. Some lenders will look at two ratios— the front end and the back end. The front-end ratio is computed by taking housing expenses and dividing them by your gross income; the back-end ratio is your total debt-to-income ratio. To determine your debt-to-income ratio, use Worksheet 3-1 on page 40. This worksheet is also provided on the companion CD.

If you recognized any of the symptoms described earlier, read Debt Management Rule #6.

Debt Management Rule #6

If you've taken on more debt than you can handle, take action immediately. Don't wait for the problem to solve itself.

The first step is admitting that you have more debt than you want, need, or can reasonably handle. But once you acknowledge the problem, there are steps you can take which will help you remedy the situation and get your finances back under control.

1. Take a close look at how you actually spend your money. Do you make a purchase and then worry about how to pay for it? Do you know why you are buying something? Do you plan your expenditures or are you an impulse buyer? Try tracking every penny you spend for thirty days. You are likely to uncover a few surprises as to where your money actually goes.

2. Understand how credit ratings work. Your ability to borrow money is heavily dependent on your credit score. Although there are several credit agencies, they all track your requests for credit, your actual loans, your payments (including their timeliness), and the number of creditors you have, along with several other factors. Lenders look at these credit scores each time they decide if they want to loan you money.

   There's an old saying that banks only loan money to people who don't need it. In reality, lenders loan money to people who demonstrate both a willingness and an ability to repay it. Making payments on time, staying under your approved credit limits, and otherwise using credit wisely will help ensure that you'll have the ability to borrow again when you need it.

   If you have never seen your credit report, you can get a copy of it from any of the agencies. Type in "credit bureaus" in any Internet search engine and you'll be pointed to the websites for the three major companies. From there you can learn more about credit scores in general and your credit report in particular.

3. Notify your creditors if you expect to have problems making your payments in the near future. Many of them will work with you to extend the payments, defer a payment or two, or even lower the interest rate. Particularly if you agree to make payments electronically, the

WORKSHEET 3-1
Your Debt-to-Income Ratio

This worksheet is also available on the companion CD.

Monthly Payments

Dollar Amount

Monthly mortgage or rent $_____

Minimum monthly credit card payments $_____

Monthly car loan payments $_____

Student loan payments $_____

Other monthly loan payments $_____

Total Monthly Debt Payments $_____ **A**

Monthly Income

Monthly gross salary $_____

Bonuses, overtime, additional productivity pay $_____

Other income(s) combined $_____

Total Monthly Income $_____ **B**

Your Debt-to-Income Ratio (A ÷ B)   _____ **C**

If your debt-to-income ratio is:

36% or less:	This is a healthy debt load for most people (the optimum, of course, is to have no debt).
37% to 42%:	Not bad, but you need to start reducing debt now, before you get in real trouble.
43% to 49%:	Financial difficulties are imminent unless you take steps to reduce debt and/or increase income.

Table 3-1

GOOD DEBT VERSUS BAD DEBT

Good Debt	Bad Debt
Affordable housing—make a plan to buy a home that has potential to hold or increase in value	Large fancy home that requires your entire net income just to pay the mortgage or rent
Modest transportation	Luxury car or expensive pickup, especially if leased
Investment in the business—your future	Vacation loans
Modest stylish clothing—not everything must be the top name brand at full retail pricing	Expensive and unnecessary clothing, extravagant club memberships, items with brand names
Consolidation of student loans to a lower fixed interest rate	Large furniture purchases with a zero down payment and no payments for one year
Refinancing a home at a lower interest rate (fixed) and using some of the equity to pay off high-interest debts (e.g., credit cards)	High-dollar recreational items that are used only once or twice a year (boats, jet skis, premium hunting equipment)

lender may lower your interest rate since they will take their payments directly from your bank account. Remember: They want their money back but they would rather not incur collection costs and legal fees to pursue borrowers who really are going to pay. Particularly if your financial difficulties are only temporary, you may find that your creditors are willing to work with you. But if your problem is chronic and your history indicates that you handle credit poorly, don't expect any sympathy or cooperation.

4. Consider consolidating your loans with a debt consolidation plan. If you have several debts with different lenders and can't make your payments, there are many nonprofit organizations as well as fee-based companies who will serve as an intermediary between you and your creditors. For a fee, they will try to settle accounts with your creditors for less than the full amount owing.

   In addition, they will ask you to make one monthly payment to them which they then distribute among your creditors. These repayment programs can be helpful in getting the total amount of your debt reduced. If you decide to work with a credit counseling agency, be sure that it is accredited by the National Foundation for Credit Counseling or Association of Independent Consumer Credit Counseling Agencies.

5. Consider consolidating your loans with a debt consolidation loan. Unlike a plan which deals with your existing debt, the proceeds of a consolidation loan pays off your old debt. You then repay the new loan, which hopefully has lower payments and a lower interest rate than your old ones. These lower payments and lower interest rates generally result from longer loan repayment periods, so that the total interest you pay over the life of the new loan may end up the same or even higher than before.

   Also, lenders constantly advertise debt consolidation loans which are tied to the equity of your home. By borrowing against your home, the lender has a much safer loan secured by real estate and can offer a lower interest rate than on unsecured debt like a credit card. But taking out this type of loan means that you are essentially borrowing the equity in your home to pay for purchases you made months or years ago. Beware of lenders who will let you borrow all of your equity—that can be very dangerous since if you had to sell your home, you would likely not have enough equity to cover expenses of the sale, let alone have any proceeds left over.

6. Consider consolidating student loans to a fixed-rate loan. The strategy and beauty of consolidating school loans is that you basically trade variable-rate loans for one fixed rate that is based on an average of your loans' current rates. In this manner, you do not have to worry about paying additional amounts when interest rates climb— an inherent risk of variable-rate education loans like the Stafford or PLUS.

Interest rates on the Stafford and PLUS loans are set once a year, in July, based on the May auction of the ninety-one-day Treasury bill. Kalman A. Chany, author of *Paying for College Without Going Broke*, indicates the best time to decide to consolidate or not is in June. That gives you a one-month window. Consolidate in June if rates look like they will rise or consolidate in July if rates look like they will come down.

MAKING YOUR CREDIT WORK FOR YOU

The key is to weigh all your financial needs with the options available to you and to not put off developing a plan. Someone else's plan may not be the best for you.

Like most of us, you will probably make a few bad decisions as you learn to handle credit and manage your debt. Fortunately, you'll likely recover from those mistakes and no permanent harm will have been done. However, if you feel at some point that your debt is unmanageable, seek out one of the nonprofit organizations that exist to help you manage your debt. They can work with you to develop a budget, consolidate your debt, and sometimes even reduce the amount you must pay.

Overall, don't lose sight of the fact that building and maintaining good credit can open doors for you in the future. Just as too much credit card debt can keep you from being able to purchase a home, carrying too much debt can also keep you from being able to purchase a practice or start one of your own. At some point in your career, you will likely need to have good credit to make a major purchase, so start developing good debt management habits now—they'll pay off handsomely in the future.

RESOURCES

Websites

Student Loans
www.FinAid.org
www.slccloans.com

Debt and Debt Management
www.myvesta.org
www.center4debtmanagement.com
www.credit.about.com

CHAPTER FOUR

Creating Your Personal Vision

Samuel M. Fassig, DVM, MA

IN THIS CHAPTER, YOU'LL LEARN:

- **How to create your preferred future**
- **How to develop achievable goals**

The things that matter most in life are often held hostage to the things that matter least. When something or someone else controls your life, you are neither happy nor productive, and you cannot experience inner peace or fulfillment. The secret to achieving inner peace lies in understanding your core values—those things in your life that are most important to you.

You can always find a consultant, a software program, or a book to help you manage your time better. However, just doing a better job of managing your time is meaningless unless you are managing it to accomplish those goals that are of the greatest importance in your life. Usually, most new associates and many employers have yet to visualize and capture in words what those goals are.

PERSONAL VISION

A personal vision defines what you aspire to become. It symbolizes your dreams and values and requires a balance of reason and intuition, which taps into your sense of purpose in life.

When faced with change, a vision can help you stay focused on your preferred future and on choices that will allow you to attain that future.

Most people's vision is simply an extrapolation of the past. This may be the main reason why so few people are able to create compelling visions of the future. A vision based simply on past accomplishments can never provide the basis for true challenge. Moreover, as every investment portfolio manager will tell you, past performance is often a poor predictor of the future.

PERSONAL VISION AND CAREER

People who enjoy enduring success have a core purpose and values that remain fixed while their strategies and practices endlessly adapt to a changing world. The ability to balance continuity and change requires discipline. People with a personal vision have such clarity about who they are, what they are all about, and what they are trying to achieve that they tend to attract people who are willing to accept and thrive under

> People who enjoy enduring success have a core purpose and values that remain fixed while their strategies and practices endlessly adapt to a changing world.

their demanding standards. Such visions should be clear and compelling. They should also fall well outside of your general comfort zone.

It is important to visualize your career as a completed picture. Is what you see yourself doing a year from now in keeping with your personal vision for your life? Can you see five years from now? Are you heading toward your preferred future and living your life the way you say you want to? What skills and talents do you need to make this happen? What additional skills do you need to acquire, and how will you get them? Setting a timetable to reach your objective will support your progress and keep you on track. It will also help you know when you have reached it. Continue to revisit the plan and revise it as new horizons appear.

Example of a Personal Vision Statement

One veterinarian has a stated personal vision that each staff member has accepted as his or her own. With some additions by the staff, it has become the vision statement of the hospital: "To treat all my patients, every one of them, as I would my own animals, which I consider members of my family. I will provide all that is possible to ensure the highest quality of life for them and appreciate the personal attributes of each individual."

The acid test of a personal vision is, does the definition of the vision make sense to a person who does not know you?

In the process of stating your vision, have you identified the potential opportunities and challenges associated with your vision in both tangible and intangible terms? Have you weighed the risks of carrying out your vision?

The Role Values Play in a Personal Vision

Values are the prevailing beliefs and opinions of individuals, groups, and organizations. Values are directly related to identity questions: Who are you? Where do you fit in? What is your role in life? Values are also a

moral force. They tell you right from wrong.

All visions must include your values. The veterinarian with the personal vision discussed previously holds the following values, which support his vision for his hospital:

- People are the key resource.

- Integrity is a way of life.

- Quality in customer service and patient care is fundamental.

- Technical excellence must guide the medical treatment process.

- There must be an element or a sense of fun in what I and the staff do each day.

The hospital staff added these values to his to create the overall vision of the hospital:

- We will create a sense of urgency in every individual on staff to take responsibility for the quality of his or her own work.

- We will create an environment where each individual can make important contributions and achieve his or her full potential as part of our team.

- We will ensure that all employees understand how their jobs relate to the success of this hospital.

- We will ensure that individual and team performance has a meaningful relationship with recognition and compensation.

- We will make timely, innovative use of available technology, emphasizing responsive, user-friendly solutions for our patients and customers.

- Our management system in this hospital, including policies, procedures, and organizational structure, will be simple, effective, and consistent.

YOUR PREFERRED FUTURE

Only you have the power to realize your potential or prevent yourself from achieving it. You can create your own future. How you live your life is up to you. Preferred futures are

> Only you have the power to realize your potential or prevent yourself from achieving it.

44

really images of potential—making choices about who and what you will be in the future. There is nothing you *can't* do.

To face your preferred future is to take a big step toward adventure, commitment, and discipline. It's a risk for a person to move from the inquiry posture of: "What is happening in my world?" and "What might happen or is going to happen in my world?" to the action posture of "What do I want to *make* happen? What future would I prefer, and what do I need to do to move toward it?"

In order to shape that preferred future, you need to hold in your mind an image of what it is that you really want. Human beings are the only creatures on earth who can project and manipulate models of ideas inside their heads. Imagination is what propels people into the future, whether by idle dreaming or by conscious intention. There are many possibilities.

If you do not imagine and begin to conceptualize your preferred future, there is less chance of things happening as you would like them to happen. You may get bored, lose energy, or become easily distracted. You may fail to recognize that the future doesn't just happen to you but rather is something you create.

The key questions to ask yourself when you create a preferred future are:

- What do you want out of life?

- What do you have to offer?

- Are you living your life the way you say you *want* to?

A preferred future is something *you* proactively create. Within the realm of all things possible:

- If you do *nothing,* which in itself is a choice, something within the *possible* realm will occur. It represents everything and anything that can occur. You will be a passive participant, and, until it happens, you will not be prepared for any consequences, and you have not taken any active role in bringing it about.

- If you do *anything,* either on purpose or inadvertently, you may set about a course of events that will alter the outcome or the direction you travel. Something within the *probable* realm

will occur that is at least minimally defined and, in general, targeted. You will have an active but unfocused role in bringing it about. You may have some idea of potential consequences, but the target remains fuzzy.

- If you lay out a strategic plan with goals and measurements, then implement it, something within the *preferred* realm will occur. You will have taken an active and focused role in creating the outcome. You will be aware of the consequences before they happen and will be prepared to act to stay on course should further action be required.

Neil Armstrong and the astronauts on his NASA team had a focused preferred future of getting to the moon and back. The fact is, they were actually off course almost 98% of the time. However, by taking a proactive and focused role targeted at creating the outcome with measurable actions, they were able to make course corrections to realize the results they aimed for and desired. And, they got back home.

In a similar manner, if you desire to, for example, be a veterinary orthopedic surgeon, and if you do nothing and operate in the realm of *all things possible*, it probably will not happen. You may be a veterinarian, and you may do some surgeries, but you will not be credentialed and recognized by your peers as a veterinary orthopedic surgeon.

If you apply for a general surgery internship at a teaching hospital, it may get you on the right road or path. Yet your goal to be a bone specialist may well remain fuzzy depending on what surgeries you get to perform as an intern. It may be *probable* that you will become a veterinarian with advanced skills in surgery, but you have left much to chance. The outcome is uncertain and it is likely you will not meet your goal.

However, if you are proactive and seek specialized internships, residencies, and work experiences on a time line that will satisfy the requirements to make you a qualified orthopedic specialist, you are now on a path to your *preferred future*. You will be able to make the adjustments necessary, measure your progress in accordance with your personal strategic plan, and reach your objective, becoming a board-certified veterinary orthopedic surgeon.

Let's work on determining what you want your life to be like in the future. For this exercise, you are to construct a vivid, detailed fantasy about your life. This is often a first step toward making a change in your life.

Take the time to complete the exercise in Worksheet 4-1 on page 48. This worksheet is also available on the companion CD.

Implementing Steps to Your Preferred Future

Creating a preferred future is about being conscious of what you are doing every day and reviewing your progress. Take time regularly to reflect and take inventory. If you are not headed in the right direction, visualize your preferred future and repeat your vision statement to try to get back on course.

> Creating a preferred future is about being conscious of what you are doing every day and reviewing your progress.

BEING FOCUSED

Staying focused and on track is chiefly a matter of looking ahead and considering the consequences of your actions. What you do now will not alter the past. Changing the future is unavoidable. Once the action is taken, the process has been set in motion and consequences from that action are inevitable. Although you cannot disconnect consequences from the actions that precipitate them, you can reliably influence those consequences by controlling your actions.

By keeping the consequences in mind, your actions will take you precisely where you want to go. This, and the visualization of your preferred future supported by your personal vision, is the blueprint that will lead you to personal fulfillment, joy, and a sense of satisfaction.

BEING AWARE OF THOUGHTS AND ACTIONS

Your thoughts are like many thin, tiny threads, woven and braided together into a heavy rope. Each individual thread would snap under the slightest of forces, yet when the threads are bound together in a large rope, they can support an enormous load.

If you think about the limitations of your past, all those thoughts will soon create a strong rope that will tie you down and hold you back. If you consis-

tently think about your positive possibilities, you create a sturdy rope that connects you to the best you can be. Your actions will help you climb the rope. Your positive thoughts will weave together to give you a clear way to reach your preferred future.

SETTING GOALS

If left to your own designs, you may set goals that are unattainable, thereby setting yourself up for failure. Here are some ideas to help you develop realistic, achievable goals.

- **Express goals in terms of specific events or behaviors**. For example, instead of saying, "My goal is to own a practice," express your goal more specifically. Define "own a practice." A goal statement might be: "I intend to be the owner of a small-animal veterinary practice that focuses on cats and exotic animals within the next five years in St. Paul, Minnesota. During my first year after graduation, I will obtain an internship at a teaching hospital, such as Angell Memorial Hospital, in companion-animal medicine and then work in a metropolitan feline-only practice for at least two years." Your desire is now clearly stated and broken down into steps. It can be managed and pursued more directly. Express your goals in terms that can be measured.

- **Assign a time line to your goals**. Instead of saying, "I want a lot of money," make the goal, "I want to achieve an income of $100,000 per year by December 31, 2007." By making a schedule or timeline, you impose project status on the goal. The deadline you have created imparts a sense of urgency or purpose and becomes a motivator. A time-sensitive goal does not allow for procrastination. Create a date to arrive at your goal, and make it realistically attainable.

  If your goal is to add 120 new clients in twenty-six weeks, your goal date is twenty-six weeks from the day you start. Working backward from that date, you can see where you have to be at the midpoint of thirteen weeks (have you secured sixty new clients?). Likewise, you can see where you need to be at six weeks and eighteen weeks. Thinking in terms of a calendar allows you to assess the realism of your plan and determine the intensity of what you must do to reach your goal. It also allows you wins along the way when you meet or exceed those milestones, which, in turn, are motivators to complete the goal.

- **Choose goals that you can control**. You can't control revenue for the practice at which you work, but you can control how many times you offer geriatric lab workups. You can't control the marketing campaign for the practice, but you can make sure reminder dates are entered in the computer for your patients.

- **Plan and program a strategy that will get you to your goal. Do not rely on willpower alone.** Say your goal is losing weight. You have the habit of coming home from work through the kitchen door right into the den of temptation. Your travel path goes past the cookie jar and potato chips in the cupboard. Change your route. Make it a point to come home through the front door and go to your study to drop your briefcase, then go upstairs and change clothes. There are no opportunities on this route to create failure. Bottom line—**make the plan, work the plan, and reprogram those things that might interfere so that they do not compete with what you really want.**

> Bottom line—make the plan, work the plan, and reprogram those things that might interfere so that they do not compete with what you really want.

- **Define your goal in terms of steps.** You do not go from 1,200 clients to 1,320 clients (120 new clients) all at once. It is unrealistic to say at the first of the year, "I will have increased the number of my clients to 1,320 by July 4." Instead, put it in a reality-based statement, such as, "I will take certain steps to add five new clients a week for the next twenty-six weeks. I will do so by 1) becoming active in breed clubs and being involved with the members, 2) sponsoring youth activities and becoming a 4-H leader, 3) encouraging my regular clients to bring in new clients with incentives, and 4) defining a very targeted direct mailing on weeks ten and twenty. By the end of that time, I will be seeing these 120 new clients as regular customers." The path is clearly stated, your movement from one point to another point is defined, and your goal is reachable.

- **Create accountability for your progress toward your goal.** Without accountability, you may con yourself, thereby failing to recognize poor performance in time to adjust and keep from falling short. Set up an accountability system that will make it impossible for you to fall short of the goal.

- **Maintain a positive mental attitude.** If each day you fill each task with positive affirmations, such as, "I am successful, happy, and learning new things today," you will indeed be successful and happy, and you will learn new things every day. The principle goes back to King Solomon and his statement: "As a man thinketh, so he is."

- **Commit entirely.** Once you have defined and visualized your preferred future, commit to nurturing it and making it happen. Dedicate yourself to those goals that are truly important to your life. Understand that the greatest obstacle to making the preferred future your reality is your own procrastination and resistance to change.

It has been said that the most overrated phenomenon in the United States is the will to win. Actually, the most underrated is the will to *prepare* to win. Because time is a limited resource, success is often directly proportionate to how you utilize your time. Goal creation, especially when you write down a goal, helps you prioritize your time.

Business consultants and personal planners often use the acronym SMART in reference to goals and goal attainment. In short, SMART in reference to goals represent the following points:

S Specific goals
M Measurable progress
A Attainable end points
R Realistic—sensible, practical goals within reach
T Time frame—specific or timed

47

WORKSHEET 4-1
A Vision of Your Preferred Future

This worksheet is also available on the companion CD.

For this exercise, have paper or a notebook ready, along with a pen or pencil.

1.   List everything you see yourself doing, having, experiencing, embracing, and enjoying in your preferred life. Include details for each of these categories:

   •   Personal (include self-esteem, education, finance, health, hobbies)
   •   Professional (job performance, career)
   •   Relationships (significant others, friends)
   •   Family (parents, children, siblings, extended family)
   •   Spiritual (your personal relationship with your higher power; your life focus)

2.   Next to each description, write a comment about how achieving this vision would make you feel.

3.   Review your work.

4.   Write a vision statement in no more than one page.

5.   Condense that page into one paragraph. Read it to yourself out loud.

6.   Read this paragraph out loud to someone you trust. Ask her to tell you what she heard.

7.   Was it clear to the listener? If not, rework it.

8.   Save the final draft and revisit it often. Continue to improve on its clarity and strength.

Now review each of your roles in your preferred future in Worksheet 4-1. Write down the steps you will take to achieve your preferred future, along with time lines. You will know exactly what to do and when you will have it done. You will know that it is reasonable and appropriate and that you are capable of doing it, and you will have an exact written deadline.

SELF-POTENTIALITY

Your beliefs are nothing but feelings of certainty about what something means. For example, if you believe you are a great surgeon, you have activated certain points of references to support those feelings of certainty. Your thoughts can back up any idea you want: that you are confident, insecure, empathetic, and caring, or egotistical, self-centered, and self-serving. According to Anthony Robbins, "The key is to expand the references that are available within your life. Consciously seek out experiences that expand your sense of who you are and what you're capable of, as well as organize your references in empowering ways."

The message is, focus on the things that empower you and that are in keeping with your vision and preferred future. Remember—the values that form your vision stem from your beliefs, which are formed by the way you interpret life experiences. You have the choice to view from the positive or the negative. Each can have a profound effect as a filter on how you interpret an experience and react to it.

The world is not doing "it" to you. You are the one who is in the active role, reacting to events and stimuli. It's okay to have anxious, scared, angry, depressed, or lazy feelings—as long as you don't let them stop you from doing what you have to do.

Seek to expand your reference base. You can easily accomplish this by networking—belonging to professional organizations and common-interest groups and through other types of community involvement. Undoubtedly, then, you will challenge your values and perhaps alter your beliefs. Out of such challenge, confrontation, and strife come growth and forward movement. Good luck on the journey, and enjoy the ride.

> The world is not doing "it" to you. You are the one who is in the active role, reacting to events and stimuli.

REFERENCES

Fassig, S. "Putting 'Essence' into Veterinary Continuing Education" (3 parts). JAVMA, Vol. 204, Nos. 8, 9, 10. AVMA: 1994.

Robbins, A. *Awaken The Giant Within: How to Take Immediate Control of Your Mental, Emotional, Physical and Financial Destiny!* Simon & Schuster, 1991.

Wlodkowski, R. *Enhancing Adult Motivation To Learn.* Jossey-Bass, Inc., Publishers, 1989.

RESOURCES

Books

The AVMA Directory and Resource Manual by the American Veterinary Medical Association.

Deliberate Success: Realize Your Vision with Purpose, Passion and Performance by E. Allenbaugh and D. Waitley.

First Things First: To Live, to Love, to Learn, to Leave a Legacy by S. Covey, A. Merril, and R. Merril.

Full Steam Ahead: Unleash the Power of Vision in Your Company and Your Life by J. Stoner and K. Blanchard.

The Magic of Conflict: Turning a Life of Work into a Work of Art by T. Crum.

Seven Habits of Highly Effective People by S. Covey.

▶ PART TWO ◀

Finding Your First Job as a Veterinarian

▶ CHAPTER FIVE ◀

Creating Your Personal Employment Plan

Samuel M. Fassig, DVM, MA

IN THIS CHAPTER, YOU'LL LEARN:

- **How to analyze your professional skills**
- **How to assess what you want in a job**

Forming a well-defined set of goals, no matter how much you hate to do it, is critical in all areas of your life. This is especially true when it comes to obtaining a job.

Sometimes, sitting down to think through your plans is difficult, especially in light of today's fast pace, society's focus on instant rewards, and an incessant compulsion to be entertained. The pressure to get immediate income now that you have graduated can make the discipline of figuring out what you really want quite stressful.

You must have a personal vision and objectives, as discussed in Chapter Four. There is no way around it if you want to be successful (however you define it) or even if you want to survive. But for veterinary students and new associates of today, creating a five-year (or longer) plan is a foreign concept. The need for a plan becomes clear, though, when you get a notice that your first student-loan payment is due.

Defining your employment objective is known as career planning. Ideally, it is tied directly to your preferred future and personal vision. You can get a more personal perspective regarding the workplace you are considering or the one in which you currently find yourself if you ask yourself this question: "Is the organizational vision of the business or the owner of the practice congruent or compatible with my own personal vision statement?"

If you are feeling friction or are uncomfortable, you may be in the wrong place. If you are feeling significantly uneasy or disturbed, is this really the road to your preferred future? Although you can rarely control what happens in the world, you can determine *how* it happens to you. The more accountable you are for your own life, the more it will work in your favor.

STEPS IN FORMING YOUR PLAN

The steps in this process include:

1. Analyzing your professional skills and preferences by identifying your professional needs and wants

2. Assessing your marketable and transferable skills—what are your attributes and skills outside of your formal veterinary training?

3. Analyzing employment options and identifying ones that fit your vision

Analyzing Your Professional Skills and Preferences

To analyze your professional skills and preferences, ask yourself the following questions:

- Do I want to work directly with animals?

- Do I want to work with people? (Like it or not, veterinarians are in the people business.)

- What species of animals do I want to work with?

- Do I want to specialize? If so, in what? Do I need more training or certification? Under what circumstances can I get advanced skills?

- What type of employer (personality, work habits, environment) do I want to work for?

- What type of business (fast-paced, casual, HMO mode, rural, metropolitan) do I want to work in?

- What schedule (weekends, evenings, emergency, travel) am I willing to work?

- What are my career short- and long-term goals? (Remember your personal vision.)

- What specific attributes regarding veterinary medicine do I already have?

A number of standardized interest-inventory tests are available to help you raise your awareness regarding your personality, your strengths, your problem-solving abilities, and your adult learning styles. These might be helpful if you are not sure what part of the profession might suit you the best or what type of organizational system will allow you to thrive. The tests are meant to provide additional self-insights, not to make you think you are being categorized. If you write down what makes you happy and full of energy, and what you really like to do (no limitations), you can usually get to the same place.

What follows is a partial list of statements that might appear on such a test. Note the ones that apply to you and your job-related interests or that trigger a response in you.

I enjoy:

- Working with things most of the time
- Working with people most of the time
- Working in an office or business environment
- Working out-of-doors in the weather
- Doing scientific and technical studies
- Doing routine or repetitive activities
- Doing abstract and creative activities
- Working with people in a helping role
- Working with machines most of the time
- Working for prestige and the admiration of others
- Seeing concrete results of my work almost immediately
- Driving to many places during the day
- Having to improvise
- Being paged or called frequently on the phone
- Working with large groups of animals and people
- Working by myself
- Having to meet deadlines
- Handling multiple projects at the same time
- Having many people depend on the outcome of my work

In veterinary medicine, you are in the people business. This is true whether you are in the clinical, academic, research, or corporate world. People are your clients. As a student, life in the academic environment sometimes shelters you from what goes on off-campus in the world of business. If, for example, you find that you do not like dealing with the retail public, it is best to

> In veterinary medicine, you are in the people business. This is true whether you are in a clinical, academic, research, or corporate world.

be honest with yourself now and make choices about your personal strategies to optimize your comfort zone, yet allow sufficient challenges. You may decide that focusing your career on pathology or radiology may be your calling. These specialties deal more with written findings and telephone consultations than they do with face-to-face interactions. Because they are specialties, you will have significant personal challenges in remaining competent and current.

Envisioning a specific workplace environment that will be rewarding and stimulating is often difficult for the new veterinary graduate. Due to a lack of actually being on the job full-time, coupled with the economic constraints of starting out, some choices can lead you into workplaces that clash with your personal values.

If you are honest with yourself about your comfort zones, you can at least start out by minimizing the emotional trauma of a "bad" choice. It has been said, "You are what you do." Consider turning this phrase around to read, "You do what you are."

Your personality, your likes and dislikes, your values and goals, and your personal vision should determine where you work, what you do, and with whom you work—not the other way around. Try to look at the big picture regarding your life—all things possible, all things probable, and all things that make up your preferred future.

Here is an exercise completed by many creative-writing students. It requires you to write your epitaph. It does not have to be a one-line composition—write as much as you want. Answer the question, "What do you want to be remembered for?" Use the time to figure out what is important to you and where your passions lie. Career development is not just looking for a paycheck.

Assessing Your Marketable and Transferable Skills

You are a whole person—a complete package. Many times, an employer will choose a candidate on the basis of her perception of the candidate's ability to fit in. The employer may be looking for a team player who has a good outward appearance and is approachable, a good listener, and confident. The employer may also look for any additional skills that you may bring to the organization beyond your veterinary medical competence.

To stimulate your thoughts about what these skills might be, use Table 5-1, Assessing Your Skills. Think in broad terms, *and* think about actual events or past examples that pertain specifically to you. Once you've identified these broad skills, you'll feel more confident talking about yourself to prospective employers.

Analyzing Employment Options and Identifying Ones That Fit Your Vision

You have worked hard and achieved the difficult goals set out for you in veterinary school. You're smart and are a hard worker. You are in one of the most challenging professions in the country. Are you poised for success, or will you try the hit-and-miss game that many veterinarians play with their careers? Will you have to sacrifice family life, income, and free time for your career?

The job search starts with a positive state of mind that comes from thorough preparation.

You are in a job market desperately in need of more veterinarians. At the same time, employers are realizing the true costs of hiring the wrong person. These costs can be up to twice the amount of your first year's salary. Thus, a situation has been created where there are many employers for each candidate, but the employers have become very selective. To get the job that *you* want, you need to present your case well.

During the assessment process it is important to follow all of the steps described below.

Know Yourself

In order for you to be happy with your career, it must match your core values. Core values can include qualities such as integrity, drive for results, client service, and emotional resilience. Refer to the work you did in Chapter Four and from that, identify your core values.

Personality profiles can help in this process, especially the Meyers-Briggs test (which should be administered and read by a professional psychologist). By studying your personality profile, you learn about yourself and your motivations, while also learning about others. Soon you begin relating to people with different personalities more easily, and you become less judgmental.

Table 5-1
ASSESSING YOUR SKILLS

Which of the following statements describe your skills? What others might you add about yourself?

- ❑ I understand and use words well.
- ❑ I do arithmetic quickly and accurately.
- ❑ I see details.
- ❑ I make precise movements quickly.
- ❑ I work well as part of a team.
- ❑ I work independently.
- ❑ I lead others when needed.
- ❑ I handle crisis situations.
- ❑ I take a position and then defend it.
- ❑ I listen to others.
- ❑ I am empathetic to another's plight, yet remain level-headed.
- ❑ I can make a decision.
- ❑ I seek counsel and mentoring when I know my limits are surpassed or I have no experience in that area.
- ❑ I am a self-directed learner.
- ❑ I am a problem-solver.
- ❑ I can manage a project or department (or multiple projects or multiple departments).
- ❑ I communicate well with coworkers and customers.
- ❑ I provide value-added customer service.
- ❑ I continually demonstrate a good work ethic.
- ❑ I share resources.
- ❑ I am honest, trustworthy, and ethical.
- ❑ _____
- ❑ _____
- ❑ _____

KNOW YOUR PRIORITIES

List your priorities for your new job in order and review them. Separate the list into items that are negotiable and those that are nonnegotiable (see Table 5-2). Priorities can include geographical location, commute distance, rural vs. urban environment, demographics of clientele, work schedule, benefits, compensation, continuing education, career development, equity (partnership/ownership), and quality of life. Knowing your priorities is crucial. For example, if you intend to "buy in" to a practice at some point because ownership or equity is important, you should negotiate that up front or you will be building value into a practice that will be more expensive for you to buy into in the future.

DEVELOP AN "OWNERSHIP ATTITUDE"

Consider that you are entering into a long-term relationship that is similar to a marriage. An ownership attitude means that you have carefully selected this job and will be a partner in problem-solving. Because the practice matches your core values and you care about the practice, obstacles do not become barriers. You care about the financial health of the practice as well as about the physical health of its patients. You are concerned about the clients and their education. You are an advocate for the pets or animals you see. You take responsibility for communicating the consequences of not delivering care to each pet. Your "ownership attitude" will land you the job in the practice you have selected and make your compensation negotiation more successful as well.

UNDERSTAND YOUR WORTH

Be able to justify your compensation expectations. Do not mention your student loans, car payments, or mortgage. Potential employers are not interested in your financial woes. Instead, be excited about the hospital's production and how you will *contribute*.

NETWORK CREATIVELY

The more veterinarians you know, the more likely they will introduce you to employers or tell you about job openings. You may even get the chance to interview *before* the job is advertised.

Memberships in your local, state, and national veterinary organizations help, because grassroots networking is the best way for you to find out about open positions. Your colleagues begin to know and trust you and will more readily recommend you for great jobs or offer you a great job themselves.

Don't wait for people to approach you, and don't fear rejection. Remember online organizations like Veterinary Information Network (VIN) and Network of Animal Health (NOAH). For example, there is a VetQuest section on VIN, and most veterinary schools have job boards on their websites. Many hospitals have their own web pages and may list positions available. Internet recruiting and job hunting are expanding rapidly. We discuss where to look for a job in Chapter Six.

PERFORM A PHYSICAL EXAM ON THE PRACTICE

Starting with an open mind allows you to explore opportunities and gather facts before you make a judgment. More options are available to veterinarians now than at any other time in history. Take advantage of the opportunities to select the right situation for *yourself*. Veterinarians are scientists who should use the scientific method in job hunting. Job hunting is really just "diagnosing the right career." Just as you would conduct a physical examination and diagnostics before treating a pet, do a thorough "physical exam" on

Table 5-2
SAMPLE NEGOTIABLE AND NONNEGOTIABLE ITEMS IN YOUR JOB SEARCH

Negotiable Items	Nonnegotiable Items
Geographical location/quality of life	Minimum $40,000 starting compensation
Paid vacation, 2–3 weeks	Some benefits provided—basic medical insurance, reimbursement for personal-liability insurance
Retirement program—participation in a 401(k), Keogh, IRA	Maximum 50-hour work week
Ability to see exotics	Equity/partnership/ownership potential
Registration fees and paid time off for continuing-education meetings	In-house lab, isoflurane anesthesia, automatic processor, reproductive ultrasound
	Paid membership in AVMA and AAHA

Note: Your table may look very different from this sample and may have the categories switched, depending on your individual career and personal needs. Be honest with yourself, and be flexible when you can.

a practice before you join it. Thorough research is needed to gather compensation information, cost-of-living analysis, work schedules, and other pertinent information. Your ideal practice may be different from that of your mentor. It can be difficult to go against what others expect of you, but it is essential for you to choose the right job for *you*, not for someone else.

Think like a detective. Tour a hospital yourself before making a judgment about its quality. This can be a good place to start your research, because hearsay is not always reliable. For example, you may hear a negative blast from a veterinarian who left the practice. When you visit the facility, you may be pleased with the hospital and the team. Their values and standards are more in line with yours, but not with the veterinarian who left.

In another example, a hospital may be advertised as "high-tech," but it fails to comply with state regulations because there is no designated surgical suite and the X-ray unit sits unprotected in the bathroom. Become clear on what your "minimum standards" are for the hospital in which you plan to build your career. Set your standards high, and don't settle for less. Ask to see new client numbers and the practice growth rate in revenues. Know that more revenue equates to better equipment and a higher quality of medicine as well as more compensation for *you*.

UNDERSTAND THE JOB

Setting and having realistic expectations before starting your new position is crucial, because most problems stem from unrealistic expectations that could have been addressed in the beginning. Communicate them before you commit to this employer. Take responsibility for asking questions that may give you the information you need about your position and responsibilities in the practice. The way to rise in your career is to start taking on responsibilities from your supervisor and doing them well.

Have a clear understanding of the employer's expectations regarding client loads, your gross or net production, and what medical and surgical skill levels are required. Not only can this prevent serious disagreements in the future but also it opens lines of communication in the beginning. If you do not feel comfortable working alone for the first three months, you need to state this up front. If you are uncomfortable with certain surgical procedures, it is imperative you let the team know this and hustle to gain experience.

HONE YOUR INTERVIEWING TECHNIQUES

Interviews are valuable sources of information that will help you analyze a potential position. Informational interviews require some preliminary background exploration, organizational preparation, and practiced questioning techniques. Be prompt and on time, whether the interview is via phone or in person. First impressions always count—big time. It may take an enormous effort to overcome a poor first impression.

You are interviewing the practice at the same time the practice is interviewing you; therefore, come well prepared with questions to ask the owner(s) and staff. Appear flexible, and be prepared to communicate your priorities so they appear reasonable. Although you have your list of negotiable and nonnegotiable items, it may be wise to let others do the initial presentations. Wait and evaluate the situation. Be familiar with the market-rate salary range for your position, and outline your strengths and what you will do specifically for this practice to add value. If you are well prepared, you will be more relaxed during the interview. The goal is to discover if you and the practice are a match, not if this is a "good" practice. Practice using personal examples to illustrate your strengths prior to the interview so that they are on the tip of your tongue. We discuss interviewing in more depth in Chapter 8.

RESOURCES

Books

Career Choices for Veterinarians: Beyond Private Practice by C. Smith, DVM.

Do What You Are: Discover the Perfect Career for You Through the Secrets of Personality Type by P. Tieger and B. Barron-Tieger.

Second Acts: Creating the Life You Really Want, Building the Career You Truly Desire by S. Pollan and M. Levine.

What Color Is Your Parachute: A Practical Manual for Job-Hunters and Career-Changers by R. Bolles.

▶ CHAPTER SIX ◀

Searching for a Job

Samuel M. Fassig, DVM, MA

IN THIS CHAPTER, YOU'LL LEARN:

- **The different ways to find a job**
- **How to contact potential employers**

For most of you, finding meaningful employment is new territory. Most newly graduated veterinarians are approaching thirty years of age and have not yet held a full-time job that must pay the bills. Searching for, interviewing for, and selecting a job can be a very scary and nerve-racking process even for the experienced. For new associates, it can be downright terrifying.

There are several basic concepts to keep in mind during the employment-search process. Remember:

- No one owes you a job.

- You can be fired or let go just as easily as you are hired.

- The key to employment and job satisfaction is the fit—your fit to the employer and the employer's fit to you. To really work, this needs to be a symbiotic relationship.

- Avoid burning bridges. Veterinary medicine is a small community. Things do come full circle—sometimes when you least expect it.

- The process may force you to deal or cope with uncomfortable feelings and irritating personalities. How you rise above that will speak volumes about your character. Your character is one of the key elements employers will be evaluating. It is one of the things an employer will ask about when checking your references.

- Employers will evaluate your worth, not by your skills alone, but by your spirit, your attitude, your compassion for others, and your sense of perspective.

- Courtesy, honesty, respectfulness, and truthfulness are essential. Creativity is fine as long as it is not a fabrication, a purposeful misstatement, or a less-than-truthful representation.

THE JOB OF JOB HUNTING

Job hunting is tough work, physically and emotionally. It is also an intellectually demanding effort that requires you to be at your best. The most logical way to manage your time during this process is to keep regular working hours. If you are unemployed, make the job search your regular job. Keeping an activity record of your contacts and the results of those contacts can be a helpful tool as you refine your search. It will facilitate organization and access to telephone numbers and referrals and help you identify the people who need a thank-you note as a follow-up.

Remember—you are creating and projecting an image as you travel through the search process. Just like your outward dress makes a statement about your values and who you are, the way in which you interact with people creates an impression on them as well. As a professional, image is *ever so important*.

Getting started on your job search is the hardest, toughest, nastiest part. It is akin to physical exercise. When you work out, usually the most difficult part is getting up out of the chair or off the bed. Once you've begun, and you start to focus on the routine, it becomes much easier. Your goals become achievable, and the world tends to be a brighter place.

Preparing Yourself Physically and Mentally

The length of time it takes to find a job is totally unpredictable; therefore, you must have a plan and be mentally and physically prepared for whatever it takes to land that job.

The longer it takes you to find meaningful employment ("meaningful" denoted as having a sense of personal value and fulfillment for you), the more you risk becoming disenfranchised, down-hearted, and depressed and having feelings of powerlessness, abandonment, hopelessness, and anger. After all, you studied hard for four years of veterinary school, and now nobody seems to want to offer you decent employment. There are all kinds of pressures on you to be successful in your employment quest, especially if you have not been as lucky as your classmates in getting offers.

Many students (about 80% of the graduating class) will have committed to a job by the time commencement arrives. The remaining students will need to work hard at keeping a positive outlook

> Getting started on your job search is the hardest, toughest, nastiest part. It is akin to physical exercise. When you work out, usually the most difficult part is getting up out of the chair or off the bed.

while they hunt for work. Here are some suggestions for staying on track during this potentially difficult time.

- Stay physically fit. If you are not fit, make this one of your goals. Be active outdoors and commit to some form of realistic self-improvement.

- If you start an angry internal dialogue, such as, "Why have they done this to me?" or "God, why are you letting this happen to me?", find someone to talk with, write it all down in a letter to yourself (which you can destroy), or find a good therapist. If you are spiritual and believe in God or a higher power, there is a point where it is important to realize God does not create these misfortunes in your life. If you find yourself in this unhealthy mindset, make healing your spirit another goal for this time period.

- Set several goals to work on during your period of unemployment. Sure, securing a job is number one. Create several more goals that are achievable. This relieves some pressure and gives you permission to be a person. Such goals might include going to the gym every day or riding your bike ten miles three times a week, reading a book a week, volunteering at a homeless shelter (for people *or* animals), or taking a class in computer skills.

WAYS TO FIND JOBS

There are a number of sources for obtaining employment information and jobs.

Direct Contact

Direct contact encompasses the cold call in person, via email, or by phone with the practice owner or manager, hoping it will turn into an informational interview. An informational interview is not the same as a job interview—in fact, it is a highly focused conversation with someone in your field that provides you with key information about your chosen career. See the list of resources at the end of this chapter for more information.

Networking

Networking involves letting people know you are available and looking for a job. According to human-resource researchers, more than 86% of all jobs are found through networking. The more veterinarians you know, the more likely they will introduce you to employers or jobs available. Join your local, state, and national veterinary organizations. Grassroots networking is the best way for you to find out about available positions. Thank everyone who has given you a lead with a timely, personalized, handwritten thank-you note.

> According to human-resource researchers, more than 86% of all jobs are found through networking.

Make it a point to attend professional events. While you are there, apply some basic fundamentals of networking:

- Set a goal for the number of personal contacts you want to make.

- Be conscientious. Spend at least half of your time in conversation with people you do not know. Maintain a positive, cordial, approachable attitude and have a genuine smile on your face. Introduce yourself.

- Be ready with a thirty- to forty-five-second, well-rehearsed infomercial about yourself.

- When you engage another person, listen and find out about him or her before you talk about yourself. Develop a rapport in areas of mutual interest.

- Write yourself notes on the back of the business cards of people you meet so that you can write follow-up notes to them later. Do this discreetly, immediately after the conversation is completed and the person moves on.

- Try to arrive at the meetings early. Stand near the entrance doors at the beginning and end of the event, and wear your name tag on your right side.

- The object is to have fun, meet new people, and be open to perspectives you might not have considered before. All the while, you are projecting the image you want the world to see.

While attending professional meetings and events is usually a highly productive endeavor, there can be a down side if you are not on good behavior and do not arrive with your purpose foremost in your mind. You may be guilty of image-busters, which include the following:

- Do not use profanity or "put-down" humor, especially at someone else's expense.

- Do not drink. If you must, set a limit and never drink too much.

- Do not monopolize any one person's time.

- Dress appropriately for the occasion.

- Do not complain or whine about your current situation or speak badly of anyone.

- Do not prejudge people by their job title.

- Never give a hard sell.

- If you promise it, deliver. Never promise something, then fail to follow through.

- Do not get too personal. Do not volunteer too much personal information about yourself or pry into someone else's life. Keep it light, professional, and cordial.

- Remember your manners. This is the time to exude subtle charm.

You also might use the AVMA directory, AAHA directory, local VMA directories, pharmaceutical-company sales agents, and distributor representatives to locate potential employers. These are excellent networking resources for finding individuals who are working in areas of veterinary medicine that interest you. Once identified, contact them to learn more about what they do. When the opportunity arises, ask how you might get hired for a job in the same area of focus. There are many excellent resources for networking protocols listed at the end of this chapter.

61

Help-Wanted Ads

Even in professional journals, help-wanted ads are often stale leads as well as fishing expeditions by employers who want to see what is out there. Less than 3% of jobs are filled via want ads, although the percentage is somewhat higher when the ads are in professional trade publications.

Employment Services

In general, employment services work for employers, not for you. If you have to pay a fee for their services, consider avoiding that company. Positions listed and filled by these agencies should be employer-fee-paid at no cost to you.

Alumni Placement Offices

Alumni placement offices serve as clearinghouses for interested companies. Remember—college professors may also have leads.

Professional Associations

Many professional associations have placement services. Sometimes these organizations have more information regarding a position than is in print. Many also offer posting boards, either at meetings or online, where you can post a message that you are looking for a job. Be brief when posting. You want to be contacted—not screened out.

Online Databases (Electronic Internet Listings)

Professional associations often link to universities and to related state and local sites. Companies may also use website links to post application forms, position descriptions, and requirements. If you apply electronically, the screening agent will see only one dimension. There is usually no opportunity to ask questions or learn more about the position. However, sometimes the service gives the name of the person to contact or the name of the department, especially for government agencies. Applying online may also mean you must have a rich text or text-only version of your resume and cover letter to send.

Visit the VetQuest section on VIN and veterinary schools' job-posting boards on their websites. Many hospitals have their own web pages and may list available positions. Internet recruiting and job hunting are rapidly expanding businesses. A short list of job sites is included at the end of this chapter. There are dozens, if not hundreds, of others that you will find if you type "veterinary jobs" into an internet search engine.

CALLING ABOUT JOB OPENINGS

How to Make the Call

For people who have something other than naturally outgoing "bubbly" personalities, making phone calls to strangers and then asking questions may be frightening. This is especially true of a cold call to a "bigwig" who has advertised an employment position.

Speaking on the phone ranks second only to public speaking as the most common phobia in business communications; don't think you're alone. You have a fear of the unknown, and you experience panic and emotional anxiety due to your investment in the outcome of the call—before it ever takes place. On the whole, it is self-inflicted pressure, including fear of rejection and movement into a zone of discomfort and the unfamiliar.

The worst that can really happen when you inquire about a position that has been advertised is that the other person will say "no" and hang up or ask you to call back later. There is very little physical danger in either of those scenarios. It is important to learn from your experiences and move on. The first few phone experiences may make you feel like you are jumping off a rock overhang into a pool of dark water. There is hesitation. You have

> Speaking on the phone ranks second only to public speaking as the most common phobia in business communications; don't think you're alone.

an idea what it will feel like and what will happen, but you also know that the reality may be shockingly different from what you've imagined. The water might be cold, but you don't know *how* cold until you actually fall in and your head gets wet. Your nervous energy rises. When you make that call, either you will talk so fast that people on the other end of the phone will have trouble understanding you or you will clam up and end the conversation before you find out all that you need to know. What a way to begin the process of trying to get a job. Good news! Practice, mistakes, and trial and error will help all that go away.

If you are apprehensive, here are some ideas to help make your calls successful:

- Always be polite and patient. If you do not get the information you want this time, you can call back. If the contact person is not available or cannot talk at this time, ask when it would be a good time for you to call back. Then, be sure that you keep your word and call back at the appointed time. Even if the party cannot talk then, this person will remember that you were diligent enough to keep your word.

- Stay focused. Know what you want and how you will ask for it before you call. Write it down and have a pad and pencil in front of you to take notes.

- Have a goal for the call. Be realistic about what you can accomplish with each call.

- If the employment opportunity has been advertised, ask to speak to someone who can tell you about the position.

- Always write, email, fax, or mail a thank-you card or note. Be sure to thank the person for taking the time to talk to you.

- What if you get an answering machine? Leave your name and number and a message as to why you called. If you say you will call back on Tuesday, keep the date and make the call.

The Phone Conversation

The primary goal of the phone call is to get an interview. Here are some tips and examples that will help you through the phone conversation.

Sample Dialogue

1. The phone rings and is answered. Say "hello" and acknowledge (also note on your pad) the name of the person with whom you are speaking. *"Hello, my name is Dr. Max Stone. What is your name please? Thanks, _____."*

2. Tell why you are calling and with whom you wish to speak. If you are conducting a follow-up call, briefly explain the previous conversation.

   "I am calling about the veterinary associate position that Dr. Joe Arlington advertised in the Texas VMA newsletter. Is he available to briefly discuss the position?" (If the person says no, ask when it would be a good time to call back.)

   Or

   "I saw the advertisement for the veterinary associate position on the Texas A&M website. Is there someone at the hospital who could tell me more about the position? Good. What is the name of that person? And the phone number? Let me make sure I am spelling his (or her) name right. Does he (or she) have an email address? Is he (or she) available now? Can you please connect me?"

3. If you were referred by someone, indicate very early in the conversation the name of the person who suggested you call.

   "Hello, my name is Dr. Max Stone. Dr. Sharon Moen suggested I call Dr. Arlington. Is he available at this time? Is there a better time to call him?" If the receptionist asks why you are calling, say: *"Dr. Moen has referred me to Dr. Arlington about a personal matter. Can I set up a time to visit with him?"*

4. In some cases a receptionist or secretary will try to screen your call and ask you to simply send your resume. Get the key individual's name because you want to send your materials to a real person in charge of the search process. Thank them. Then, call back later. Ask for the key person by name.

5. If you have applied previously, assess the status of your candidacy, confirm if your fax, email, or

mailed materials were received, and identify the next steps in the selection process. Take a polite but assertive approach. Now is the time to request a job interview or an informational interview. If you are not speaking to the person who can make that appointment for you, ask this person for suggestions regarding the next steps, or ask to speak to the person who can schedule an appointment for you with the key person.

"Recently, after speaking with Dr. Arlington, I emailed a letter of interest and my resume to him. Would it be possible to briefly speak to Dr. Arlington? I would like to confirm that my resume was received and that he was able to open the attachments okay." (Also either ask Dr. Arlington for an appointment or tell the person on the phone, *"I would also like to schedule an appointment with Dr. Arlington."*)

Requests for an appointment for an employment interview or informational conversation can also be in this type of format:

"Yes, I understand that final candidate-selection decisions regarding formal interviews will not be made for several weeks. In the meantime, could you refer me to one of the other associates currently working in the clinic? I would like to informally learn a little more about what it is like to work there and ask some questions about their experiences. Who would you suggest I speak with? Is she available so I can make an appointment?"

6. Always thank the person with whom you are speaking. Confirm the spelling of names and the correctness of phone and fax numbers and email addresses. Thank the person for his or her time.

"Thank you so much, _____ (person's name—remember, you wrote it down). You have been quite accommodating. If I have any further questions, is it all right to call you, or is there someone else I should ask for? Thank you again, _____ (person's name), for taking the time from your busy day to help me. I really appreciate it. Have a great afternoon. Good-bye."

Asking for the Interview

You must ask for the interview. It may take several times. Here is a sample conversation used to overcome initial rejections that you can modify to fit your tastes. It may not work every time, and you may not want to use it every time. However, practice it a few times and keep it in your tool kit:

You: *"Dr. Arlington, thank you for visiting with me on the phone today about your hospital. I would really like to learn more about how one could become an associate on your staff. Would it be possible to come in and interview or visit with you in person?"*

Employer: *"As I said, I really do not have any positions open now."*

You: *"That's okay. I would still like to come in to talk with you about the possibility of future openings."*

Employer: *"I really don't plan to hire anyone within the next six months or so."*

You: *"If it would be all right, I would still like to come in to your hospital and observe you and your staff on a typical day. Your practice sounds so forward-thinking and in touch with your clients. I would really like to see how a progressive practice flows. I am looking for ideas on how to join such a practice and growing my career in such a setting. Is there some arrangement we could make?"*

If the person agrees to your coming in (remember the goal was an interview), arrange a specific date and time. In this case, wear attire appropriate for the work setting (no jeans, no sneakers). Wear a professional smock with your name on it (or name tag). Prepare for this meeting just like you would for a formal interview, and be professional. Mingle, meet the staff, and approach the situation as if you *were* being interviewed, because in a sense, you are.

When an Interview Does Not Make Sense

There will be times when your better judgment tells you not to ask for an interview at this time. Perhaps the person is not helpful, you may have caught the person at a bad time, or you got a mixed message during the phone conversation. If so, take a different approach.

- **Ask for a referral**—Inquire if the person knows the names of others who might be able to help you. Find out how to contact them. Ask permission if you can use this person's name as a means of introduction. (Never name drop without permission.)

- **Ask to call at a later time and get an appointment**—Perhaps the contact is busy right now. Ask if it is okay for you to call back. Get a specific time and day. Put it on your calendar, and be sure to make the call.

- **Ask to keep in touch**—Ask your contact if you could call back from time to time in case the employer hears of an opening, or if additional information has surfaced that could be helpful.

- **Write thank-you notes**—Besides good manners, this is the tried and true method for people to remember you. Thank them for their time in talking with you. If they gave you a referral, let them know how it came out. If they gave you a suggestion, send a note that you appreciated it and how you followed up on it. Be brief. Handwritten notes are best, and penmanship counts.

SELF-ANALYSIS

Other chapters of this book address personal vision, goals, and career development, which are important elements to consider and keep in mind when you are searching for a job. After all, you are looking for a fit. All career counselors will tell you, and rightly so, that the search and interview process is a selling effort. You are selling yourself and what you bring to the business.

One other key element that you might want to consider while searching the job pool, besides stating what you can do for the practice, is what the practice will do for you. Sometimes there will be clear answers and obvious choices. Then again, because it is too easy to focus on key items during the job search, you might miss the overall picture. To get a broader view, ask, "Will I be happy working in this particular business for the short term? For the long term? Will it meet my needs?" If the answer is "yes," keep it on your list of possibilities. If the answer is "no," be prepared

to cross it off and move on. Before you do this, ask yourself, "Do I need more information? Have I tested my assumptions?" Make the effort to get appropriate information before you discard a potential opportunity completely. Revisit the practice if necessary. That way you can avoid second-guessing and asking the "what if" questions regarding your choice. With clarity comes peace of mind.

RESOURCES

Books

A Foot in the Door: Networking Your Way into the Hidden Job Market by K. Hansen.
Job Hunting for Dummies by M. Messmer.
Masters of Networking by I. Misner and D. Morgan.
101 Ways To Get From Here To There by N. Feingold and M. Feingold.
Power Networking: 59 Secrets for Personal and Professional Success by D. Fisher.
10 Insider Secrets to Job Hunting Success! Everything You Need to Get the Job You Want in 24 Hours—Or Less! by T. Bermont.
What Color Is Your Parachute?, 2004: A Practical Manual for Job-Hunters & Career-Changers by R. Bolles.

Websites

AAHA Job Bank
www.aahanet.org
Click on Job Bank to see ads placed by veterinary practices across the United States and Canada. Also click on Online Classifieds to see ads placed in *Trends* magazine.

AVMA Career Center
www.avmaorg/vcc/default.asp
Search jobs, post a resume, and sign up for email notification of new jobs.

Monster Jobsite
www.monster.com
View all types of veterinary jobs, including those in industry.

Veterinary Information Network Classifieds
www.vetquest.com/classifieds/
Free access to posted jobs.

CHAPTER SEVEN

Resumes, Cover Letters, and References

Samuel M. Fassig, DVM, MA

> **IN THIS CHAPTER, YOU'LL LEARN:**
>
> - How to construct a good resume
> - What type of resume is best for you
> - The importance of a cover letter and what it should include

RESUMES

What Is a Resume?

A resume is a one- or two-page synopsis of your skills, background, training, experience, accomplishments, and education created to grab a prospective employer's interest. It is your image-marketing tool, designed to get you an interview. A poorly constructed resume will cause a potential employer to sort you out, regardless of your talent or capabilities. And remember—a resume is not an autobiography or a place to report your every experience. It is a written report of your qualifications related to a specific position. Keep it brief and to the point.

A resume is used when you apply for a new job, because it:

- Communicates your experience and skills

- Shows your education related to a specific position

- Reflects your interest in specific aspects of the job or areas of expertise

- Provides insights into your leadership talents and capacity for assuming responsibility

How Long Should a Resume Be?

Your resume should be as long as it needs to be. Today's guideline is that a resume should be long enough to entice the person who is sorting or making hiring decisions to call you for a job interview.

The simple rule is that a maximum of two pages covers the last ten years of experience. Three pages are permissible in the rare case where the employer has specifically asked you for a detailed resume, or you apply for a senior position and have more than ten years of relevant experience.

Volumes of "how-to" texts have been written on this subject, and many of the best are listed at the end of this chapter. This chapter will cover the basics, but we encourage you to read other references as well.

Pointers for Constructing a Good Resume

USING SELF-HELP TEXTS

When you use a self-help, how-to text regarding resume construction, use one that is less than five years old. Although many timeless techniques are still valid, we have entered the age of scanned, emailed, and faxed resumes that might make an older book outdated.

MAKING YOUR RESUME APPROPRIATE TO THE POSITION

When you begin to compile information for your resume, keep in mind that this is *your* document. You can do anything with it that you think is appropriate for the position you want. Employers usually want to see how qualified you are and how you convey your specific qualifications in writing.

MAKING YOUR RESUME EASY TO UNDERSTAND

Be persuasive, clear, and truthful. Remember, you are trying to sell yourself and your abilities. Make your resume easy to understand so that the reader will not struggle to find pertinent information. Make no assumptions, such as, "Well, they should know that if I did 'x,' that means I also can do 'y.'" Spell it out in simple, concise terms with adjectives, verbs, numbers, and adverbs to reinforce the pertinent points.

CUSTOMIZING YOUR RESUME

When it comes to your resume, the "one-size-fits-all" approach doesn't work. It is very important to tailor your information to fit a particular position with a particular employer at a particular time. When you lose that opportunity, such as with an online job application, the return rate (reply) is considerably lower than when the material is customized to an employer. Certainly, some parts of the resume will fit any employer. However, the more tailored your resume is for a specific employer, the more you are able to demonstrate key points that mesh with her requirements and needs.

> When it comes to your resume, the "one-size-fits-all" approach doesn't work. It is very important to tailor your information to fit a particular position with a particular employer at a particular time.

Customizing your resume for a specific audience or reader helps you personalize the document and make it relevant to that reader. If you do not have a specific target in mind, the document might be too general or vague or may include too much information. Tailoring your resume allows it to have a better agreement of purpose and style and makes the reader feel more involved.

Understanding the Two Basic Types of Readers

You should tailor your resume to the two basic types of readers—skimmers and cynics.

SKIMMERS

These are the readers who are usually pressed for time. They glance over the document, speed-reading for key words or phrases, numbers, and highlights. To help this kind of reader, state the main point clearly up front. Place the most important information in the first and last sentences of a paragraph. Highlight key dates or figures. Skimmers prefer bulleted points, plenty of white space surrounding concise text, and crisp, easy-to-read fonts.

CYNICS

These readers are the disbelievers—the skeptics who are cautious and doubtful. They tend to read a document carefully, questioning validity, truthfulness, and, ultimately, the writer's claims. They also tend to be sensitive to a writer's sincerity. To satisfy a cynic, it is necessary to support your statements with sufficient detail and evidence. They prefer specific examples, dates, numbers, names, and percentages.

Example

Instead of saying: "I performed near the top of my class."

State: "On the Dean's list for 11 of 13 quarters, with a GPA of 3.89 upon graduation; I was ranked seventh overall in a class of 92 graduating veterinary students."

Making Sure Your Resume Has a Professional Appearance

Very small print is extremely challenging to read. Use clear, easy-to-read font sizes and styles. Check for typing mistakes, grammatical errors, and misspellings, as well as smudges, food stains, and stray marks. Use the spell check function on your computer frequently. Have a friend read a draft to find mistakes you might have missed and to see if the text flows. Make revisions and repeat the process as many times as necessary. Let the resume sit overnight, then revisit it. Does it still say what you want it to say? Does it look professional?

When you think your resume is ready, get a friend (if possible, someone who works in advertising or who was an English major) to critically review your grammar, punctuation, and overall usage of terms. Ask another friend to proofread. The more people who see your resume, the more likely your misspelled words and awkward phrases will be corrected.

These tips will make your resume easier to read or to scan into an employer's database.

- Use white or off-white 8½ x 11-inch, high-quality paper.

- Print on one side of the paper.

- Use a font size of 10 to 14 points.

- Use nondecorative typefaces.

- Choose one typeface and stick to it.

- Avoid italics, script, and underlined words.

- Do not use graphics or shading, and minimize horizontal and vertical lines.

- Do not fold or staple your resume.

- If you must mail your resume, put it in a large envelope so that you don't have to fold it.

Understanding a Resume Versus a Curriculum Vitae

The person who reads your resume is looking for a quick summary of what you have done, but only in just enough detail to get an idea of the extent of your skills and a hint of your background and training. Everything else will surface in the interview.

Usually you are being screened to be sorted out or excluded. To make the "included" pile, your key search criteria must be clearly evident and be quickly visible to the eye.

A curriculum vitae, more often than not, is reserved for academic pursuits. It is for employers who want an expanded view of everything. They want to know what you have studied, written about, taught, researched, exhibited, demonstrated, published, and projected to your peers, colleagues, and the profession. They want to know what awards and honors have been bestowed upon you, by whom, and for what reasons. They are also looking for leadership traits, contributions, and roles played that would distinguish you from your peers. It is a way to see how you stack up (on paper) against others in your field.

Unless you are applying for a job in academia or research, the curriculum vitae will be something you probably don't need to worry about to get your first job. However, it is always a good idea to keep a running log in a file somewhere of all the dates, times, projects, and subject matter in which you have had a hand in writing, presenting, or assessing, in case you do need this information for some future use.

It is also good practice to apply this same strategy for logging continuing-education courses. You may need this information for licensing and for future resume development.

Drawing Attention Away From Lack of Experience

If you do not have a considerable amount of applicable work experience pertaining to veterinary medicine as a clinician, consider listing your education and relevant courses taken, work-study experience, and special projects near the top. Also include focused areas of interest with any special programs attended, certifications, or assistance you have given as part of a project being conducted by a faculty member. This is the place where you can showcase or highlight other experiences you know the employer is looking for. When your work history is weak, include internships, class projects, independent study programs, summer clinic jobs, and any work you did on investigator grants to show your experience.

Table 7-1
WORDS AND PHRASES THAT CAN MAKE YOUR RESUME STAND OUT

Designed, developed, and delivered

Conducted a needs analysis

Consult and counsel clients about grief, loss, and the human-animal bond

Write client take-home instructions and handouts

Revamped staff training program

Designed and implemented

Facilitate problem-solving meetings

Facilitated discussion

Managed a five-person team

Coordinated scheduling for six other students on work study

Assisted director of Veterinary Teaching Hospital with the AAHA-accreditation site visit

Proctored and scored freshman anatomy lab practical exam as an instructor assistant

Assessed student needs and presented findings to faculty council

Chair of SCAVMA Pet Week program

Assisted the Dean's office with coordinating off-campus events

Represented the College of Veterinary Medicine at . . . .

Implemented student lounge improvement program

Oversaw use of grant funds to purchase new equipment

Managed the veterinary student bookstore—ordered textbooks and supplies in timely manner, recruited and managed staff, prepared financial reports for review with the Dean . . . .

Enlisted the support . . .

Formed a committee . . .

Sold, budgeted, improved, increased, maintained . . .

Using Action Verbs and Phrases

Table 7-1 presents a summary of some sample words and phrases that will help make your resume stand out, and Table 7-2 lists action verbs that can make your resume "pop." Use these words to help project energy and ability into your resume and cover letter.

Being Specific

It is important to use dates and to tailor your objectives to a given position. Demonstrate relationships between a skill and a particular position,

or leave it out. Note how example 2 achieves the objective of linking skills to the position, while example 1 does not.

Example 1

2001–2002 work-study. Supervisor Professor Roger P. Allen. Veterinary Teaching Hospital. Helped with dogs in clinical study.

Example 2

September 2001–May 2002. While on work-study, assisted Professor Roger P. Allen,

Note: Text continues on page 74 following Table 7-2.

Table 7-2
ACTION VERBS TO MAKE YOUR RESUME POP

A

accelerated	addressed	anticipated	assembled
accompanied	administered	applied	assessed
accomplished	advanced	appraised	assigned
achieved	advised	approached	assisted
acquired	advocated	arbitrated	attained
acted	aided	arranged	attracted
activated	amplified	ascertained	augmented
adapted	analyzed	asked	authored
added	answered		

B

| balanced | broadened | buffered | |
| bargained | budgeted | built | |

C

calculated	changed	collected	contributed
canvassed	channeled	combined	convinced
captured	checked	composed	coordinated
carried out	choreographed	compressed	corresponded
cataloged	circulated	computed	counseled
catheterized	clarified	conceived	counted
centralized	classified	conceptualized	created
chaired	coauthored	conducted	cultivated
challenged	collaborated	constructed	

D

debated	delivered	devised	distinguished
debugged	demonstrated	diagrammed	distributed
decided	described	directed	diversified
decreased	designed	discounted	documented
defined	determined	discovered	doubled
delegated	developed	displayed	drafted

E

earned	encouraged	established	expanded
edited	engaged	evaluated	explained
effected	engineered	examined	exposed
elected	enhanced	exceeded	extended
eliminated	enriched	exchanged	extracted
employed	entered	executed	extrapolated
enabled	equalized	exercised	

Table 7-2 (continued)
ACTION VERBS TO MAKE YOUR RESUME POP

F

facilitated	fit	formed	framed
familiarized	focused	formulated	fulfilled
fashioned	forecasted	fortified	functioned
fielded	formalized	founded	furnished
figured			

G

gained	gave	governed	greeted
gathered	generated	graded	grouped
gauged	gentled	granted	guided

H

handled	held	hosted	
headed	hired		

I

identified	induced	instilled	intubated
illuminated	influenced	instituted	invented
illustrated	informed	instructed	inventoried
implemented	initiated	insured	inverted
improved	innovated	integrated	investigated
improvised	inquired	interfaced	invited
inaugurated	inspected	interpreted	involved
increased	inspired	interviewed	isolated
incurred	installed	introduced	issued
indexed	instigated		

J

joined	judged	justified	

L

launched	led	lobbied	located
lectured	lightened	localized	

M

maintained	measured	minimized	monitored
managed	mediated	modeled	motivated
mapped	merchandised	moderated	moved
marketed	merged	modernized	multiplied
maximized	met	modified	

N

narrated	negotiated	noticed	nurtured

Table 7-2 (continued)
ACTION VERBS TO MAKE YOUR RESUME POP

O

observed	opened	ordered	originated
obtained	operated	organized	overhauled
offered	orchestrated	oriented	oversaw
offset			

P

perceived	polled	prioritized	promoted
performed	prepared	probed	prompted
persuaded	presented	processed	proposed
phased out	preserved	procured	proved
pinpointed	presided	produced	provided
pioneered	prevented	profiled	publicized
placed	priced	programmed	published
planned	printed	projected	purchased

Q

qualified	quantified	quoted

R

raised	rectified	renegotiated	restored
ranked	redesigned	renewed	restructured
rated	reduced	reorganized	revamped
reacted	referred	repaired	revealed
read	refined	replaced	reversed
received	regulated	reported	reviewed
recommended	rehabilitated	represented	revised
reconciled	reinforced	requested	revitalized
recorded	rejected	researched	rewarded
recovered	related	resolved	routed
recruited	remodeled	responded	

S

safeguarded	shaped	staffed	substituted
salvaged	shortened	staged	suggested
saved	showed	standardized	summarized
scheduled	shrank	steered	superseded
screened	signed	stimulated	supervised
secured	simplified	strategized	supplied
segmented	sold	streamlined	supported
selected	solved	strengthened	surpassed
sent	spearheaded	stressed	surveyed
separated	specified	structured	synchronized
served	speculated	submitted	synthesized
serviced	spoke	substantiated	systematized
settled	stabilized		

Table 7-2 (continued)
ACTION VERBS TO MAKE YOUR RESUME POP

T

tabulated	tested	trained	transported
tailored	testified	transformed	traveled
targeted	tightened	translated	treated
taught	traced	transmitted	tripled
terminated	traded		

U

uncovered	unified	updated	upgraded
undertook	united		

V

validated	verified	viewed	

W

weighed	widened	won	wrote
welcomed	witnessed	worked	

chair, endocrinology, OSU College of Veterinary Medicine, in research study of female poodles with Addison's disease. Was responsible for collecting blood samples weekly from colony of 38 dogs and tabulating results of their blood chemistries, focusing especially on liver enzyme levels and serum electrolytes. Was also responsible for weighing food and charting medications given each day, performing complete physical exams on each of these animals monthly, and administering Percorten-V® at frequencies determined by study protocol.

Avoiding Optional and Personal Information

Do not send optional items such as transcripts, letters of recommendation, copies of awards and citations, or examples of your work unless you are specifically asked to do so. Bring this supplemental material with you to the interview if you want to use it to demonstrate a point during the conversation.

Personal information (age, race, family, hobbies, marital status, children, physical description, or outside sports activities) does not belong on a resume for use in the United States. The exception might be if an aspect pertains directly to your experience in veterinary medicine.

Example

"As a breeder of AKC Champion Brittany spaniels, I have studied artificial insemination in dogs in depth. I applied my knowledge and skills, in concert with Robert T. Kline, DVM, to produce two field-trial champions in the past three years through these techniques."

ELEMENTS OF THE RESUME

Employers take about thirty to forty seconds to look at a one-page resume before deciding to keep it or discard it. Human-resource professionals may take only fifteen seconds to decide if you make it to the "maybe" pile of prospects. To get past that initial screening, you should design your resume and place the copy so that employers can read the document easily and process the information quickly.

If you conform to a more conventional style, employers are conditioned to look for certain information in certain places. They also read from left to right and top to bottom. Think of your document as being sectioned into four equal quadrants. Creating a document that is balanced (equal text and white space) in each of the four quadrants will ensure ease of eye movement and about the same amount of time spent in each section. Because the reader usually starts in the upper left-hand quadrant, this is where you should place your most important information or anything the reader needs to see first.

In order to write an effective resume, you must take the time to make a self-assessment. Collect, identify, and write down all of your personal data, skills, attributes, and experiences. Don't worry about order or the final format at this stage. Your main intention is to identify relevant information and accomplishments. Gather sample job descriptions that pertain to the position you want to apply for, especially if the employer is not able to provide one. See where your strengths match up. Hone the list to create as many corresponding items as possible. Once you have determined what to include on your resume, it will be easier to choose a format that best highlights your relevant skills and experiences.

The information you will need is:

- Career or job objective/professional objective
- Education
- Work experience
- Interests (pertinent to the position only)
- Activities (pertinent to the position only)
- Awards and honors
- References

Contact Information

All resumes should include contact information either in the header or upper-left quadrant unless they are being posted on a website.

Example for a Senior Veterinary Student

Mariana Delgatto

After 5/28/2003	Before 5/26/2003
12434 East Broadway Avenue	673 North Oval Drive #2A
Union, New Jersey 07083	Columbus, Ohio 98765
Phone: (908) 629-8844	Phone: (304) 788-9534
Email: MJDelg@hotmail.com	Email: MJDelg@hotmail.com

Example for a Graduate Veterinarian

Mariana Delgatto, DVM

12434 East Broadway
Union, New Jersey 07083
Home Phone: (908) 629-8844
Mobile: (823) 989-6673
Fax: (980) 629-8812
Email: MJDelg@hotmail.com

Objective

There are conflicting opinions as to whether or not an objective is necessary and professional. Objectives are considered by some to be acceptable only when you are young and/or inexperienced. Others think an objective clarifies what kind of job you're looking for. But this can also be done by listing the target position at the top of your resume. For example, you could have your name at the top left of the resume and Associate Veterinarian at the top right.

This section is designed to give the employer an idea or brief glimpse of your qualifications and how your skills will benefit the company. Avoid telling employers what they can do for you. Demonstrate what you can do for them. The best objective statement is one that emphasizes your qualifications and goals while appealing to the employer's expectations.

Example

Not this: "I seek a position where I can gain experience in veterinary dentistry."

This: "Seeking an associate clinical position in which I can contribute my background in the research of canine periodontal disease, advance my skills in veterinary dentistry,

75

promote client education, and work toward reaching diplomate status with the American Board of Veterinary Practitioners.

This is *not* the place for a flowery or overused general statement like: "I am seeking a challenging and responsible position enabling me to contribute to the goals of the business while offering me an opportunity for growth and advancement and promoting the development of new technologies in veterinary medicine and honoring the human-animal bond." All a statement like this does is waste space. Rather, since you are on a career track as a new professional, consider replacing the objective statement with a professional goal or tagline that says what you want and what you bring to the practice.

Example

Professional goal: A position as a veterinary associate in a progressive practice where I can use my business background and training as a computer programmer to successfully manage the business aspects of a progressive veterinary practice.

Education

Employers are not interested in details of your primary schools. If you are given an application form, list your high school (date of graduation, city, and state). Have copies of college diplomas and transcripts, as well as your state license, available in case you need to present them during the interview. Most practitioners do not want transcripts. They are more focused on trying to determine if you can do the work—not how well you took a test.

The education section of your resume will usually contain (with most recent data first):

- Name of college, dates of attendance (GPA may or may not be needed—if lower, consider leaving it out unless specifically asked for)

- Related applicable coursework, special projects, and academic awards

- Professional or occupational qualifications

- Advanced academic courses postgraduation, including certifications; you may want to consider including focused continuing-education wet labs if they directly pertain to proficiency

- Training courses

- Military service schools, rank, and leadership roles

- Include your degree(s) (BS, BA, MS, MA, DVM, MPH, MBA, JD, etc.), your major, the institution attended, and your minor or concentration if it relates to the job

New graduates without much work experience should list their educational information first. But if you have work experience that directly relates to the job specifics, list it first.

Examples

The Ohio State University
Doctor of Veterinary Medicine: May 2002
GPA (4.0 scale): 3.67

Or

Washington State University
Bachelor of Science: May 1998
Major: Animal Science
Minor: Computer Applications in Industry
GPA (6.0 scale): Major 5.6; Overall 5.27

JOB-RELATED COURSES

If you are a student or new graduate, there may be times when you want to emphasize certain aspects of your college training by listing course names (not catalog numbers) that may be particularly beneficial to the position for which you are applying. List those courses apart from the crowd (not English 101 or Introduction to Sociology, which are courses everyone must take).

Examples

Statistics (4 quarters)
Technical Writing
Molecular Biology
Plant Physiology
Environmental Engineering
    (6 semester credit hours)
Individual Studies—Animal Nutrition
    (2 semesters)

Work Experience or Career History

List all jobs held—full- or part-time, paid or unpaid. It is usually preferable to list your most recent job *first*, then work backward. For each job, identify the skills you used or learned. Indicate the level of responsibility and if you supervised anyone.

In reality, the past four years of veterinary school have been your primary employment. If you worked on grant programs, completed a work-study program, or were employed during college, consider listing them, especially if they can add a positive dimension to your overall impression on the employer. Be mindful that a potential employer may talk to past employers; therefore, be sure you have a general idea if the former employer would speak highly of you. Lapses in employment may not be as critical just after graduation as they will be if you have been out of school for four to five years and have gaps in your work history.

Employment information usually includes:

- Dates of employment for each company and each position within a company

- Employers' city and state

- Job title

- Your key tasks and responsibilities

- Accomplishment statements (see page 78)

This is the most complex section of the resume. You have a great deal of freedom in how you choose to present the information. Keep it easy to read and applicable to the position.

As you develop the descriptions, try to see your experiences as a professional would. Which is the more professional description?

This: Answered telephones

Or this: Served as a liaison between clients and the four veterinary clinicians

Employers say they are impressed by job candidates who have excellent communication skills, good grooming habits, and relevant work experience. Veterinary businesses indicate they want trustworthy new hires that can move right in, get along with their coworkers, and get the job done without having to be babied at each step. As you start to assemble your resume, remember to address, by example, the top ten qualities employers seek (see Table 7-3).

Table 7-3
TOP TEN QUALITIES EMPLOYERS SEEK

Self-confidence

Communication skills
(verbal and written)

Interpersonal skills
(relates well to others)

Teamwork skills
(works well with others)

Honesty/Integrity

Motivation/Initiative

Strong work ethic

Analytical skills

Flexibility/Adaptability

Computer skills

IDENTIFYING YOUR SKILLS

"Skill" is defined as the ability to use your knowledge effectively and readily in the execution of learned tasks, especially as a result of experience. It is the learned power of doing something competently. Most skills are transferable to other work settings and can be grouped in many ways. There are two types of skills that employers look for:

- Functional or technical skills in working with people, data or information, and things or objects

- Intellectual, attitudinal, creative, leadership, and problem-solving skills (also known as "soft skills")

TECHNICAL SKILLS

Sometimes termed "hard skills," these demonstrate your ability or knowledge base. They describe what you can do; for example, computer languages, years of management experience, and tools utilized. When you mention an element of a job, such as, "Supervised three other students,"

77

ask yourself what you could have learned by doing this and what skills you developed.

SOFT SKILLS

Soft skills are conveyed as a result of your accomplishments, such as leadership, communication, and interpersonal skills. Soft skills are best illustrated when transformed into accomplishment statements (see below).

Assessing and identifying your skills is the most time-consuming part of preparing your resume—it is also the most essential. It is a key preparatory phase for the interview. Putting what you know about yourself down on paper will heighten your awareness and help you quickly recall important information about yourself during an interview. It will be the basis upon which you can give a powerful impression of yourself and link your talents to the needs of the employer.

> Assessing and identifying your skills is the most time-consuming part of preparing your resume—it is also the most essential.

Here are some questions that may assist you in identifying your soft skills:

- Did you implement a new method or procedure?

- Did your leadership role help a student organization communicate with the college administration?

- How did you save money on behalf of the organization? How much did you save?

- Did you increase the output or benefit? By how much? Did you develop a new technique for getting a procedure done more efficiently or more effectively?

- Did you provide some value-added service?

- Were relationships with the community enhanced by what you did? How?

Creating Accomplishment Statements Using the PAR Method

By collecting personal data, you now have a list of skills, abilities, and activities. You can use the Problem-Action-Results (PAR) method to help develop accomplishment statements. In order to

do this, you will need to complete several steps:

1. Think of a problem you experienced in school or in a work setting. What types of challenges did you face? Choose an area where you knew things could be done better. Write this down.

2. Recall what actions you took to overcome and solve that problem, and what skills you employed to arrive at the solution. Write them down.

3. Now, write down the results of your effort(s). How did your performance benefit the school, company, or organization?

When creating accomplishment statements, describe your actions positively and accurately, without modesty or exaggeration. Use quantities, amounts, and dollar values when they enhance the description. Typical areas of accomplishment are:

- Analytical/problem-solving

- Flexibility/versatility

- Interpersonal skills

- Oral/written communication

- Organization/planning

- Time management

- Motivational skills and leadership

- Self-starter/initiative

- Team player

When you design accomplishment statements for your resume, use a combination of paragraphs and bullets. Accomplishments can be prefaced with a heading such as "Key Accomplishments" or "Significant Contributions." For each employer, provide a short narrative detailing the scope of your responsibilities. Then create a bulleted list of your top contributions. Bullets draw attention to your accomplishments while giving the eye a chance to rest. However, if you just used bullets, they would tend to blur duties and accomplishments, diluting the impact of your achievements.

In a like manner, if you used just a narrative, it would be difficult and cumbersome to find the salient points.

Example

Leadership Ability: As vice-president of SCAVMA, I coordinated three fund-raising Pet Week activities on campus with the goal of raising $1,200 for a gift to the local Guide Dog Foundation.

Key Accomplishments
- The dog wash earned $455.
- Under my leadership, a total of $1,889 was raised. After expenses, SCAVMA was able to present a check for $1,450 to the Guide Dog Foundation, exceeding the goal by $250, or 21%. SCAVMA members talked with 123 dog owners about preventive measures for flea and tick control. The university cited SCAVMA as an outstanding community citizen.

Interests

This is your chance to introduce a human element into your resume. These are your hobbies, travel experiences, and special talents. They can give insight into your community involvement, social skills, leadership abilities, and ability to be well rounded. Remember, though—*do not clutter your resume*. Use only what is pertinent to the job.

Ascertain the impression others get from reading your resume. If you do not need to include some information, do not use it. More is not always better. If you list your interests, they *must* promote you in a positive light and must add, not detract, from your overall presentation. They must be *directly related* to your ability to do the job.

Activities, Affiliations, College Organization Memberships

You can include this section if you have available space and feel it lends some value. Incorporate social or civil activities, and health, fitness, or sports activities only if they directly relate to your ability to do the job.

Think about the image you are projecting. Once again, less may be more.

Let's say, for example, that you want to include your volunteer work at the local humane shelter. However, you may want to "walk softly" with regard to your involvement with an animal shelter if the prospective employer is embroiled in a dispute with the city that is subsidizing a full-service clinic right down the street in direct competition with his hospital. On the other hand, you may want to include shelter experience to emphasize your knowledge of the challenging treatment protocols for control of respiratory diseases in closely housed animals.

Perhaps you have strong religious, political, or pro-life/pro-choice convictions. Certainly, you are entitled to your beliefs. If you use your resume to advance those causes, the consequences may not coincide with the outcome(s) you envision. Depending on what you want to happen, this may or may not be the best time to reveal in a descriptive statement or paragraph that you are the "new-member" recruiter for your church, a district political organizer, an anti-abortion rally coordinator, or strong advocate of animal rights. Controversial and sensitive issues can be addressed during the interview if you so choose. Depending on your intensity, they may still bring unfavorable consequences at that time.

The employer, if she sees this information while glancing through your resume, may get the sense that if you were to get the job, you would try to convert every client who comes into the clinic—on the employer's time. She may think you will not project a favorable image of the business, that your main focus is not veterinary medicine, or that you have other agendas that will divert your time and energy away from work. Without even meeting you, she may leap to the conclusion that you are too controversial and will not be a team player. Subsequently, your resume hits the round file!

Or even worse, your reputation in the community may be impaired, especially if this potential employer disagrees with your stance. The employer may network with other employers in the area, and without

Your resume is a one-dimensional, black-and-white look at you and should not raise more questions than answers.

your knowing why, you may be effectively black-balled in the community with a reputation of being a "potential troublemaker."

Your resume is a one-dimensional, black-and-white look at you and should not raise more questions than answers. The resume is the primary tool you have to get the interview.

Avoid strong philosophical statements, contentious issues, and arguments. Once you know the people better and are on more secure footing, there may be the opportunity for friendly debates.

Awards and Honors

Be sure to list awards that relate to the kind of job you are seeking. List scholarships, class standing, special recognition, and academic achievements.

TYPES OF RESUMES

There are some basic styles used to format resumes. Each has its own particular application. Once you have collected, listed, and sorted personal data, you can decide which kind of resume style best fits your needs. All of the resumes, the cover letter, and the reference list are also in editable documents on the companion CD.

Chronological Resume

A chronological resume focuses on your previous work experience and responsibilities. Employers, when viewing a chronological resume, notice the dates first. They are looking for gaps in your employment history, length of employment with each employer, and stability. This format starts with the present or most recent job held, then moves back in time (see Figure 7-1).

A chronological resume is effective if you:

- Have a good work history

- Have no time gaps in your past work history

- Have not experienced numerous job changes

- Are looking for another job in the same field

- Have worked for a prestigious company that carries some weight in your community

ADVANTAGES
- Traditional and widely accepted among employers

- Very easy to read and follow

- Illustrates your job stability

- Shows steady growth and increasing levels of responsibility

- Emphasizes your job titles and company names

- Describes your duties and accomplishments

DISADVANTAGES
- Tends to emphasize job-hopping and prominently displays gaps in employment

- Often allows employers to infer too much about your age

- Highlights any lack of experience

Functional Resume

A functional resume focuses on professional skills and experience as a result of employment, formal education, and training and illustrates transferable skills and knowledge you have acquired. It is well suited for people who have had internships or cooperative experiences.

Resumes that are not chronological may be called functional, analytical, creative, or some other name. The differences are less important than how they are similar. They all stress *what you can do*. The employer can see immediately how you will fit the job.

This format also has advantages for many job hunters because it camouflages gaps in paid employment and avoids giving prominence to irrelevant jobs. You can list the company name first or the title of the position. Be consistent and use the same format throughout the resume. You may skip jobs and work periods that do not apply to the job, and you do not have to put entries in chronological order. In fact, it looks better to put the most impressive job first, then work downward in order of importance, regardless of dates of employment. See Figure 7-2 for a sample of a functional resume.

Note: Text continues on page 84 following Figure 7-2.

80

Figure 7-1
EXAMPLE OF A CHRONOLOGICAL RESUME

This document is also available on the companion CD.

David Allen Wagner, DVM
Rural Route 2
Aurora, Nebraska 68790
(402) 665-1223

CAREER OBJECTIVE
To develop my skills as a companion-animal clinician and eventually become an owner of a progressive practice.

EDUCATION
Colorado State University College of Veterinary Medicine
Doctor of Veterinary Medicine (DVM) May 2002

University of Colorado
Master of Business Administration (MBA) June 1998

University of Nebraska
Bachelor of Science, Animal Science (BSc) May 1996

WORK EXPERIENCE
Great Plains Animal Hospital, Aurora, Nebraska   **June 2002–Current**
Companion-animal associate veterinarian. Responsible for patient care, marketing small-animal services, and promoting specialty services such as dental prophylaxis and geriatric care. Oversee staff accounting functions and determine cash-flow projections for the practice. Assist practice manager. Oversee bookkeeping functions.
  • Generated additional $10,000 in fees compared to year before.
  • Provide after-hours emergency services for companion animals.
  • Track performance of the seven major profit centers I established for the practice.

Westfield Animal Clinic, Fort Collins, Colorado   **June 1998–April 2002**
Veterinary Duties:
While a veterinary student, started as kennel person, then progressed to technician and surgical assistant duties.
Business Duties:
Tracked patient responses to reminders and call-backs to determine financial impact on clinic. Kept financial and other management records. Prepared preliminary quarterly tax reports for clinic owner. Participated in marketing client education programs and the clinic's Pet Week activities.
  • Designed a comprehensive marketing program for clinic.
  • Increased new clients by 10% in one year.

Barney, Ralston and Gender CPAs, Denver, Colorado   **October 1996–June 1998**
During my MBA program training, worked 30 hours per week as a general accountant. Was the designated account manager for a local medical outpatient-treatment facility as well as several hospital-supply companies, each with annual gross revenues in excess of $18 million. Handled new client orientations and setups for computer-generated reports.
  • Decreased client orientation time by 25% by improving quality of supporting documentation.

Burlington Northern Railroad, Lincoln, Nebraska   **August 1993–May 1996**
Part-time on-call freight handler. Member of four-person work crew responsible for servicing refrigeration railcars and off-loading produce.

HONORS AND ACTIVITIES
Pi Alpha Alpha—Business Management Honor Society
Alpha Zeta—Honorary Agricultural Fraternity

Figure 7-2
EXAMPLE OF A FUNCTIONAL RESUME BASED ON WORK EXPERIENCE

This document is also available on the companion CD.

Michael Q. Robinson, DVM
2233 East Hampden Road
Denver, Colorado 80112
(303) 623-3876

EMPLOYMENT OBJECTIVE

A position in which I can use my research background and training in bovine reproductive physiology to contribute to the success of your company and fulfill my qualifications for diplomate status with the American Board of Veterinary Practitioners.

EDUCATION

University of Missouri, Columbia, Missouri
Doctor of Veterinary Medicine (DVM), May 2002
Bachelor of Science in Animal Science, June 1998, Distinguished Student Program

EXPERIENCE

Preparation of Recipient Cows
Work Study Special Project, University of Missouri, Reproductive Physiology, October 1999–May 2001
Coordinated ovulation program for recipient cows. Responsible for preparation of embryo-transplant media and equipment. Assembled research data regarding clinical examination of recipients and associated blood work parameters of the investigative protocol.
• Improved data collection protocol to save 15% of time previously required.

Bull Stud Management
COBA/Landmark Genetics, Appleton, Wisconsin, June 1998–September 1998
Worked in bull stud collection facility as a bull handler. Responsible for feeding, exercising, and collection for nine premier bulls and training of four junior bulls just starting on the genetic improvement program. Assisted with management of collection schedules, collection, handling, and storage of semen. Involved with filling client orders, packaging, and shipping of frozen semen.
• Reduced average order fulfillment time by 10%.

University of Missouri College of Veterinary Medicine, Columbia, Missouri, Winter 2001
Took eight private client producer bulls to Rocky Mountain Select Sire Services for collection during National Western Stock Show in Denver. Used production records and scoring to rate bulls. Assisted staff with training bulls to teaser and with first collection semen evaluations.
• Successfully integrated bulls into producer's herd bull rotation program.

Page 2

Michael Q. Robinson, DVM

Artificial Insemination

ABS Training Program, Lansing, Michigan, June 1996

- Completed certification course as Artificial Insemination Technician

Kansas State University Animal Science Center, Manhattan, Kansas, March 2002

Student assistant for Dr. Mark Heider and the Kansas Animal Health Institute's Artificial Insemination Basic School (5 days) to train field inseminators. Prepared recipient cows, managed materials for the course, and assisted in preparation of student workbook.

- Used experience as base for an independent study credit. As part of that course, I wrote a training design program using adult learning styles for the continuing-education sequel to Dr. Heider's basic course.

Other Bovine Clinical Experience

Coleman Veterinary Hospital, Jefferson City, Missouri, June 1995–May 1998

Worked as an assistant for farm calls and in clinic on food-animal side. Documented and maintained animal health-management records; discussed treatment directions and withholding times for pharmaceuticals with clients. Assisted with veterinary procedures performed by Dr. Coleman at the sale barn.

- Assisted during more than 200 surgeries, especially C-sections and surgeries related to foot disease in cattle.

University of Missouri College of Veterinary Medicine, Columbia, Missouri, Spring 2002

Took two extra elective blocks in ambulatory food-animal medicine (eight weeks total). Focused on spring calving and dystocia calls.

ADDITIONAL ACTIVITIES

Student Council Advisory Committee

Treasurer, Student Chapter of the American Association of Bovine Practitioners

83

You begin writing a functional resume by determining the skills the employer is looking for.

- Study the job description.

- Review your experience and education to see when you demonstrated the abilities sought.

- Prepare the resume itself, putting first the information that closely relates to the job.

A functional resume is effective if you:

- Focus on skills rather than length of employment

- Are reentering the job market after an absence

- Have time gaps between employment intervals

- Have numerous job changes

- Think your age is a barrier (too young, too old)

- Have had several unrelated occupations

- Are a mature individual with numerous areas of expertise

- Are a new college graduate

- Have skills and abilities other than those you are currently using and you desire to make a change or are looking for a job in a very different field or industry

- Have extensive military background and experience

- Are self-employed and operate your own business

ADVANTAGES

- Underscores accomplishments and strengths

- Allows flexibility to organize the presentation of your skills in a way that best suits you

- Eliminates repetition and redundancy of similar jobs

- Highlights diverse volunteer experience, interests, and skills that have not been a part of your past employment

DISADVANTAGES

- Downplays specific job titles and companies for which you worked

- Leaves out some employment experience

- De-emphasizes longevity

- Shows a limited number of job duties

Skills Resume

A skills resume is also considered a type of functional resume. This resume will have headings such as "Engineering," "Computer Languages," "Communications Skills," "Foreign Language Fluency," or "Sales and Marketing Experience." These headings will have much more impact than the dates that you would use on a chronological resume. Figure 7-3 is an example of a functional resume based on skills.

Remember, skills can be categorized three ways:

- Acquired skills as a result of past experience and education (knowledge-based skills)

- Skills you bring with you to any job (transferable or portable skills)

- Personal traits—characteristics unique to you that make you who you are

THE RECENT-GRADUATE DILEMMA

If you have graduated recently, you will most likely be competing with a peer group that has similar education, experience, and perhaps more clinical or related work experience. If you do not have much actual work experience, emphasize your recent education and training to include pertinent course content as well as participation in applicable continuing-education programs, workshops, and wet labs.

> If you do not have much actual work experience, emphasize your recent education and training to include pertinent course content as well as participation in applicable continuing-education programs, workshops, and wet labs.

You can approach your time in school as an equivalent to work experience. It did require that you exercise self-discipline and self-directed learning. It also required you to complete a variety of tasks and other activities that mirror those

84

required in many workplace settings. You can present a wide range of points that are directly job-related in a skills resume in much the same manner you might present work experiences in a chronological resume.

If it is truthful, you can also play up the fact that you have been taught and exposed to the latest in trends, techniques, and technologies relevant to veterinary medicine. You will be able to bring these with you and be able to readily share them on your new job. In addition, because you are already conditioned to studying and learning new things, you are better prepared to adapt and learn the new job quickly.

The skills format will also enable you to demonstrate how proficiencies you acquired by working other jobs (like being a waitress), which are not related directly to veterinary medicine, are actually a source of adaptive and transferable work-experience abilities. You can use military experience, involvement with student clubs, and volunteer work to illustrate leadership and responsibility roles. For example, being a waitress might have better prepared you for handling customer complaints and delivering value-added customer service to clients. It instilled a sense of teamwork, because you had to get along with the cook and with those who cleared the tables.

Combination Resume

The combination resume is in a chronological format that lists accomplishments in functional skill areas. The chronological resume lists jobs in order, starting with the most recent job you held, working backward. Functional resumes group accomplishments under specific areas of skills and abilities. The combination resume utilizes both chronology and function. Figure 7-4 is an example of a combination resume.

A combination resume is effective if you:

- Have a clear, specific job target and know what you are looking for

- Have no direct work experience in a specific area, yet are skilled and capable of doing that type of work

- Are currently employed by the same company that is offering this position

ADVANTAGES
- Confirms that you have a clear understanding of what you want to do and the related skills necessary to do the job

- Highlights important accomplishments

- Gives you flexibility and creativity when marketing your skills

- Targets your resume to a particular job or employer

DISADVANTAGES
- Requires multiple versions of your resume, each one specific for a particular employer

- Eliminates some information about your skills and experience, which may exclude you from being considered for another job within the same company

The Scannable Resume

Today, many employers incorporate the latest computer document-imaging technology to scan a resume to a database, which allows them to search for applicants. Like a traditional resume, this document is a personal summary of your professional history and qualifications. It includes information about your goals, education, work experience, activities, honors, and special skills or certifications.

There are a few adjustments that you should consider making to enhance the quality of your information for a scannable resume. The use of key words and phrases, proper format, and traditional type styles is critical to ensure that the sensitive computer software captures your assets.

FORMAT
- Justify the entire document to the left.

- Minimize punctuation marks and avoid them altogether if possible. If a computer is conducting a word search, it may not recognize a word with a comma and may reject or scramble the word or phrase, leaving a portion of your resume garbled and unreadable.

Note: Text continues on page 90 following Figure 7-4.

Figure 7-3
EXAMPLE OF A FUNCTIONAL RESUME BASED ON SKILLS

This document is also available on the companion CD.

Barbara Ann Wilson

Permanent Address:
2019 North Channel Road
Pleasanton, South Carolina 29805
(816) 555-1897

Current Address (until May 24, 2003):
341 Swan Street #3D
St. Paul, Minnesota 55110
(612) 555-6244

PROFESSIONAL GOAL

A position in veterinary medicine that involves client educational services and that makes use of my considerable background in animal nutrition. My goal is to promote nutritional aspects of good health and well-being for animal patients and become board certified by the American College of Veterinary Nutrition.

EDUCATION

University of Minnesota College of Veterinary Medicine
    Expected graduation: May 2003

Cornell University
Bachelor of Science   Major: Food Technology   Minor: Public Relations   June 1999
    GPA (4.0 scale)   Major 3.83   Minor 3.48

SKILLS

Veterinary Medicine
- Worked as technician on a special investigative project in the physiology department regarding malabsorptive disorders related to pancreatic enzyme deficiency in dogs. Grant program by means of Dr. Trevor Scythe (2000–2002).
- Current GPA (4.0 scale) is 3.79.
- Have been selected for eight-week externship block in epidemiology with U.S. Cooperative Extension Service to work on wasting disease in deer in Fort Collins, Colorado, spring 2003.

Customer Service
- Student internship (ten weeks), The Iams Company, June 2002–August 2002. Presented eighteen in-clinic service presentations to veterinary technicians and lay clinic staff regarding "How to Feed the Geriatric Patient" with company representatives. Helped prepare clinic handout materials for the product manager for Iams® geriatric diets.
- Hill's Pet Nutrition® student representative (University of Minnesota), September 2000–May 2002. Distributed Science Diet® samples and literature to end users (faculty and students). Arranged for company speakers for animal nutrition seminars on campus.

Figure 7-3 (continued)
EXAMPLE OF A FUNCTIONAL RESUME BASED ON SKILLS

Page 2

Barbara Ann Wilson

Customer Service (continued)
- Waitress, Hillside Café (four years, part-time as undergraduate, 2000–2003). Waited tables, took orders, and ensured that the customers enjoyed their meals and were satisfied with the restaurant service.
- Telemarketer, KanDo Windows (two years, part-time, 1998–2000). Contacted homeowners in a designated territory regarding purchase of replacement windows and installation.

Nutrition
- Received in-depth training on animal diet formulations, digestive physiology, and product applications from the Iams Company and Hill's Pet Nutrition.
- Co-authored Dr. Scythe's findings regarding pancreatic enzyme physiology, draft of which has been accepted by *Journal of Veterinary Research*.
- Trained and acted as a Weight Watchers' counselor (1997–2001) and group discussion leader.
- Elective courses in animal nutrition (eight hours, Cornell); physiology (six hours, Minnesota).
- Earned achievement certificate as Level II Pasteurization Technician during work-study at university creamery, Cornell University.
- Have participated in six national continuing-education workshops on stress physiology and the impact of nutrition on physiological parameters in health and disease at the University Medical Center, St. Paul, Minnesota.

Public Relations
- Planned, organized, and obtained funding sponsorship for the St. Paul Summer Festival Queen Pageant (2000–2003) for the St. Paul Chamber of Commerce.
- Coordinated Pet Week student activities on campus (2000–2003).
- Volunteered as on-air host (twelve air-time hours) for KCSP, a local radio talk show, during the month of Pet Week to promote SCAVMA activities in St. Paul area.
- Current vice-president, Student Chapter AVMA.

Figure 7-4
EXAMPLE OF A COMBINATION RESUME

This document is also available on the companion CD.

Donna Marie Jackson, DVM
4620 West 64th Avenue
Seattle, Washington 98034
(290) 455-1212

PROFESSIONAL GOALS

I am seeking a position where I can contribute my advanced ASIF bone-plating skills and focus on advancing my orthopedic surgical expertise. I plan to achieve diplomate status in the American College of Veterinary Surgeons within two years.

EDUCATION

Clinical Residency: Orthopedics, Washington State University
        July 2000–September 2002
Clinical Internship: Orthopedics, Ohio State University
        June 1999–May 2000
DVM, Ohio State University, College of Veterinary Medicine
        May 1999
Master of Science, Major—Pathobiology, Purdue University
        May 1995
Bachelor of Science, Major—Animal Science, Purdue University
        June 1993

WORK EXPERIENCE

September 2002–Current: Animal Surgical Specialists Center, Bellevue, Washington

Management Skills
• Coordinator for outpatient services

Clinical Skills
• Investigator—pharmaceutical company clinical trial; evaluation of alleviation of clinical symptoms using post-hyaluronic acid therapy in joints of giant breeds.
• Orthopedic clinician—on average, manage twenty-four referral cases per week.

July 2000–September 2002: Surgical Residency, Companion Animal Orthopedics, Washington State University

Management Skills
• Supervised two orthopedic surgical interns.
• Co-wrote new grant proposals for the university.
• Assisted with administration of program for practitioner referral cases.

Figure 7-4 (continued)
EXAMPLE OF A COMBINATION RESUME

Page 2

Donna Marie Jackson, DVM

Clinical Skills

- Grant study on retrospective look at anterior cruciate ligament repair techniques in dogs. Published in *JAVMA*, August 2002.
- Clinical case rotation, performed 561 orthopedic surgical procedures; assisted in 134 orthopedic surgeries as team member.

Teaching Skills

- Presented at North American Veterinary Conference, January 2002; review of repair techniques for sixteen of the most difficult canine joint reconstruction cases at the veterinary teaching hospital.
- Lectured and monitored clinical teaching laboratories for veterinary students during their orthopedic clinical rotation in both static and survival procedures.
- Provided continuing-education to WSVMA and local VMAs on the topics of clinical orthopedic surgical approaches and referrals.

June 1999–May 2000: Surgical Internship, Companion Animal Orthopedics, Ohio State University

Clinical Skills

- Graduate, ASIF bone-plating basic and advanced courses.
- Clinical focus, reconstructive joint repair.
- Assisted in 211 orthopedic procedures; performed surgery in 102 cases as clinician in charge.

Teaching Skills

- Assistant instructor—teaching veterinary students basic orthopedic procedures in static laboratory.

September 1995–June 1999: College of Veterinary Medicine, The Ohio State University

Clinical Skills

- Took four elective blocks in orthopedics and one in veterinary companion animal anatomy.
- GPA 3.9 (4.0 scale).
- Work Study—assisted in preparation of orthopedic specimens and worked as an assistant for ASIF courses taught by Department of Surgery at Ohio State for practitioners (four workshops).

- Do not use vertical or horizontal lines, graphics, or text boxes.

- Use white, 8½ × 11-inch paper and provide a laser-printed original if possible.

- Do not fold or staple.

- A one-and-one-half- or two-page resume is acceptable.

- Your name, with standard address format below it, should be at the top of the page.

- If you have more than one address, place one on top of the other in complete versions, including a name line with each.

- List each phone number on its own line.

- Try not to abbreviate. If you do, use standard industry terms associated with veterinary medicine.

- Use more nouns than action verbs: For example, instead of "design continuing-education programs," try using "continuing-education program designer" or "designer for continuing-education programs."

KEYWORDS

Keywords can be used in the body of your experience section, or you can create a keyword section summary at the end of the resume. Keywords are words or short phrases that are used commonly in a particular industry. They are what an employer may use in a query. For example, in veterinary medicine, you might use words like "biosecurity," "zoonotic disease control," "regulatory affairs," "clinical research," "animal welfare," "humane shelter," "clinical practice," "treatment," "practice management," "anesthesia," "surgical procedure," or "dentistry."

Remember—the scanner more readily identifies nouns. Therefore, try to use items like these when possible: "humane shelter volunteer," "clinical research assistant," "practitioner," "clinician," "student clinician in charge of biosecurity," "clinic supervisor," "treatment specialist," "practice manager," "anesthesiologist," "surgeon," or "dental assistant." Also, place your keyword summary at the end of your resume.

Example

Keyword Summary: veterinary medicine • doctor of veterinary medicine • DVM • companion animal practice • regulatory affairs • anesthesia • anesthesiologist • practice manager • clinician • small animal practitioner • biosecurity experience • humane society • animal shelter • soft tissue surgery • dentistry • animal health

FONT OR TYPESTYLE

- Use a 10- to 12-point font size.

- Use standard typefaces such as Times New Roman, New Century, Courier, Schoolbook, Georgia, Garamond, Geneva, Universe, Helvetica, Futura, or Arial. Remember—you do want to project a warm image, not a standoffish or "cold" document. Try different fonts and get other people's first impressions.

- The key to using fonts is to be consistent. If, for example, you use Times New Roman for the section headings, use the same font for all section headings throughout the document.

- Avoid fancy font styles, including italics, shadows, 3-D effects, underlining, and word art.

- Boldface and capital letters are appropriate as long as the letters do not touch each other. If they do, the scanner may not be able to distinguish the word.

- Provide white space between words and number groupings. For example, separate the area code of a phone number with spaces rather than with parentheses and include an extra space on either end of the dash of the number (i.e., 712 675 - 9984). Put several spaces between a zip code and the state unless you put the zip code on its own line.

THE COVER LETTER

A Vital Strategic Connection

The cover letter is your primary opportunity to make a great impression. It is a personalized piece of correspondence that:

- Is your letter of introduction

- Shows you are serious about your job search and career and have researched this employer

- Presents your intentions, qualifications, and availability to a prospective employer

- Displays your writing and communication skills

- Explains to the employer why he or she should consider you for the position

- Serves as a teaser to get the employer to explore your accompanying resume

- Acts as a targeted sales instrument designed to lure the reader to contemplate selecting you, rather than countless other applicants, to come in for an interview

- Provides clues to your level of professionalism, character, personality, and ability to pay attention to details (e.g., Are there spelling, typing, and other errors in the letter?)

- Is absolutely necessary; your resume should never show up without one

The Importance of Focus

Be clear on your objectives. Are you:

- Applying for a specific job?

- Trying to get an interview?

- Exploring opportunities in general with this employer?

In each case, the cover letter should capture the employer's attention, show why you are writing, indicate why your employment will benefit the company, and ask for an interview. Information that must be included is very specific and targeted. This means that you must write each letter individually.

Your typing needs to be perfect; therefore, the use of word-processing software, along with spell and grammar checks, is strongly advised. Frequently, only the address, the first paragraph, and the specifics concerning an interview will

vary and can easily be changed in a word-processing document. It is wise to change the wording of the text a bit for each hospital to which you are applying, especially if the hospitals are in the same locale. Some employers pass around applicant resumes with colleagues in the area—so you might want to make each letter unique.

Sections of the Cover Letter

A classic cover letter generally contains several sections that are each about a paragraph in length. These include the salutation, the opening, the body, and the closing.

SALUTATION

Address your cover letter to the person with decision-making authority. This is most likely to be the person who will actually supervise you once you start work. Call the clinic or hospital to make sure you have the correct name, and take great pains to spell the name correctly and use the correct title (Mr., Ms., Dr., Mrs.).

OPENING STATEMENT

The opening statement should appeal to the reader, cite the position for which you are applying, and state how and where you learned of the opening. Cover letters are sales letters. As such, the opening statement becomes a preview to the rest of the letter, letting the reader know how your qualifications fit the requirements of the job.

Capture the reader's attention by talking about the company rather than yourself. Mention a favorable comment recently published about the clinic, what you know they are noted for, and why you are attracted to them as an employer. If you are answering an advertisement, you can refer to the details of the position announcement. If through your networking someone suggested that you write, it is okay to use his or her name as a source (but only with permission).

> The cover letter should capture the employer's attention, show why you are writing, indicate why your employment will benefit the company, and ask for an interview.

91

BODY OF THE LETTER

The body of the letter will briefly organize and describe three to five of your top qualifications in a manner that best suits you for the position and that would be valued by the employer. If your on-the-job experience is your strongest qualification, discuss significant elements. If your work experience is relatively weak, reference your educational training and exposure to some advanced feature of veterinary medicine or technology you had as a student—one that ties to the orientation of the practice. This section needs to refer to the resume, where the reader will see more detail.

Ultimately, one strong qualification that a reader can envision you performing on the job can be enough. If you have two or three other strong areas and they apply to this position, develop them in one or two additional paragraphs. Make the pitch strong enough to convince your reader you are a worthy choice for the job, but don't make it so long that you turn the reader off.

Never include any negative information, salary requirements, salary history, or relocation information in the cover letter. If the employer requests that you include a comment regarding salary and/or relocation, it would be in your best interest to indicate that salary and relocation are negotiable. Save those discussions until *after* you have been offered the job.

CLOSING STATEMENT

Take a proactive posture. At the end of the letter, courteously request a personal interview. Propose a date or range of dates (day, not time) for the appointment. Be specific about how an employer can contact you. Indicate that you will be following up to confirm what might be convenient for the employer. You can place your home, work, email, and/or cell-phone numbers in the close of the letter. However, it will be more difficult for the employer to find them if the reader wishes to call you. State that you will follow up on this letter to make available any additional information the employer may want.

Use a standard complimentary close as the first part of the signature block, such as "Sincerely" or "Sincerely yours." Leave two to four lines for your signature, height being proportionate to font point size, and type your name below. Do this either as:

Dr. Stacy M. Katz or
Stacy M. Katz, DVM, MS

Do not mix the title "Dr." with academic degrees. Use either one format or the other. Do not include Dr. or DVM or other degrees in your signature (see Figure 7-5). It is preferable to type your phone number and other contact information as part of the header of your letter, instead of taking up space in the closing paragraph.

Rules for Writing Cover Letters

- Target your reader.

- Present more of what you can do for the employer than what they can do for you.

- Express focused career goals. *Never indicate you will take any job they have, even if you would.*

- Be specific, be precise, and cut to the chase—do not ramble.

- Back up any claims with examples.

- Keep copies of all letters you send (mail, fax, etc.) so that you can follow up with the employer and refer to them for creating other letters.

- Use paper and font choices that are similar to what you use on your resume.

- Keep the letter brief and under one page. Keep paragraphs short, with two to four sentences.

- State that you are enclosing your resume.

- Do not repeat information contained in the resume, except in the briefest, most introductory manner.

- Send only originals. Never send photocopies.

- Include only information you can easily explain and work to your advantage in an interview.

- Be professional. Remember—readers "deselect" applicants because of the appearance of the letter and/or the accompanying resume.

- Seek advice. Have at least one critical reader go over the draft of your document. Ask the reader to check your letter for mistakes and first impressions and to make suggestions for improvement before you revise and send your letter.

- Remember to sign your letter. Black ink is preferred.

An example of a cover letter is presented in Figure 7-5.

APPLICATION FORMS

Some large employers, such as corporate practices and government agencies, make more use of application forms than of resumes. Human-resource people find information more quickly if it always appears in the same place. Creating a resume prior to filling out an application form will help you organize your information and bring to mind skills and abilities you can highlight with short words and phrases.

You can use a cover-letter format and include a resume when you send a letter to an employer inquiring about a position. You can submit a resume even if an application is required, because it will spotlight your qualifications. Information on your resume will serve as a handy reference in case you are required to fill out an application form quickly. No matter how rigid the form appears to be, you can still use it to show why you are the right person for the job.

At first glance, application forms seem to be inflexible and give a job hunter no leeway. Remember that the attitude of the persons reading the form may not actually be, "Let's find out why this person is unqualified," but, "Maybe this is the person we want." Use all parts of the form—experience blocks, education blocks, and others—to show that the person they want is *you*. In most cases, especially for small blocks for which you have a lot of information, you can write: "Please see attached sheet" and use a supplemental page. Be sure to identify what block and which subject material is being answered with each response.

Rules for Completing Application Forms

- Request two copies of the form from the employer so that you can prepare rough drafts.

If only one is provided, photocopy it before marking on it.

- Review the entire form before you start to complete it.

- If several divisions within the same agency, company, or organization use the same form, prepare a master copy. Leave the specific job applied for, date, and signature blocks blank on the master copy. Complete that information on the photocopies when you submit them.

- Type the form if possible. If it has lots of little lines that are hard to type on, consider typing the information on a piece of blank paper that will fit in the space. Paste the paper on the form, and photocopy the finished product. Such a procedure results in a much neater, easier-to-read page.

- Fill in all the boxes with information or comments; enter n/a (for "not applicable".) when the information requested does not apply to you. This tells people checking the form that you did not simply skip the question.

- It is a good idea to carry a resume and a copy of other frequently asked information (such as previous addresses) with you whenever you visit potential employers in case you must fill out an application on the spot. Whenever possible, however, fill out the form at home and mail it in with a resume and a cover letter that highlight your qualifications, abilities, and strengths.

REFERENCES

Employers may ask for letters of reference or a list of your references they can contact. In general, any reference needs to be a person who is familiar with your character, the type of person you are, the quality of your work, and your achievements, especially those accomplishments you have claimed on your resume. An employer may request a list of references or require letters of reference prior to or during the interview or as part of the application process. Usually it is best to wait to be asked to produce your list of references rather than volunteer it ahead of the interview.

93

Figure 7-5
EXAMPLE OF A COVER LETTER
This document is also available on the companion CD.

Thomas H. McMurray, Jr., DVM, MS
28 Court Street
Wapakoneta, Ohio 45895
(419) 555-1212
thmcm2@hotmail.com

May 26, 2006

Dr. Adrian L. York
York Animal Hospital for Orthopedic Surgery
728 Wilson Street
Dayton, Ohio 45429

Dear Dr. York:

Dr. Robert Rhodes, a professor of mine at The Ohio State University College of Veterinary Medicine, suggested I contact you about a possible position at your hospital. I am seeking an associate intern position in a private progressive referral hospital such as yours. I am aware that the York Animal Hospital for Orthopedic Surgery is one of the most advanced animal orthopedic facilities in the Midwest.

I have a special interest in orthopedics, having done significant extracurricular work with bone-plating and grafting techniques in Dr. Rhodes's department while a veterinary student. In addition to assisting him with basic and advanced bone-plating courses for practitioner continuing-education programs, I was fortunate enough to be on work-study and was assigned to Dr. Alice Cramer's orthopedic research project for the past two years. As you may know, her work was highlighted in an article in the OSU alumni magazine, *The Speculum*, this spring. As a result of this work experience, I am proficient in bone-marrow transplant methods and have learned regenerative stem-cell relocation techniques. I have performed 127 procedures under her direct supervision.

One of my professional goals is to become a diplomate of the American College of Veterinary Surgeons and work as a clinical specialist in a professional group practice. I believe I have much to contribute to your hospital and surgical patient care as an intern. Given my background, I feel confident I would be able to matriculate rapidly into your work rotation.

Since I live only a short distance from Dayton and am already in the area, would it be possible for me to visit with you at your hospital sometime during the week of June 21 at your convenience? I am excited about learning more about your vision regarding the specialty practice of orthopedic surgery and to explore the possibility of working with you. I will contact you next week to schedule an appointment. Thank you in advance for your time and consideration.

Sincerely,

Thomas H. McMurray Jr.

Thomas H. McMurray, Jr., DVM, MS

Enclosure: resume

Letters of reference are used and requested by academic institutions, government agencies, and employers who have many candidates with very similar qualifications. In these situations, the letters of recommendation add valuable information to your profile that a resume is not capable of illustrating. Recommendations from teachers or professors carry little weight unless you are in an academic setting. Employers also may contact these individuals to determine if the letter is authentic or if the applicant actually wrote or provided written copy to the reference to be used in the application process.

Today, many employers have replaced formal letters of reference with a telephone interview with whomever you provided as a reference on your reference sheet. In this format, the employer or his agent is really verifying and elaborating on your professional experience, which you mentioned in the work-history section of your resume.

Selecting References

Out of courtesy, always contact the people you wish to use as references before you list them. Explain what you are applying for and ask their permission to use their name and contact information. Be mindful that some persons you contact may decline to become involved.

It is a good idea to call your potential references first. Then, once you have permission to use their names, follow up by sending each of them a copy of your current resume, a copy of the job description of the position for which you are submitting an application, and a sheet of bulleted highlights of your accomplishments targeted for the job(s) for which you are applying. Include on this piece of paper some details or abstracts of specific examples in support of each accomplishment as a memory jog for your references.

Some may be leery and may want you to provide everything for them, including the finished letter they should sign and send in as if they wrote it. Don't do it.

For others, you may have to reintroduce yourself or bring them up-to-date on what you have been doing in the more recent past. This is particularly true if you have not spoken to them for a while. Do not assume they will remember events the way you have projected them to the employer.

In any case, be prepared to help any potential reference get ready to answer typical questions an employer may ask. Stress what impression you need the employer to come away with. Take time to ask them typical questions and listen to what they say. Then, like an attorney might do with a witness, provide a little coaching to help ensure you get the results you expect. Remember—a poor or lukewarm reference can sometimes cost you the job you want.

When you send prospective references your information packet (resume, job description, updated work history with accomplishments), write an accompanying cover letter. In such a note:

- Reintroduce yourself if necessary. Remind them about the situations the two of you were involved in together.

- Summarize your qualifications and experience.

- You may want to state your professional goals and plans for career development and review your areas of specific focus and interests in veterinary medicine.

- Formally ask to use the person as a reference.

- Be sure they understand that if you do not hear otherwise, you will assume they do not mind being listed as your reference.

- Be sure to thank them.

The Reference List Format

When creating a list of references, just as with the cover letter, pick fonts that are easy to read. Use the same fonts you used on the cover letter and resume. Position information on the page in a pleasing manner that your eyes can follow with ease (see Figure 7-6 on the next page for a sample format of a reference sheet). List three to four references unless the employer specifies a different requirement. Include the following information:

- Your name and contact information at the top

- For each reference person include

  —Name
  —Name of company he/she works for
    (if applicable)
  —Title/Position

Figure 7-6
EXAMPLE OF A LIST OF REFERENCES

This document is also available on the companion CD.

Kasper White, DVM
222 Watkins Road
Gold Ridge, Colorado 80122
(970) 666 - 5210
kasper@hotmail.com

REFERENCES

Jason S. Roberts, DVM
White River Veterinary Hospital
123 Main St.
Ft. Collins, Colorado 80331

Work Phone: (970) 666-5555
Home Phone: (970) 662-1818

Employer while I was a student at Colorado State University College of Veterinary Medicine (1998–2002).

Alda E. Burnside, DVM, PhD
Professor, Orthopedic Surgery
Colorado State University,
College of Veterinary Medicine
Veterinary Teaching Hospital
Ft. Collins, Colorado 80323

Work Phone: (970) 667-1212
Mobile Phone: (970) 889-4554

Work-study supervisor. Worked on grant project for Dr. Burnside for three years while a veterinary student.

Elliot N. Ness, DVM, MS
Senior Livestock Agent
Cooperative Extension Service
Colorado State University
Administration Building #31
Ft. Collins, Colorado 80343

Work Phone: (970) 663-1227
Home Phone: (970) 555-9090

Dr. Ness was my Future Farmers of America advisor in high school, has assisted with my family's farm livestock production programs for the past eight years, and was my coach on the CSU Livestock Judging Team.

— Address
— Telephone number(s)
— Email address if reference wants to be contacted that way
— Brief statement as to how you know this person and/or the relationship you had/have with them (e.g., previous boss, former professor, coworker)

A Lasting Impression

Your resume, along with a cover letter, is often the first chance you'll have to introduce yourself to a potential employer. You must point out your strengths, skills, and experience and how you can contribute to the employer's success all in a well-organized and concise manner. Furthermore, resumes are self-evaluation tools—composing and updating your resume can help you determine what you have to offer an employer as well as help you make career goals. But like it or not, first impressions are lasting ones, so never underestimate the power of a good resume.

RESOURCES

Books

Best Resumes for $75,000+ Executive Jobs, Second Edition by W. Montag.
Cover Letters That Knock 'Em Dead by M. Yate.
How to Say It in Your Job Search by R. Kaplan.
101 Best Resumes for Grads by J. Block and M. Betrus.
175 High-Impact Cover Letters by R. Beatty.
Resume Magic: Trade Secrets of a Professional Resume Writer by S. Whitcomb.
Resumes for Dummies, Fourth Edition by J. Kennedy.
The Very Quick Job Search by M. Farr.

Websites

Most web providers, like *AOL.com, Yahoo.com,* and *MSN.com,* provide links to career development sites. Also, employment sites such as *Monster.com, Employment911.com, hotjobs.com, careerbuilder.com,* and many others provide access to articles, commentary, and self-help files that will provide examples for resume and cover letter formats.

Many universities have websites sponsored by the English department that provide handouts and general information regarding resume and cover-letter construction with examples.

97

▶ CHAPTER EIGHT ◀

The Art of
the Interview

Samuel M. Fassig, DVM, MA

IN THIS CHAPTER, YOU'LL LEARN:

- Interview preparation tips and techniques
- What to expect during interviews
- How to handle typical interview questions
- What happens after the interview and how to follow up

An interview is a meeting that gives the employer a chance to put a face with the resume. Resumes list your experience, education, and skills. The interview breathes life into those words. How you handle the interview determines whether you are offered a position or your resume goes to the bottom of the pile.

PREPARING FOR THE INTERVIEW

The most important elements of any interview are *preparation* and *practice*. Preparation will enable you to be confident, overcome interviewing inexperience, and help you sell yourself and your qualifications. As part of your preparation, make some study lists—for your eyes only—that have key elements and facts about you, what you have accomplished, and what you have learned. State your strengths and how they link to your experiences and training. Be specific when describing results. Review and study this guide often during interview season. Refresh the list after every interview,

building it in response to questions you were asked but felt you answered inadequately.

If you are inexperienced, interview often, even if you may not really want that particular position. You can always tactfully refuse the job at the appropriate time. Practice will help you become more at ease in showing your capabilities and talking about how you approach challenges as a professional. Hold mock interviews and videotape them. Have good friends, your student advisor, and other colleagues critique you and offer constructive ways to improve.

Find out as much as you can about the interviewer(s) with whom you will be meeting. Do some investigative work regarding the practice and the position for which you're interviewing. Is this a new position, or are you replacing someone? If someone left, why did they go? Is the practice expanding? Prepare for the questions they are likely to ask you, as well as the questions you would like to ask them. Formulate an objective—i.e., getting a job offer and learning enough about the practice, its people, and its reputation in the community to help you decide if you want to work there.

If you are well prepared, you will be more relaxed during the interview. Remember—the common goal is to discover if you and the practice are a match, not if you are a "good" veterinarian or this is a "good" practice.

To be well prepared, follow these steps before your interview:

- Keep track of all career-related correspondence, written and verbal. Use a notebook or some other means to log employment activity with each prospective employer. Jot down names of people when you talk to them on the phone, and log in each time you mail something with a description of what was sent, to whom it went, and how you followed up.

- Identify what you will wear as your basic interview wardrobe (see the next section on "Appearance"). If it is dry-clean only, take it to your overnight or one-hour cleaners a day or two before the scheduled interview.

- Polish your shoes the day before the interview.

- Get a haircut about one week before the interview. This will keep it neat but not make it look like you just had it cut.

- Clean out and run your vehicle through the car wash. Invariably, about the time you do not, someone from the clinic may walk you out to your car after the interview. If it is filled with old pop cans, clothing, and a disorganized array of "stuff," it may send a message that you are not a detail-oriented person and really do not care about your public image. Besides, arriving in a clean car can help make you feel good that day.

- Prepare an interview folder to bring with you. It should contain several copies of your resume in folders or plastic sleeves, reminders for yourself about your skills and abilities, a pen, some paper, and business cards if you have them.

- It is always a good idea to have a crisp, clean business card with your name, address, and contact information to give each person with whom you are interviewing. Get theirs as well so that you can follow up with a thank-you letter.

- Know in advance where you are going. If possible, check out the location, where to park, and the layout of the neighborhood the day before your interview. If you are coming from out of town, this is especially important.

- Get a good night's sleep before the interview.

- Be sure to fill your car with fuel. It is best to do this the night before the interview; that way, you will not get your interview clothing dirty.

- As you get ready on the day of the interview, visualize yourself sitting in the interview feeling calm, poised, and confident. Picture yourself handling the questions well.

- Eat a light meal an hour or two before the interview. Interviewing on a completely empty stomach may make you feel uncomfortable or restless, and your stomach may growl loudly. Interviewing on a completely full stomach may make you less energetic or sluggish, as will a high-sugar hit. It is best to eat light and avoid excessive sugar and caffeine.

- Bring the names of the people with whom you are meeting, the address with directions, and the phone number with you to the interview.

- If you have a cell phone, put it in the car fully charged.

- Bring a comb or hairbrush, tissues, and breath mints. Use the mints before entering the building for the interview.

- If possible, make a "pitstop" in a restaurant or other convenient place somewhere near the location before entering the building.

- Physically leave home (or your motel) with plenty of time to get to the place of the interview. Always be prompt or just ahead of time to the interview. Try to be early, but not by more than a few minutes.

- Leave enough margin for error to avoid any possibility of being late. First impressions always count—big time. No one will remember your excuse for being late—only that you were late. It may take an enormous effort to overcome a poor first impression; therefore, maximize your effort to control as much of the

100

process as possible. If you are unavoidably late, offer a sincere apology just once, then let it drop.

Appearance

Every business or organization, large or small, has its own culture. This is likely to include a dress code for appropriate attire and grooming (e.g., length of hair and use of cosmetics, perfume, and jewelry). Although you may end up working in scrubs, smock tops, and jeans, *none of those are appropriate for an interview.*

The factors that you have control over, and that can influence the interviewer who is developing his or her first impression of you, are your appearance, your communication skills, your body language, and your mastery of interviewing techniques.

What you wear and how you look speak volumes to an employer. You should be dressed two steps higher than the job for which you are interviewing. Dressing well shows consideration, respect, and a level of professionalism that honors this veterinarian as a businessperson.

Many interviews for associate positions last several hours. If the interview is held at the clinic, it usually includes a tour of the facilities. If you

> The factors that you have control over, and that can influence the interviewer who is developing his or her first impression of you, are your appearance, your communication skills, your body language, and your mastery of interviewing techniques.

expect this will be the case, wear clothing that will look neat all day and comfortable, including footwear. Bring a brush or comb and whatever other paraphernalia you may need to maintain a neat appearance. If it's raining, protect your ensemble with dependable rain gear. Never, under any circumstances, allow yourself to appear disheveled. Employers make the connection—sloppy appearance often equals sloppy job performance. If this person cannot take care of herself, how will she take care of the clients?

Common sense and a little attention to detail will go far in helping you set a positive first impression. Women should refrain from excessively low-cut outfits and men from flashy or trendy clothing. Interviewers always respect conservative attire, even if they themselves are trendy.

Listed in Tables 8-1, 8-2, and 8-3 are some basic traditional guidelines for dressing like a professional when you go to an interview.

You also need to maintain poise, confidence, good posture, and a relaxed natural smile. During the job interview, even *one* of the following items can negatively affect the first impression you make on a potential employer.

- Chewing gum, smoking, or using other tobacco products

Table 8-1
DRESS GUIDELINES FOR WOMEN

- **Dresses, suits:** Conservative business suit, pantsuit, or dress of a natural or woven-blend fabric in a dark or soft color that complements your skin tone and hair color. Skirt length should be at least to the bottom of the knee but not past mid-calf. You want to look businesslike yet approachable. Have some friends comment on your selection.
- **Blouses:** Avoid frilly styles and low necklines. Use simple, conservative styles.
- **Shoes:** Wear sensible shoes—polished pumps or low to medium heels that match your outfit.
- **Nail polish:** Use a clear or conservative color.
- **Makeup:** Wear moderate makeup—no strong colors.
- **Jewelry:** Keep it simple and minimal.
- **Purse:** Avoid carrying a purse if you can—it may detract from your professional image.

Table 8-2
DRESS GUIDELINES FOR MEN

- **Suit:** Still the traditional standard for an interview; dark blue, gray, brown, or very muted pinstripe; a good-quality woven blend of natural fibers that looks professional is a good choice. Suits should be properly tailored, freshly dry-cleaned, and the best quality you can afford.
- **Shirts:** A good-quality, white button-down shirt is preferred. Most importantly, be sure the shirt is pressed.
- **Ties:** Silk or high-quality blends only. Wear conservative ties that complement your suit. The tip of a tie should fall near the center of the belt buckle.
- **Shoes:** Highly polished black, brown, or cordovan shoes and dark socks. If you must wear boots, make them solid-color conservative dress boots, highly polished and complementary to rest of the outfit. Colorful snakeskin and exotics, although often expensive, may be viewed as a negative.
- **Facial hair:** No beards. Many employers view a beard as a sign that the individual has something to hide. If you have a moustache, make sure it is trimmed neatly. Nose and ear hair should be clipped.
- **Jewelry:** No bracelets, chains, bands, or necklaces showing. Multiple rings (other than wedding and college rings) and multiple earrings may be viewed negatively.

Table 8-3
DRESS GUIDELINES FOR MEN AND WOMEN

- Well-groomed hair
- Clean, manicured fingernails
- Interviewers often consider the condition of your shoes as a way to tell if you pay attention to detail. Avoid unshined shoes or those with run-down heels.
- Be sure to bring a watch, pen, and pad of paper for taking notes.
- A briefcase or portfolio, if you have one, will help complete the look of professionalism.

- Tapping your fingers, rattling change in your pocket, clicking pens, bouncing your legs, tapping your feet, making noises with your mouth, or displaying other annoying physical habits

- Smelling of body odor, strong perfume, or cologne

- Displaying visible tattoos or body piercings on the tongue, nose, eyebrows, or lips

- Having torn or patched clothing or runs in stockings

- Displaying unusual hair—spikes, heavily bleached hair, odd colors

- Wearing too much jewelry

- Having worn or unpolished shoes or wearing gym shoes

- Being poorly groomed

- Using foul language or off-color comments or jokes, even to same-sex staff when you think no one of importance is listening

Your Attitude

The best way to approach an interview is with enthusiasm and an open mind. Treat everyone you meet with courtesy. If you decide during the interview that you don't want the job, or that you may not be sufficiently experienced or qualified to receive the offer, chalk it up to experience.

Continue to present yourself in an upbeat and professional manner. If they are giving you the courtesy of their time and consideration, the least you can do is respond in kind. Practice manifesting a positive attitude before each interview—it's a good habit to develop and maintain.

If you are unsure of your abilities, then you need to learn to appear competent and confident. Of course, feeling confident doesn't automatically make you competent, but it does create an atmosphere that is conducive to success. Remind yourself that:

- **There is no question you cannot answer with a positive response.** You have your list of skills, experience, and abilities and know to tie your answers to them. You have practiced answering typical questions. You have prepared.

- **You are well suited for the position.** You are a licensed veterinarian. You have researched the practice and you are looking for an employment fit.

- **You would be an asset to the practice.** You know what you bring. You know the interview is a time to sell the attributes you have that the employer is looking for.

TYPES OF INTERVIEWS

There are three primary types of interviews:

- Face-to-face
- Comprehensive online prescreening
- Phone

Face-to-Face Interview

This type of interview is the one you traditionally think of in which you sit down face-to-face with an employer or his or her agents at the employer's site. You are expected to provide responses to rounds of questions. Hopefully, you will be asking questions as well. Face-to-face interviews are discussed in detail throughout this chapter.

Comprehensive Online Prescreening Interview

In an effort to weed out potential candidates, more companies and corporate employers are moving to this prescreening method. The concept is: Why waste precious time interviewing a slew of candidates when undesirable applicants can be weeded

out by using a comprehensive online interview? Employers set the criteria with the help of the questionnaire designer.

Before an interviewer ever shakes your hand, he or she knows all about you, your employment history, your grade point average (GPA), and whether or not you are a team player, a problem solver, or executive material.

Here are some typical questions you will be asked in an online interview:

- Would you rather have flexibility or structure in your job?

- How often do you forget important details?

- How often do your decisions result in unexpected consequences?

- What approach have you taken in the past to solve difficult problems?

- How do you react to working without direct supervision? Can you set your own goals and meet them?

- In what type of work environment are you most productive?

- In the past, when you have been assigned numerous tasks with little or no direction, how did you react?

- Do you like to work alone or in the company of others?

- Do you like routine, repetitive tasks?

- Do you like handling many projects at one time?

According to Brian Stern, a psychologist and managing director of SHL Group, a human-resource consulting company, determining the right answer is not easy. Stern says most candidates assume that a right answer is what a company wants to hear, and that a wrong answer is what a company does *not* want to hear. He says it does not work that way. He thinks the preassessment technique "casts a wide net" and captures qualified candidates based on the criteria set by employers. He claims that some 25% of applicants get jobs when screened in this manner, although there is no specific data regarding veterinarians.

According to Stern, the way to ace these tricky assessment interviews is to be honest. Do not try to tell the companies what you think they want to hear. Stern advises: "It is important to be candid. There are trap questions that are designed to see if you are responding in an overly socially responsible manner (fudging). The last thing you want to do is paint a picture that is not you."

Phone Interview

Plain and simply put, employers want to do things as efficiently and cheaply as possible. Therefore, many conduct their first screenings on the telephone. For some, this interview may not be with the actual decision maker, but rather with someone who determines if you are to be considered further. Basically, this screening is to determine if you are worthy of taking up the boss's time in a future interview.

POSITIVE ASPECTS

For a phone interview, you can prepare notes and keep them in front of you while you talk. You aren't dressed in a suit, which should make you more at ease. Treat the phone interview as an information-gathering time. Have a list of questions at hand. Listen to the responses given. Whenever possible, tie your responses to one of your strengths.

NEGATIVE ASPECTS

Without interacting with someone face-to-face, many interviewees lose their energy. There is no body language to read as an indicator of whether or not this person is following along with your responses. Without eye contact and facial expression, it may also be difficult for you to demonstrate your passion and get your message across.

Use the same "winning" visualization technique described in Chapter 10, Mastering Negotiation (page 154), to help you become energized ten minutes before you get the call. By focusing on a time when you were really successful and felt "pumped up" as a result, your enthusiasm will boil over into the conversation.

Another technique is to complete a moderate physical workout at home. Then, take a quick

> Treat the phone interview as an information-gathering time. Have a list of questions at hand. Listen to the responses given. Whenever possible, tie your responses to one |of your strengths.

shower, finishing fifteen minutes or so before you are scheduled to get the call. Have a drink of water by the phone in case you need it. By then, your heart rate should have returned to near normal and your cool-down should be complete. Often your endorphins have kicked in and you have some zip in your step. You may exude the high-energy feeling of accomplishment, have eased any tension in your voice, and come across as relaxed, yet energized. You will also be awake.

The Lunch Interview

The business lunch is making a comeback, especially in hectic veterinary practices. The boss may want to get away from the phones and interruptions at some point during the course of your interview. Commonly, it may be set up so that you and the interviewer, or you and the other veterinarians in the practice, go out to lunch together.

Here is a refresher in dining etiquette:

- Don't make the group wait for you. Decide quickly on what you are going to order.

  - Avoid those hard-to-eat or messy dishes like corn on the cob, super-tall triple-decker club sandwiches, and barbeque ribs.

- Try not to choose items that take a long time to prepare. People may have to wait for you to get something to eat. The whole lunchtime may be consumed without anyone having a meal because yours has slowed up the table order. And once it does come, everyone must hurry to eat in order to get back to work. They stop listening to what you are saying.

- Do not choose the most expensive item on the menu.

- Abstain from huge portions. Remember—you are going to do most of the talking during the lunch break.

- Drink to the right. Eat to the left. This should help you avoid eating someone else's bread or taking a water glass.

- Napkins go on the lap, not under the chin or on the table or anywhere else.

- Knives and forks go on the plate after you first use them and remain there until the next bite.

- Avoid licking your fingers or brushing crumbs off the table with your hand.

- Strongly consider avoiding alcohol altogether. If you feel you must drink alcohol, nurse one drink.

- The host, or whomever arranged for the interview appointment, should pay the check. If you feel it is appropriate, you can offer to pay for *your share*. Only make the offer to pay your share one time. Do not argue about whether to pay the check. *Never* offer to pay the entire tab. After all, they asked you to come.

Just like interviewing in the office, interviewing over a meal consists not only of what you say, but observations regarding what you do. Consider this case in point:

A large corporation on the East Coast was interviewing a young man. He was a newly graduated PhD-level chemist with a couple years of experience in the industry with a competitor. This was the final interview for the job. It was down to him and one other candidate. Part of the interview included going to lunch with a group of five chemical engineers and three other project leaders from what would be his work group.

They were in a very nice restaurant, and everyone got the blue-plate lunch special: Porterhouse steak and the trimmings. When he was served, he picked up the salt shaker and salted his meat and mashed potatoes like he always did at home, then passed it to the right. Distracted for a moment when someone asked a question, he then took his first bite and reveled in the juiciness of the steak, which he could cut with his fork. He thought there was great conversation at the table and everyone seemed to relate well to his responses. He was really excited and felt great about his performance. The day after the interviews were over, he was informed

he did not get the job. He politely inquired as to the reason he was not selected, especially since he felt it had gone so well.

The response he got made him sit up and take notice. He was told he did not get the job because at lunch he salted his food before he had even tasted it. Worse yet, in their observation, they concluded that he did so out of habit, almost unconsciously. In their review of the impression he left on the group, they (four of the interviewers commented about this to the decision maker) thought it was a bad habit, especially for a chemist, to assume that something was the case without checking it out first. To make assumptions out of habit was a red flag.

They were concerned he might approach his work in the same manner he had approached his steak. In this case, taste first and adjust later would have been the more appropriate approach to something unknown. If he would easily make assumptions about a meal in a restaurant he had never eaten in before, would the way he approached his work be too great of a risk for many of the sensitive projects they were dealing with?

In this case, unconscious actions spoke volumes and cost this person the job offer. Be very careful about your every action because you are on stage.

The Dinner Interview

Having dinner with a prospective employer is sometimes part of the interview, especially if you have come into town from somewhere else. It may include you, your spouse, the employer and his or her spouse, and other staff members and their spouses.

The dinner interview may be informal, semiformal, or formal; therefore, it is important to ask (if not presented in the initial invitation) and dress accordingly. Even if the dinner is billed as an informal get-together, remember that you are being watched, observed, and critiqued. The same is true of your spouse. The lunch principles apply. Be very careful about alcohol consumption and use common sense in all things.

If you are invited to a dinner interview in business attire and your potential employer is not dressed accordingly, it will not be taken as a negative. In fact, being dressed professionally rarely, if ever, hurts your ability to be seen as someone employable. Being too casual, on the other hand, does hurt you.

TYPES OF INTERVIEWERS

There are different kinds of interviewers with different goals. A human-resources professional or personnel manager will usually screen you to prevent wasting the decision maker's time. You do not need to impress this person, and you certainly can't snow him or her. This person simply wants to ensure that you have truly and accurately represented yourself in your job application and resume.

When a screener interviews you, answer the questions as clearly and accurately as possible, but do not volunteer additional information except for specific points that highlight your skills and abilities as they pertain to that question. A screener does not need to like you. The screener's job is to decide that you are a candidate worth passing along to the decision maker.

The decision maker, on the other hand, wants to feel comfortable with you and be certain that you can do the job. This is where you put your best foot forward, discuss more personal interests, and talk shop. Usually, and especially if it is a one- or two-veterinarian practice, the decision maker does not have a lot of experience conducting interviews and may be uncomfortable. If time goes by and she is doing most of the talking without asking you questions, you may have to take control of the interview process to illustrate what it is you can do for the practice. Remember—your job in this process is ultimately to get a job offer.

How to Interview With Different Types of Decision Makers

Job interviews are negotiations. The person being interviewed (you) is attempting to sell a product (yourself) to a potential customer. The job interview is not unlike the sales process that a good sales representative would use. Many of the same principles you would use to sell a product apply. Successful salespeople are careful to

"qualify" prospective customers. They research whether what it is they are selling meets their customer's needs.

Good salespeople also understand that different players in the business speak different languages, and that there is a hierarchy of power and authority. These people can be ranked, top to bottom in authority, as the leader, captain, or CEO; the manager or director; the analytical intellect; and the consumer/end user. During the interview, you may encounter individuals from some or all of these groups. Understanding the reasons for their questions will give you considerable information about the potential employer. Answering their questions appropriately will win them over.

LEADER, CAPTAIN, OR CEO

This is the top-ranking individual who has the leadership, credibility, passion, ego, power, control, willingness to take risks, and decisiveness to champion his or her vision. In some cases, this may not be the owner. This person is also most concerned about the image of the business and the admiration of colleagues and wants measurable, tangible results. No doubt about it, this is the power position—the boss. This person establishes the business culture and how the business operates.

This person needs to know about *benefits*. By hiring you, what will you bring to help the company realize its fullest potential, and what impact will you have in a positive manner on the bottom line?

In conversations with the leader, do not hedge. This is not a time for smoke and mirrors or half-truths. Be straightforward and present a clear picture of how you can help the company realize its full potential and what you can do to impact the bottom-line results. Ask what the leader's specific goals are. What are this person's criteria for a good employer-employee relationship? What will it take for the leader to "do business" with you (hire you as an employee)? What do you need to show the leader to meet his or her criteria?

Leaders like to look at tangible results, such as measurable improvement in the business, increased market share, and progress that leads to new opportunities. When talking with a leader, share something about how you will contribute to increasing clinic revenue and business volume, decreasing overhead, capturing a larger market share, and developing innovative ways to market the business.

A leader also looks at intangible benefits. How will hiring you help reduce his or her risk or worry? How might you provide the business with increased customer loyalty, a higher standing in the community, ability to set new trends, an improvement in staff morale and motivation, and an ability to ease the completion of daily tasks for the staff?

MANAGER OR DIRECTOR

This is the person who takes the leader's visions and turns them into workable policy objectives. This might be the hospital manager, the medical director, or the chief of staff.

This person needs to know about *advantages*. What can you do for the department or a particular aspect of the business? What leading-edge solutions and experience will you contribute to help the business distinguish itself in the community or with competitors?

When dealing with a manager, try to establish that person's needs for the current department or the part of the business for which he or she is responsible. Ask about present and future objectives and priorities. How have they been doing up to now with the current use of an associate(s) in the role for which they are hiring? Has that person met their needs? What do they see that they need now?

ANALYTICAL INTELLECT

This is the person who is concerned with the data—usually the financial data. The analytical intellect looks at solutions in terms of technical capabilities to meet his or her real or perceived needs, which may not be those of the business. Perhaps this is the office manager, the bookkeeper, or a senior technician in charge of keeping the place stocked. It is often the gatekeeper who controls the clinic's relationship with distributors and sales representatives.

This person needs to know about *features*. How do all the elements of what you bring fit together? The analytical intellect wants to know what makes you tick. In an analytical way, what makes

your character? If this person was buying a car, he or she would be the one checking under the hood to inspect all the component parts.

When dealing with an intellect, take everything with a grain of salt. Ask, and then be prepared for a long answer: "If you could solve the problem or were in charge of hiring, what do you think the perfect solution or employee for this associate position would be?" Realize that this person is not a decision maker; therefore, do not ask who makes the decision.

CONSUMER/END USER

This is the person who actually uses what you are selling—the coworkers and lay staff in the trenches, as well as the pet owners.

This person needs to know about *functions*. What solutions will you contribute in the workplace to help make this person's job easier? When you are dealing with a consumer, find out what the person is doing now. How is this person getting by? Are there any serious problems? What have been the previous solutions? Find out from this individual who's who in the business.

Interviewer Personalities

Although you experience interviewers because of their authority position in the business, how they act during the interview can give you additional insights regarding how you should handle yourself in their presence.

THE STUDIOUS INTERVIEWER

The studious interviewer tends to show little emotion and does not share personal feelings. He or she may seem formal and will tend to focus on facts.

- **Interviewer's body language**—Indirect eye contact; limited gestures; slow and deliberate speech; soft-spoken, often speaks in a monotone voice

- **Interviewer's office appearance**—Well organized and functional; his or her walls will be bare except for diplomas

- **How you can adapt**—Answer questions with specific facts when possible; be reserved but not cold; avoid being emotional or threatening; be conscious of time, but do not be hurried; expect to negotiate

- **Your follow-up letter**—Should be organized, brief, and to the point, with measurable facts where possible

THE FRIENDLY INTERVIEWER

The friendly interviewer tends to focus on feelings and people. In a slower-paced atmosphere, he or she will conduct a relaxed and informal interview.

- **Interviewer's body language**—Makes frequent eye contact; hands move freely

- **Interviewer's office appearance**—Neat, fairly well organized; may use warm colors and personal photos

- **How you can adapt**—Stress human issues, perhaps including the human-animal bond; give the interviewer reasons to trust you

- **Your follow-up letter**—Use a friendly tone that is not strictly business; add a personal touch; stress client and staff relationships

THE ENTHUSIASTIC INTERVIEWER

The enthusiastic interviewer focuses on ideas, concepts, and the future. He or she will often jump from one thought to another. This person tends to be a risk taker.

- **Interviewer's body language**—Quick movements; uses hands to talk; makes frequent eye contact; speaks quickly and controls the conversation; laughs easily; will often express personal feelings and responds with enthusiasm

- **Interviewer's office appearance**—May not be well organized; creative works may be displayed

- **How you can adapt**—Show enthusiasm and support for the interviewer's ideas; control the flow of the interview by asking questions; summarize as you answer questions; demonstrate your creative side

- **Your follow-up letter**—Use a friendly, optimistic tone; emphasize your futuristic ideas

THE SERIOUS INTERVIEWER

The serious interviewer appears hurried and impatient. He or she acts quickly, appears forceful, and maintains a formal atmosphere.

- **Interviewer's body language**—Has an air of confidence; uses limited gestures; is formal and deliberate in voice pattern

- **Interviewer's office appearance**—Organized; tends to display trophies and awards; has conservative decorations

- **How you can adapt**—Be friendly, yet reserved; present facts; be brief and organized in your responses and avoid becoming defensive

- **Your follow-up letter**—Use action words; demonstrate that you are a doer; make it brief and to the point in an organized, logical fashion.

WHAT TO DO AND SAY DURING THE INTERVIEW

Rather than looking at an interview as a time to put on a performance or demonstrate all of your talents, it may be better for you to learn more about the expectations of the potential employer. If an employer is looking for experience, find out whether there are other creative ways to substitute additional qualities for years of experience. How might your involvement with student clubs, social events, publications, or other outside schoolwork appeal to the interviewer?

> Rather than looking at an interview as a time to put on a performance or demonstrate all of your talents, it may be better for you to learn more about the expectations of the potential employer.

A good applicant should think about *why* an interviewer asks certain questions. Not only can this help you determine where the interviewer fits in the authority hierarchy of the business, but it can help you use the questions to exude self-confidence without seeming arrogant in your responses.

You are interviewing the practice at the same time the practice is interviewing you; therefore, come well prepared with questions to ask the owner(s) and staff. Appear flexible, and be well prepared to communicate your priorities. Practice feedback and use of personal examples to illustrate your strengths prior to the interview so that they are on the tip of your tongue.

Although you have your list of negotiable and nonnegotiable items, it may be wise to let others do the initial presentations. Wait and evaluate the situation. Be familiar with the market-rate salary range for your position, and outline your strengths and what you will specifically do for this practice to add value. *It cannot be stressed enough that you should not discuss compensation before you are offered the job.* However, it is important to have some idea of employment market statistics at hand in case such a discussion arises. You will be prepared to then talk in terms of ranges, survey results, and what is typical for your peer group.

> It cannot be stressed enough that you should not discuss compensation before you are offered the job.

Typical Interview Questions

Although you may be asked a variety of questions, here are some of the more typical ones, along with possible answers. Table 8-4 lists additional questions that you should be prepared to answer.

THE CHALLENGE

Interviewers are quick to notice inconsistencies, hesitations, and uncertainties in your responses, including shifts in body position, change in eye contact, and nervous mannerisms. They may challenge something you say just to see your reaction. If you back off, change, justify, qualify, over-explain, or retract what you said earlier, they may suspect that you have been exaggerating or lying to them. If that is the case, they likely will probe deeper.

If someone responds to a statement you make with a skeptical look, a pause, or a comment like "Really?" you need to maintain your composure. Consider smiling politely, nodding, and waiting for the person to continue. Try not to be reactive. It is best to respond with a sense of confidence, such as

(depending on the question), "Yes, that has been my experience with it." Fortunately, this does not happen often. Remember—employers are people, too. The conversation or some other matter may have actually triggered some unrelated thought. Their response or body language may not even be directly related to you or the interview.

If, however, the interviewer is making this challenge by design, he or she is usually trying to get insight into your character. The person is trying to figure out how you will fit in. How will you respond to a challenge of your authority or position of expertise?

Example

Situation: You are asked to assume that you are the attending clinician on a bloat/torsion bowel case. You make a statement about the diagnosis and treatment protocol for this Great Dane. The interviewer's response to your statement is, "Really?" in a bit of a questioning tone.

Outcome: Are you going to be rattled? If so, how rattled? How threatened are you by a challenge from a person in power? Are you going to give a ten-minute dissertation out of the *Merck Veterinary Manual* on twisted bowel syndrome? Are you going to panic and retract your statements? Do you fear confrontation and being discounted by the interviewer? Are you going to reaffirm your position and exude a sense of confidence? Are you just going to ignore it? Are you going to get angry?

You do not need to know all the answers. You do not have to be absolutely right. How you handle interactions and what you project about your ability, values, and self-confidence to the interviewer are the important points.

If you find yourself in a "pregnant-pause" situation or become uncomfortable during the interview, engage the interviewer. Each time you ask a question of the interviewer, wrap your response with something about your skills and abilities.

Keep putting your message forward. To break the ice during those times of unexpected silence, ask questions like:

- What has been your experience with (whatever the subject was)?

- Do you see this often in this practice? How did the staff approach it the last time?

- This is one of the reasons I was interested in applying to this practice. I wanted to be able to continue developing my abilities in oral surgery. I think that my background charting patients' mouths for Dr. Smith in his dental-referral practice at the U of X teaching hospital last summer really spurred my interest in dentistry.

- Was there anything else you wanted me to talk about?

- Are there other aspects of (whatever the subject) that you would like me to provide more detail about or comment on?

Whatever the interviewer's response, you can tie what you say next to those things you have on your interview-preparation sheet. Keep thinking about what you are selling, to whom you are selling, and why they should offer you this job above anyone else. Imagine in your mind the interviewer being asked by the boss to describe three things about you that he or she remembers. What is the "take-home" message you wish to instill in the interviewer?

THE NUMBER-ONE QUESTION— "TELL ME ABOUT YOURSELF"

Most interviews include a form of this vague question. Usually it means, "Tell me about your qualifications," although it could also mean "Tell me what kind of person you are," or, "Tell me about your attributes," or, "Tell me what you have been doing since graduation," or, "Did you actually learn anything in veterinary school?" or, "What makes you think I would consider hiring you?"

In the interview-preparation process, you should have arranged a five- or ten-minute answer describing your training and work experience. This would be a comprehensive response that encompasses your skills, abilities, interests, and achievements.

To help set the stage, primarily because you are not sure what the interviewer really wants to hear or cares about, a safe way to approach your response is to qualify your answer.

Example

"Certainly, Dr. Alexander, I would be happy to tell you about myself. I am sure you want to hear about my work experience and my areas of interest in veterinary medicine. Let me share with you some of the highlights of the past few years and how I believe they relate to the position you are seeking to fill. I can start with my most recent experience if you would like."

When you take this type of self-qualifying approach, you give the interviewer plenty of opportunity to respond and direct the conversation to the path of his or her real area of interest. In this manner, you can avoid talking for ten minutes about all the "wrong" things. This prevents you from "volunteering" information this interviewer may not only *not* want to hear but that could be viewed less favorably than you might desire.

You may also wish to have a well-rehearsed action story prepared to emphasize some important aspect. If you fail to tell a memorable story, do you think the interviewer will remember the conversation? People remember good stories far more readily than the content of a "one-way" conversation. One of your goals is to be remembered favorably. Sharing a story is a great way to achieve this goal.

PERSONALITY QUESTIONS

"Are you creative?" "Would you describe for me what kind of manager you are?" "How do you get along with people?" " Would you rather work with a group or by yourself?" "Give me an example of an experience with a supervisor that worked particularly well for you and an example of one that did not work well for you and how you handled those situations."

These types of questions are used to determine if you have the qualities the employer is seeking. Your best response may be to answer these in a straightforward manner and use examples of past and present experiences as proof of your claims. This is also a good opportunity to interject how

110

you might approach problem solving in a creative way using an example to further document it. Demonstrate your people skills with examples.

Example

"Describe how you get along with people."

"I would say that my leadership and communications skills are excellent. My role as committee chairperson for SCAVMA Pet Week is a typical example.

"The SCAVMA membership voted to have four activities during Pet Week. As committee chair, my role was to coordinate, facilitate, plan the logistics for the overall program, and motivate each of the four activity leaders to ensure that everything was accomplished on time. I was successful in delegating the details to each leader while ensuring that all aspects of the project were accomplished on time and within budget. Each leader was given responsibility for achieving his or her individual goals. This provided them with autonomy to perform their functions and yet empowered the SCAVMA team as a whole to reach the objective. The Pet Week events yielded a 31% increase in attendance over last year and generated $1,234 for the Veterinary College Library fund. I publicly rewarded each activity leader in a recognition program attended by all veterinary students during a lunch sponsored by a local veterinary distributor."

CASE STUDY QUESTIONS

Case interviews are used to test your ability to problem solve. Several corporate veterinary practices use these as part of their qualification-assessment procedure. Although case interviews can be in a written format, they are usually oral questions asked with one or more interviewers present.

You may be given a bit of a history regarding an animal—fairly typical of what may actually happen when you go into an exam room to evaluate a patient. You will get to ask questions and will receive answers but no interpretations. You receive points for the validity and appropriateness of the types of questions and test results you request. However, your score may be reduced if you ask for information (test results) that would not be in keeping with where the average practitioner would or should be progressing with the case as discoveries are made. In addition, points are deducted if you fail to take certain steps, akin to the standard of practice, and just guess at a diagnosis or treatment program. You may need to justify any medications prescribed and the dosages and follow-up you would use.

Sometimes, though usually reserved for business-oriented case interviews, interviewers may ask questions like: "Why are manholes round?" or "How many square yards of pizza are eaten by college students in the United States each year?" without giving you any data. They might also ask something like: "Ford is considering releasing a new model of SUV. What does the company need to think about?" These questions are designed to test your ability to problem solve and think around corners without having any real data.

If you are ever confronted in this manner, and you are not a logical thinker, you will have a tough time. The clinical case study is comparable to the clinical competency test in many aspects. You may be prepared for it by just following your training, which will reflect a fair representation of your abilities. Try not to rush through it. Focus, visualize, and address it in a straightforward manner. The problem may not have a right answer. There may not be sufficient time to reach a diagnosis. For the most part, it is the thought process you use in addressing the problems presented that is of interest. The employer is looking for a fit and is trying to decide if the way you approach challenges will be in harmony with the rest of the team.

Read some business books on case-interview techniques, or ask a local consulting firm how they might approach an answer. For the most part, other than clinical case workups, case interviews are commonly used for applicants considering consulting, finance, or executive positions in larger companies.

BEHAVIORAL QUESTIONS

The behavioral interview is used to cut through today's inflated egos and "creative resumes." Think of it as the "show-me" conversation.

Employers want to have evidence to back up any claim you make, especially those that they

111

think are exaggerated or overstated. They may ask you to relate an incident that actually happened.

If you say, "I have great people skills" or "My management abilities are excellent," have two or three well-practiced examples to back up that claim. For every positive statement you plan to make about yourself, prepare a STAR analysis:

S = name a SITUATION facing you or
T = a TASK you had to complete
A = describe what ACTION you took
R = tell the RESULTS of your actions

112

Be specific, clear, and well practiced. When describing results, state them in both tangible and intangible positive terms, preferably with *measurable components*.

Example

By implementing the new process for handling chemistry test reagents for FIP studies, the pathology laboratory on campus was able to save $1.15 per test. With 2,367 tests of that nature performed last year, I was able to help the teaching hospital save $2,722 in costs on that one test alone. The lab technicians reported that the procedure saved them four or five minutes per test as well. Those extra minutes (197+ hours a year) helped unburden them, and they seemed a bit more cheerful or at least more willing to run the tests.

If you are caught off guard when an interviewer asks you to relate a specific time when you faced a certain situation, take your time and think of an actual example. Don't be afraid to sit and think for a minute—silence while you think of an example is far better than making up something. Be honest.

MOTIVE QUESTIONS

"Describe your ideal job." "Would you prefer to work for a large or small company?" "What did you like most and least about your last job?" Motive questions are used to determine if you would enjoy the job. Your best approach to answering these kinds of questions is to be specific and emphatic. Tie your responses directly to your

education, experience, and background, or to the position in question.

Example

"Describe your ideal work situation."

"The type of environment in which I like to work has a learning component and is results oriented. I look for work that challenges my clinical skills, especially in live-stock production systems and reproductive physiology. My training in genetic identification from Rocky Mountain Select Sires while a student at Colorado State University helps me with strategic planning for clients. I'm a team player, and I enjoy having the opportunity for some self-direction and responsibility. I also like being a part of a small group. I like it best when my boss is also part mentor, helping me to learn new skills on the job, answer questions, and guide me toward possible solutions to situations that arise. I like working outdoors part of the day and enjoy variety and handling several projects at one time. I'm a 'people person'—several of my classmates and I have been volunteers at the local nursing home with our dogs each Saturday morning for the past two years. I take pleasure in listening to the patients tell their stories as they visit with our pets."

ETHICS QUESTIONS

Questions regarding ethics establish your character, your values, and your perspective on right versus wrong.

> Questions regarding ethics establish your character, your values, and your perspective on right versus wrong.

Example

"Give me an example of a real-life situation in which you encountered an ethical dilemma. How did you handle it, and what was the outcome?"

"The question of ethical behavior really first notably came to my attention when I was a first-year student in veterinary school. As in all professional programs, we were on the honor system and had been given a lecture on that subject by the Dean during orientation.

Table 8-4
ADDITIONAL INTERVIEW QUESTIONS

- What makes you think you are qualified for this position?
- What abilities do you have that will help us in our practice?
- Why us?
- Who can you give us as references—people that are aware of your clinical skills?
- Why haven't you found a job so far?
- What is the biggest failure you have had?
- What is your management style?
- Do you consider yourself a leader? If so, why?
- What are some examples of your leadership skills?
- How do you think your coworkers describe you?
- What are your outside interests?
- What attracted you to this position?
- What has been your most difficult clinical case?
- What was your biggest accomplishment at your last job or in veterinary school?
- What types of decisions do you like to make? What are your least favorite?
- Have you ever had to fire anyone? Have you ever lost your job?
- Tell us about an experience with a dissatisfied client. How did you handle it?
- Where do you see yourself in five years?
- Do you have any interest in owning a practice of your own?
- If you could travel anywhere in the world, where would it be? Why?
- Describe a time when you had a disagreement with a colleague. How was it resolved?
- What is your biggest fear?
- What brings you the most joy?
- Have you ever had to report to a woman boss? How did you handle that relationship?
- What professional organizations do you belong to? What are your contributions?
- Can you tell us about a time when you did not know the answer to a client's question?
- Describe a time when you were involved in the death of a client's animal. How did you handle it?
- Why were you originally attracted to veterinary medicine as a career?

"Midway through the first term, my anatomy lab partner had written answers for a test on her arm under her sleeve. I remember being very surprised when I happened to glance up and saw it during the quiz. At first I did not know what to do. I was torn, knowing that I did not want to get anyone in trouble, yet I felt bound to report it—not only to protect myself, but to uphold the principles and values of the school and maintain the integrity of our class. What she was doing violated the honor code and might have given us all a bad name.

"I decided to confront the individual and let her take the initiative to report herself before I did. I expressed my concerns and indicated that if she did not come forward voluntarily, I would file a complaint with the SCAVMA president and ask for action by the student council. My persuasive efforts must have been compelling, as she did turn herself into the professor and took a failing grade for that quiz. We are still friends, and she graduated in the top 25% of the class."

WHY US QUESTIONS

"What is it that attracts you to this position?" "Why do you want to work here?" "Why would you leave Colorado to come to work in Wilsonville, New Jersey?" This type of query often becomes the "lump it all together, catch all" question used by the nonexperienced interviewer. Many employers are not very good interviewers. They are unable to fully express their expectations about a position to potential candidates. They are not sophisticated enough to sort through other types of questioning or sift through answers to find accurate meaning; therefore, they lump everything together in this question. It is akin to "Tell me about yourself," because you have little clue as to what the real "hot button" might be for this employer. This type of question requires an all-encompassing answer and is an attempt to test your resolve and commitment.

The question goes to how motivated you are for this specific job at this time, with this group, in this geographic location. The interviewer is exploring the fit. To answer this kind of question, incorporate your drive, enthusiasm, training, personality, personal vision, and where you see yourself going with your career. This is one of the questions to answer in your preparation phase. Your answer will need to be rehearsed and polished. This is also a good time to show that you have researched this practice and know a little about its history. You can share what you know about the practice's leadership role and standing in the professional community.

Example

"Why do you want to work here?"

"I am attracted to this position at Glenwood Springs Animal Hospital because this is a progressive practice. My uncle lives here near Sunlight Ski Area. You may remember me coming here with him before I started college. I spent many happy summers on his ranch as a teenager. He has always spoken favorably of the service Dr. Woods has given him and his quarter horses and working dogs over the years.

"What I see as a good fit for me is that the practice has continued to spend considerable resources on good equipment and staff training and is growth oriented. The employees appear very happy, knowledgeable, and forward thinking. My background with breeding and raising champion field-trial dogs, advanced training and interest in ultrasound techniques, and laboratory diagnostics could prove to be strong assets to the practice and for possible expansion of services to the region. In addition, my skills as a horsewoman will allow me to help cover for Dr.

Woods' equine part of the practice, now that he is looking to semi-retire.

"Since starting veterinary school, I have envisioned myself working in the mountains in a smaller community as part of a predominantly small-animal practice with some equine. I already know this is a great place to raise a family. I have maintained relationships with a few of the ranchers and some of the local merchants in the area. My husband, who comes from a small town in Idaho, likes this area as well. I see this as a wonderful opportunity for us as a family and am enthusiastic about the potential working relationship with Dr. Woods and the other clinicians."

SALARY QUESTIONS

"What salary are you looking for?" Premature discussions about money can be a real deal breaker. Moreover, the more excited an employer is about you, the more likely he or she will be willing to negotiate salary.

Example

"Before we get too far into this, I would like to know how much money you are looking for."

"Dr. Roberts, if we can agree that my experience and training fit your needs, I do not believe we will have much problem regarding compensation. My concern is whether your needs call for someone with my interests, skills, and background."

Another response might be:

"Dr. Roberts, I could talk more intelligently about my circumstances after I know a bit more about the job and other contributions I can make to your practice. For example, what opportunities exist for added income potential? How are emergency calls handled? What about overtime? What additional client services and profit centers are there to explore?"

A third reply might be:

"For my part, Dr. Roberts, I am most certainly interested in the situation, the people I would be working with, and my role in the

114

overall effort of the hospital. While money is important, I am not locked into a specific figure because of these considerations." (Here, you remain gracious but avoid a specific dollar figure or direct answer. Cite things like the chance to learn more about xyz, deal with the challenging cases, or improve your skills in abc.)

If it looks like the session will go nowhere unless money is discussed, try to get the interviewer to reveal a salary range before you commit yourself. If all else fails, give a range surrounding your estimate of what the job should be paying. Realize the employer will likely be looking at the low end of what you state.

Indicate that the entire compensation package, including the value of benefits, needs to be considered in your decision. For that, you will need to learn more about this employer's expectations and vision for the position. Be prepared to cite salary-survey studies plus the cost-of-living figures you have researched in case you sense the employer's knees buckle at the range you just cited. If there is no negative body language on the interviewer's part, or you feel it is safe to move the conversation in other directions, save discussions regarding salary specifics and actual determination of compensation until the negotiation phase.

The cardinal rule is: *Do not negotiate compensation until the employer is completely sold on you and you have been offered the job.* Practice responses for every approach to money you think the employer will throw at you. The more you practice, the more comfortable you will be talking about compensation when the time comes.

Say you are presently employed in a clinic. This is an interview for a new job and you are asked, "What salary are you currently making?" Always answer this carefully. One approach is to state that the new job, while in line with your skills, cannot compare to your current position. Therefore, your present salary is not a good criterion for compensation in the new position. You can put it this way: "What I am making now is less important than whether or not my skills, talents, and abilities are what you need for your practice. I am confident the compensation range will be fair. We can work that out after I learn more about your vision for this position."

WEAKNESS QUESTIONS

"What is your biggest weakness?"

One possible reply is:

"I really do not feel I have a weakness that affects my working ability. Sometimes a coworker may say I occasionally push people too hard to get a task completed. I remember once I was riding the technicians a bit to get some blood samples run. They complained but ran the tests. The owner, who was transporting the animals across state lines, came in early for the health certificates because the flight had been changed. By having the tests completed, the clinic looked good and the owner was thrilled. Although I agree we all have opportunities for improvement and personal growth, sometimes what appears as a negative can prove to be a positive in the long run. In this case, it created a winning situation for everyone."

TALK-ABOUT-YOUR-BOSS QUESTIONS

"What do you think about your boss?"

Don't talk negatively about anyone at any prior place of employment. You don't have to be dishonest, but you do need to talk about *something* positive. A response could be:

"She's great, and I have really enjoyed working with her and have learned some good approaches to case-management."

HOW-LONG-WILL-YOU-STAY QUESTIONS

"How long will you stay with us?"

You may not think this is a fair question, but you need to say *something*. You could say something like:

"As I mentioned before, I am looking for the right career opportunity. I will be here as long as we're both meeting our goals."

WHY-ARE-YOU-LEAVING QUESTIONS

"What is wrong with your current job? Why do you want to leave it?"

As with "your previous boss" questions, do not say anything negative. It just makes you look bad. Say:

"I really do not feel there is anything wrong with my current job. I have enjoyed working there and the staff has taught me a lot. It is a good practice. However, I am ready to handle additional responsibility now and would like to explore the opportunity for career growth."

WHY-SHOULD-WE-HIRE-YOU QUESTIONS

"According to your resume and information packet, you look pretty impressive. If you are this good, you ought to be able to solve most of our problems. Tell us, Mark, why should we hire you?"

This is a bit of a left-handed compliment, and you know they do not believe you are that good. If you begin to talk about why they should hire you, you run the risk of missing what it is they really want to know and spending time on attributes they could care less about. One way to handle difficult questions is to turn them around. One such approach might be:

"Dr. Craig, in answer to your question, I have a lot of training and background that would be of considerable value to your clinic operation. However, it might be a bit presumptuous of me to tell you what you need before I have heard what you think the priorities for this job are. If you would be kind enough to share some of your thoughts with me at this time, perhaps I could give you a more intelligent answer regarding what I have to offer and how that fits in."

Your Turn—Ask the Right Questions

This is your interview. That means you are also interviewing the employer, who will expect you to have pertinent questions of your own. Your questions provide an employer with a sense of what is important to you. Develop and carry your list of prioritized questions with you in a portfolio or notebook. At the appropriate time, you can review the list or jot down key phrases of the employer's response.

How you time your questions is critical. It is best not to ask too many questions at once. A good time for some question asking may be just after you have answered one of the interviewer's questions. Here you can get additional clarity and then tie your response to one of your qualities or strengths.

Another good opportunity to ask questions is while taking a walking tour of the facility. Be sure to let the interviewer answer your question before you ask another. Stay attentive to what is happening.

TYPICAL QUESTIONS YOU SHOULD BE PREPARED TO ASK THE INTERVIEWER

- Why has this position become available? What happened to the last associate?

- If I were given this position today, what are the biggest challenges I would face?

- Would you please show me a copy of the job description?

- To be successful, what qualities does a person in this position need?

- What do you see as the top three priorities for the person in this position to accomplish or address in the next six months?

- What do you see as opportunities for career growth in this position?

- What role does someone in this position play in staff training? Supervision? Profit-center management?

- How long have you been associated with this practice?

- What is the time frame for you to make your selection?

- Will you notify all the final candidates that a decision has been made?

AFTER THE INTERVIEW IS OVER

Critique the Interview

Make a list of questions you remember being asked and how you responded. Then, jot down ideas about how you might improve your performance. Try to identify any objections particular interviewers may have had. How well do you think you did in overcoming them? What questions did you ask? How were they received? Did they get answered? Would there have been a better way to get the information? What did you leave out? What impression did you leave with the interviewers? Imagine them in a room all together talking about you. What do you think they got as a "take away" message about you? What do you need to reinforce or address in your thank you letter?

Evaluate the Experience

Evaluate your experience in terms of the practice and the business. Make a list of the positives and of the areas of concern you observed, encountered, or had an intuitive feeling about. What do you feel needs to be done about them? What additional information do you need to test your assumptions?

Write a Thank-You Letter

Any time a company has invested time in you, write a thank-you note as a sign of appreciation. Be disciplined. Within one or two days after the interview (preferably within twenty-four hours), prepare and mail a thank-you letter to each person with whom you interviewed. In such a letter, keep the tone courteous, polite, and appreciative. Consider including the following:

• A thank-you for their time, conveying your gratitude for being selected for an interview

• Reinforcement that you have interest and enthusiasm for the position

• A few key qualities you have that make you ideal for the job

• Clarification of a response, providing information you promised you would get for them, or briefly supplementing your answers

• An analysis of your visit to the clinic or of the interview

• Any new information about your qualifications or education since the interview

• A comment that you look forward to hearing from them in the near future

If multiple people interviewed you, make each letter a bit different, and use the information regarding personality temperaments to guide how you frame the letter. The follow-up thank-you letter will show the interviewer that you are thorough

and are sincerely interested in the job (whether you are or not). You can always decline it later. It will also make you feel good and develop confidence in yourself if you get an offer of employment. Now is not the time to burn bridges or prematurely take yourself out of contention. Writing the letter helps you wrap up your application to this employer. It is also the last chance to tie up any loose ends. See Figure 8-1 for an example of an interview follow-up letter.

When You Don't Hear Back From the Employer

You interviewed, sent a follow-up thank-you letter, and several weeks have gone by—no word from the employer. The next follow-up letter you may use, when you receive no response to an interview, is the subtlest of all the follow-up letters. You will normally consider using it if the practice you interviewed with is painfully slow at decision making, or you have other offers pending and you want to hurry the decision along.

Consider the following points when writing this letter:

• Address the letter to the decision maker.

• Restate the position for which you interviewed.

• Make specific reference to your visit at the hospital or to your interview.

• If you were given a date or deadline by the interviewer as to when a decision would be forthcoming, state it. Consider stating that you have deadlines from others, and reaffirm your interest in this hospital. (*Use caution here because you do not want to be excluded, especially if you have nothing else firm in the works.*)

• Request that action be taken to inform you of the status of your application, when a decision can be expected, or if the situation has changed.

It is so important to use an appropriate tone when writing this letter. If you have a genuine interest in this practice, you do not want to tip the scales against you. At the same time, the inaction and inability to reach a decision speak volumes about management of the business, especially if you were told a date the decision would come, and that date is long gone.

Remember—you may still have to go through a negotiation phase once they make you an offer. Always have a plan B. At the same time, it is good business to show you are still interested, but concerned at some level because they have not gotten back to you. Projecting this in a considerate manner can be extremely challenging. There may be good reasons for the delay. Always test your assumptions.

When You Are Rejected

Even though you are turned down for a position with a certain employer, consider writing a letter when you receive the rejection notification. You may at some other point in time, when you have gained additional expertise, training, and responsibility, want to apply to that practice again. You can also consider making this contact by phone, especially if you want more information, as to why you were not selected. Keep a file on this employer with your application for future use.

A letter might be a better approach than a phone call, because an employer may keep a letter in his or her file with your application, especially if he or she is contemplating future openings. Your phone call will be forgotten. It may have been there was a more qualified candidate than you for this position at this time. When a new position opens, many employers review their files of previous applicants as a starting point for filling the new job. Once again, their choice is based on the image you projected, the interest you expressed, your professionalism, and your attention to detail.

In either case, by letter or phone, consider including in your correspondence or conversation the following:

- A thank-you for considering you for the position

- A short discussion of your positive impressions about the practice, the staff, and the facility

- Mention of the fact that you would like to stay in touch and possibly reapply at a later date

When You Reject a Job Offer

You interviewed for a position, and the next week in the mail comes a letter offering you the job. For whatever reason, you do not want this job. A polite refusal is your responsibility as an applicant as well as a professional courtesy to this employer. In this manner, you are letting the employer know you are not interested or available to accept his or her offer at this time, allowing the employer to continue the search for an employee as quickly as possible. By ending the negotiation on a positive note, you have kept the door open to future job opportunities at this practice. If you are in a town in which many clinics network with each other, you have helped to protect your reputation as a professional as well.

Make it a point to respond in a timely manner. Don't put it off. Although it is no longer crucial to you personally, it is important to the employer and to others who are under consideration for the position you are refusing. Getting out of the way helps someone else get the placement.

It may be a good tactic to use an indirect approach when wordsmithing the refusal letter. In this manner, you would give reasons before you say "no." The purpose of the letter is to reject the offer. If you do not want to negotiate any further, it is also permissible to say "no" firmly. Follow these guidelines:

- In the opening paragraph, thank the employer for the offer. If you are using an indirect approach, give a few reasons why you do not think there is a close fit. Convey that although you appreciate the offer, you are unable to accept the position.

- Give the employer reasons for your refusal. If there is a problem in the practice, the employer may need to know that before offering the next applicant the job.

- Always end your letter on a positive note and thank them for the time they invested.

It might be preferable to use a letter rather than a phone call to refuse a position, especially if you do not want to get into a discussion on the phone about your impressions of the practice, or if you don't want to face the possibility of the employer "upping the ante." This is particularly true if you have decided you do not want to work there based on criteria other than compensation.

When You Need to Negotiate Further

You had a great interview, the hospital is all you were hoping for, and the staff seemed happy. Ten days after the interview, you receive a letter with a job offer. Unfortunately, the compensation package is below what you need or expect based on previous conversations with the owner. Now what? Assuming you still want the job and you are willing to put more energy into this, it is time to write a letter to ask for negotiation. (Actually, either side can instigate negotiations regarding responsibilities, work schedules, benefits, wages, and incentives. For the purposes of this example, you are the one who wants to negotiate.)

This letter is similar to both the acceptance and refusal letters except it will contain one, or possibly several, "if" clause(s). You might say that you would most likely accept the offer if certain conditions are met or addressed (*see* Chapter 10, Negotiating Techniques and Skills).

Do the following when you write a letter to request further negotiation:

- Thank the employer for the offer. Reinforce your interest in the practice.

- Make a request for further negotiation, or write out a conditional statement.

- List the points of your contract that require negotiation and state the reasons why. Briefly cite your strengths and what you bring to help support your views.

- Suggest that the employer contact you with his or her opinions about your points of negotiation.

- Ask to set an appointment, and invite the employer to continue the dialogue in a face-to-face meeting to further discuss the items in question.

- Be polite and professional. Review and sharpen your negotiation tools.

- If you have other offers pending, communicate a sense of urgency to this employer because you need to make a decision in the near future.

This is a fragile negotiation. You already know that this employer wants you. Now you have to convince him or her how much you are worth and what value you bring to the business. Set your limits and the point at which you'll walk away.

Polish the salesperson within. Approach the adventure in a positive manner from a position of power. Even if you have no other offers and desperately need this job, you will most likely become disgruntled if you do not try to negotiate for what you really need. You may become resentful and dissatisfied and therefore may not want to stay there for very long.

What could be worse is that by taking a job without negotiating for what you need, you are taking yourself off the market for a relatively short period of time and may not be able to use this employer as a reference. The next employer to which you apply for a job may ask about the time lapse in your employment history or why you only worked a short time at this position. If you are a new graduate, most likely you must account in some fashion for what you did in the time after graduation.

When You Accept a Job

The employer should have sent you a written job offer that briefly reaffirms the offer. It is their way of completing the legal contract between you and the business. For many hospitals today, enclosed with the offer letter may be a contract for you to complete, sign, and return.

If there is a separate work agreement, you can send your letter of acceptance pending review of the contract by your lawyer. State that to be the case in the body of your letter.

It is your responsibility to confirm that you understand the details of the offer. As far as the contract goes, be prudent and have an attorney you trust review it. If your attorney approves it, then you are ready to send the letter of acceptance. Otherwise, you may be sending a letter of refusal or a letter requesting further negotiation.

Include the following statements in an acceptance letter:

Figure 8-1
EXAMPLE OF AN INTERVIEW FOLLOW-UP LETTER
This document is also available on the companion CD.

James L. Boston, DVM
3456 Santana Boulevard
Santa Rosa, California 77555

July 8, 2005

Mr. Don Alton
Regional Director
Cooperative Extension
University Of Nebraska
Northeast Regional Office
106 "O" Street
Lincoln, Nebraska 68447

Dear Mr. Alton:

This is just a brief note to say how much I enjoyed meeting you and extension agent Dr. Jim Smith and interviewing for the position of Extension Agent (Livestock) over the past two days. Not only does it seem you have built a great team at UNL, but there is also a very supportive and active producer advisory panel I enjoyed meeting with on the second day of the interviews.

Because of my 4-H background in agriculture on the family farm, my work as National Vice President of FFA, and my experience being the secretary of the student chapter of AABP at University of California-Davis the past two years, my leadership skills and ability to work with people are excellent.

I approach client service from a value-added perspective and am comfortable communicating with people at every level, whether in black tie or blue jeans. From what I have learned through the interviews, I believe these attributes will be strong assets for success in this position. Based on my abilities, especially with up-and-coming younger producers, I will bring innovative ideas, a strong network, and the leadership, facilitation and team building skills you need to get the job done.

Thank you for your consideration. I am excited about this opportunity and look forward to hearing from you in the near future.

Sincerely,

James L. Boston

James L. Boston, DVM
Phone: (719) 555-1212
E-mail: jlbtoughguy@yahoo.com

- Thank the author of the letter and the practice for the offer.

- Accept the position.

- Reaffirm the terms of the contract (this may include salary, benefits, work location, etc.). If you need clarity, request clarification in your acceptance letter. State exactly and explicitly what you are agreeing to. Address any item that remains vague. If you are having your attorney review a written employment contract, indicate that you are conditionally accepting the position contingent on your attorney's approval of the document. State that you will complete, execute, and return the work agreement as soon as your attorney has finished his or her review and has advised you to proceed.

- Repeat any instructions given to you by the employer. These might include your starting date, your work schedule, and terms for conditions of employment (e.g., successfully passing a drug screen, granting permission to run a credit report, having an acceptable driving record, passing a criminal background check).

- Express your happiness about joining the practice and state that you will be contacting them in the near future for more details on fulfilling the conditions of employment (like the drug screen).

"They want me; they really want me!" Of all the types of letters in the employment process, the acceptance letter is one of the most pleasant letters to write.

RESOURCES

Compensation & Benefits by AAHA Press.

Case in Point: Complete Case Interview Preparation by M. Cosentino.

Executive Job Search at $100,000 to $1,000,000+ by B. Gerbert.

How to Market Yourself: A Veterinary Technician Placement Program by V. Howard.

The Interview Rehearsal Book: 7 Steps to Job-Winning Interviews Using Acting Skills You Never Knew You Had by D. Gottesman and B. Mauro.

Job Interviews For Dummies® by J. Kennedy.

Knock 'Em Dead by M. Yate.

Landing the Job You Want: How to Have the Best Job Interview of Your Life by W. Byham and D. Pickett.

More Best Answers to the 201 Most Frequently Asked Interview Questions by M. Deluca and N. Deluca.

101 Great Answers to the Toughest Interview Questions by R. Fry and R. Fry.

Power Interviews: Job-Winning Tactics from Fortune 500 Recruiters, Revised and Expanded Edition by N. Yeager and L. Hough.

Selling to Vito: The Very Important Top Officer by A. Parinello.

201 Best Questions to Ask on Your Interview by J. Kador.

Vault Guide to the Case Interview by M. Asher and E. Chung.

CHAPTER NINE

Compensation: Salary Models and Options

Samuel M. Fassig, DVM, MA

Charlotte A. Lacroix, DVM, JD

Thomas E. Catanzaro, DVM, MHA, FACHE

> IN THIS CHAPTER, YOU'LL LEARN:
>
> • **How to assess your worth**
> • **The different types of compensation, with examples**
> • **Typical benefits for associate veterinarians**
> • **How to quantify the value of each job offer**

According to a 2001 AVMA survey of graduating students, 74.7% of graduates sought employment in the private sector. In addition, the same survey revealed that 91.8% of graduates seeking employment received a mean of 2.7 job offers each. It stands to reason, then, that employers are complaining there are not enough associates to fill open positions. These data contradict the findings of the KPMG Megastudy, which states that the supply of veterinarians has grown considerably faster than demand and may exceed demand until sometime between 2004 and 2009.

There is a problem with fuzzy logic here. Employers who complain they cannot find help should stop blaming the number of job openings and take a look at their own management skills, how they integrate and reward associates for commitment to the practice, and their flexibility and willingness to improve pay levels and compensation models. Depending on how well they treat associates, and to some extent the geographic location of the practice, it may take a week or several years to fill a position. This amount of time is, for the most part, unrelated to the number of jobs open or the number of applicants who apply for any given position.

In a talk for the American Association of Equine Practitioners 10th Annual Practice Management Seminar in Keystone, Colorado (August 2002), Lowell B. Catlett, professor at New Mexico State University, was discussing the economic future of equine practitioners. Professor Catlett cited that the U.S. economy is forecasted to create 19 million new jobs during the next decade. There will be only 14 million people to fill them (one-half of the jobs will be filled by immigrants to the United States). His point, which is a message to all employers, is, "Treat your current employees really well." But there are several factors to consider:

• The employer must select an associate that fits his/her needs for quality and hours worked per week.

- The hiring veterinarians need to determine how much time they can spend mentoring the new hire.

- Employers want self-motivated employees.

These elements are the basis for employment contracts and the beginning of the compensation-and-benefits equation.

Professor Catlett went on to say that "all employees must be treated the same but differently," because each employee will demand to be treated individually. From this statement, we can assume that the associate employee will demand a specific, custom contract tailored to her particular circumstances. Such contract negotiations will likely become the norm. Employers unable or unwilling to flex to accommodate this demand will surely wait two years or more when filling an open position.

ASSESSING HOW MUCH YOU'RE WORTH TO THE PRACTICE

While it's always nice to have an extra pair of hands in a busy practice, some attributes are more important than others. Enthusiasm is one such attribute. Employers want somebody who is interested in the work, who is going to work hard on her cases, and who will work to make the practice better, not someone who will just do the minimum and go home. Practitioners want someone who is committed, dedicated, and happy about the job because that person is going to make the practice profitable. This brings up that most important question—what are you worth as a new associate? Here are a few things to consider:

- New associates have all the latest information. They are generally enthusiastic and eager to do a good job.

- New associates, while precise and particular about their work, are typically slow to get a job done.

- A new associate's value to a practice depends on the type of practice in which she works. The kind of doctor an associate is going to be depends on who trains the associate when she first gets out of school. Working with one or more doctors who care enough to go over cases and really teach and mentor makes a huge difference.

- The contribution an associate makes to a one-doctor practice, now becoming a two-doctor practice, has additional value in taking the burden off the owner, providing relief and more flexibility for the employer.

- Many new associates see veterinary medicine as a calling, not just a career. In general, new associates are passionate regarding helping animals and recognizing the human-animal bond. They enjoy the respect of clients and a professional standing in the community and tend to subordinate personal financial rewards to other goals and values.

While many practices start by paying associates a flat salary, there is a trend, supported by some practice-management consultants, that the fairest way to approach compensation is to pay a base salary plus a percentage of what the associate generates. Note the use of the word "compensation" in place of "salary." Some practices may not offer the highest salary but may provide retirement plans, health insurance, dental insurance, and other benefits that should be taken into account when considering an offer.

So, what are you worth?

> While many practices start by paying associates a flat salary, there is a trend, supported by some practice-management consultants, that the fairest way to approach compensation is to pay a base salary plus a percentage of what the associate generates.

From the Employer's Perspective

The employer first considers what you bring to the practice and the additional revenue you may generate. For the most part, unless your negotiation skills are excellent, it is the employer who initially decides how you are to be compensated. Thus, there is the need for clarity on what you are expected to do while you are representing the practice. There are hidden costs associated with your compensation as well: the employer's share of Social Security, unemployment insurance, and other taxes; your inexperience (which is also an insurance risk); and whatever other liabilities you may bring with you.

From Your Perspective

As the employee, you are looking for a payback or repayment for the use of your time and efforts. The payback must enable you to meet your living expenses and support your life plans. You want to be compensated for the effort you make and be appreciated for being there. Thus, there is the need to be clear on exactly what it is you are expected to do while working in the business. How do you fit into the business plan and goals of the employer? How will you be compensated (wages, benefits, bonus, percentages)? Recent veterinary-school graduates need to earn enough to service their student loans, have a semblance of a personal life, and ward off starvation.

COMPENSATION MODELS

Serious job applicants need to know the compensation that is paid to other starting associate veterinarians with similar skills in the geographic area where they are seeking employment and for the type of activities they will be performing. A number of publications contain starting salary information, as well as a deeper analysis of compensation and benefits. Consult the Resources section at the end of this chapter for further information.

It is important to understand and maintain a realistic budget. Like all salaried persons, veterinary associates must deal with the incredible shrinking paycheck phenomenon. According to the AVMA, the 2001 mean starting salary for new graduates employed in private practice was $44,547. Mean salaries for equine practitioners were much lower at $33,985. According to AAHA's *Compensation & Benefits*, the 2003 average salary for all companion-animal associates with less than five years' experience was $59,279.

Types of Compensation

FLAT SALARY

125

The flat salary (a fixed amount of compensation per year) is still the most common form of associate compensation for new graduates. According to *Compensation & Benefits*, 49% of all full-time associates and 67% of all part-time associates are paid by this compensation method. It is a fixed-level salary that provides you with the security of a predictable income. A predictable, guaranteed income is often needed, for example, to assure a bank that you will have the funds each month to make a car payment or fulfill other loan obligations. It is the simplest form of payment for record-keeping purposes. Unfortunately, there is no way you can increase your compensation with a flat salary—no matter how much income you generate for the practice, how hard you work, or how many hours you spend at work. Many new graduates do not like the flat-salary arrangement, especially if they are looking for the opportunity to increase their compensation in exchange for generating more revenue for the practice.

STRAIGHT COMMISSION OR PERCENTAGE OF INCOME

The straight-commission or percentage system of compensation replaces the flat salary with a commission equal to a predetermined or defined

---

TIPS FOR MAKING MORE MONEY

- Join a practice that pays you a percentage of the revenue you generate.
- Work additional shifts or moonlight at another practice, especially if it is a high-paying emergency clinic.
- Take on night emergency work, because it pays better than nonemergency day work.

percentage of the gross revenue you generate. AAHA's *Compensation & Benefits* study reports that 14% of all full-time associates and 13% of all part-time associates are paid with only a percentage of personal production. It is a plan that links the dollars you earn with your contribution to practice revenues. Because practice revenues and the associated commissions will vary from month to month, you may find it more difficult to manage your living expenses, repay your student debt, and participate in a retirement or savings plan. Moreover, you need to be crystal clear about how much income you are capable of generating, how the in-clinic scheduling system works, and how you will be credited with working on established client accounts. You also need to understand whether you will be earning different percentages for different types of revenue (e.g., pharmacy, food, surgery) or the same percentage for each type.

Straight commission is also more difficult to use in loan applications because you have no history of consistent earnings. Therefore, in addition to the stress of dealing with a new work environment and learning myriad facts and skills regarding medicine, surgery, and everything else you need to become a "real veterinarian," you may also have to worry about whether you will earn enough each month or quarter to make ends meet. The straight-commission/percentage system is not for the faint of heart.

BASE SALARY PLUS PERCENTAGE OF PRODUCTION

Under a hybrid compensation system, veterinary associates are paid a guaranteed base salary plus a percentage-of-production bonus equal to the percentage of the revenue they generate in excess of a certain target. The base salary provides much-needed security for beginning associates, as well as a predictable income stream to offset debts and monthly obligations. This is a significant advantage over the straight-commission system.

AAHA's *Compensation & Benefits* reports that 37% of all full-time associates and 20% of all part-time associates are paid a base salary plus a percentage of production. The base-plus-percentage compensation system is designed to motivate you to pay attention to and be sensitive to the practice's finances, which is in everyone's best interest. Practices and associates cannot continue to provide veterinary services unless the practice is profitable and the associate receives compensation that allows her to live within a realistic budget. This cycle occurs in private practice only as long as pet owners are willing to patronize the practice. In order for that to happen, a sufficient number of clients must be satisfied with the services rendered.

A 1998 study in New England found that practices using base-plus-percentage compensation produced 26% more revenue than practices that did not, and that veterinary associates paid this way generated 14% more revenue than those on a flat salary. The conclusion is that veterinary associates are more likely to make more money when there is an element of pay-for-production involved. In such systems, the associates pay attention to the level of service they provide, thus building a healthier practice and providing more and better service to the clients and patients they serve. In addition, if he wants someday to own a practice, an associate working in a production-based system is much more aware of the operations and costs associated with owning a practice and is more informed when making decisions that lead to ownership.

Elements of the Base-Plus-Percentage Compensation System

Base Salary. The first component of a hybrid system is the fixed base salary. While there are no precise rules to set this number, some veterinary-management consultants estimate that the base salary should be about 80% of an employee's total compensation. Practice owners want it to be low enough so that an associate is motivated to earn percentage of production and will generate sufficient revenue to earn the base salary.

Percentage of Production. The income-production bonus or percentage-based component is

> AAHA's *Compensation & Benefits* reports that 37% of all full-time associates and 20% of all part-time associates are paid a base salary plus a percentage of production.

usually equal to a percentage of the gross revenue generated by the associate's efforts. The base salary is deducted from the total amount earned under the percentage-of-production scenario. Some practices define revenue generated by the associate as only the revenue that is *collected*.

Example 1

The base salary is set at $35,000. The percentage used to calculate percentage-of-revenue-earned compensation is 20%. The veterinarian's percentage-of-revenue bonus will apply only to revenue generated in excess of $175,000 (20% of $175,000 = $35,000). Another way to state this concept is to say that the associate will be paid the higher of $35,000 or 20% of revenue generated.

Example 2

Dr. Associate negotiates a $30,000 annual base salary, plus 25% of service revenue and 10% of pharmacy, food, and other revenue. In one year, Dr. Associate generates revenue as follows:

$185,000 service revenue
$65,000 other revenue

Dr. Associate has earned $52,750 ($185,000 × 25%) + ($65,000 × 10%). The $30,000 base salary is paid in equal monthly installments of $2,500. The excess of $22,750 ($52,750 - $30,000) is paid as it's earned.

When considering and comparing an employer's offer, there are several things to watch for:

- Comparing compensation packages is complicated by the fact that some practices deduct payroll taxes and employee benefits from their veterinary associates' compensation. This would mean that the highest percentage might not be the best deal for you.

- Some practices use complex systems that apply different percentages on the income collected depending upon the type of service rendered by the veterinarian. High-margin, highly profitable services such as diagnostics,

surgery, and examinations are compensated with higher percentages (e.g., 26 to 28%), whereas low-margin, less-profitable services, such as lab work, are assigned lower percentages (e.g., 2 to 5%) and sometimes nothing at all.

- Low or no commissions are also applied to products and services when veterinarians have little influence on a pet owner's decision to consume products or services.

Income Collected Versus Income Generated. For purposes of calculating percentage-of-production earnings, the percentage does not necessarily apply to all revenue generated by the associate. Rather, it may be applied only to the revenue generated by an associate that is actually collected from clients. Translated, this means that no earnings are paid on accounts receivable. The client must pay the bill before the income counts toward the production bonus. If the client does not pay, the corresponding income does not count.

Uncollected billings can be a greater problem in large-animal practices, where billing is more common, than in companion-animal practices, where payment is normally obtained when services are rendered. Additionally, if the payment is not received for 90 or 120 days after billing, some or perhaps all of the entire percentage-of-production earnings are lost to the associate, even if the client does finally pay. In the same manner, bad checks and the cost of collection can be deducted from the production earnings, penalizing the associate.

The rationale behind giving credit only for collected income is to force you to pay close attention to the client's solvency and willingness to pay. The thinking is that, of all the clinic personnel, perhaps the attending veterinarian is in the best position to assess these factors. However, the Megastudy proves that veterinarians consistently underestimate clients' ability and willingness to pay, so this reasoning may not be valid.

PRODUCTION-COMPENSATION PITFALLS
Although production-compensation plans usually permit new graduates and associates to increase their compensation, the systems do have problems. By asking for clarification and taking a close

look at practice operations, you can be better prepared to avoid these pitfalls or at least reduce their impact.

- **Receptionist gatekeepers**—Not all cases are equal when it comes to the potential for revenue generation. To detect favoritism, you need to take a hard look at how cases are assigned among the veterinarians on staff. Usually, this means determining if the receptionist has been given instructions in this regard or if she is likely to favor some veterinarians over others. Be cautious of situations in which the receptionist or gatekeeper is the spouse, partner, or relation of one or more of the owners.

- **Staff efficiency and leverage**—You can increase your production bonuses by maximizing revenue-generating activities (which count for bonus purposes) and reducing non-revenue-generating activities, consistent with providing high-quality veterinary services and keeping the client happy. To accomplish this, the practice must have a sufficient number of well-trained and motivated support staff persons to perform as much of the non-revenue-generating activities as possible and to assist in generating revenue as appropriate. The idea underlying leveraging staff is that veterinarians should stick to diagnostics, treatment, prescriptions, and surgery, and support staff should do everything else. Maximum efficiency is achieved when as many tasks as possible are delegated to someone who costs the practice less than a veterinarian. Proper staff leveraging and efficiency are critical to the success of most practices. A leading expert in veterinary-practice management puts it this way: "In general, staff leveraging makes or breaks percentage-based compensation." You must therefore evaluate the quantity, quality, and attitude of the staff of the prospective practice. Very busy (and profitable) practices may have a higher-than-average ratio of four or more support staff per veterinarian.

- **The importance of a balanced doctor schedule**—It is important to ensure rotation between inpatient and outpatient appointments.

- **Cherry-picking cases**—Ensure that the client-relations team schedules all doctors fairly and that some new clients are assigned to you.

- **Not all doctors are motivated by money**—Employers need to know the "hot buttons" of each person on staff. You must communicate the rewards that are important to you, and negotiate with the employer.

- **Repeat business is important**—Employers tend not to reward anyone for *not* bringing patients back into the practice. Repeat visits and contacts are important.

- **Data processing and definition issues**—Production-compensation systems, particularly when variable percentages are applied, are bookkeeping nightmares. Producing production figures daily or weekly will motivate you more, but this procedure tends to raise the practice's costs.

- **Competition and distrust among veterinarians**—Perhaps the biggest problem is that production-based compensation exacerbates competition among veterinarians for high client volume and lucrative cases (rich clients or clients for whom money is no object when a pet's health is at stake). Distrust among veterinarians blooms when actual or perceived unfairness or favoritism exists in assigning cases, or if some veterinarians (such as owners) receive higher percentages than others. Basic fairness dictates that practice owners compensate themselves using the same formula that is used for associates.

A Compensation Example

The following example provides a picture of what a new graduate can expect in the first two years of employment as an associate veterinarian.

THE FIRST YEAR
The new graduate (in 2004) expects to earn $45,000 a year or more and to commit forty hours per week to a veterinary practice. This is without emergency call or overtime and with two days off each week. This is perhaps a bias you learned in veterinary school.

Many employers expect to subsidize a new graduate for six months and do not anticipate this individual to be a producer during that time. For three to six months, the graduate is often given an extra ten minutes per client per appointment, with the expectation that she will come into alignment with the practice's philosophy regarding appointment time before the six months are up. These employers are prepared to pay $1,875.30 twice a month for six months, without concern, then shift the new doctor to 20% of her personal production or base, whichever is greater. As the doctor earns more than the guaranteed base, the owner is ready to pay more.

A typical compensation model for year one is as follows. It is a starting point for negotiation.

- Base salary divided into twenty-four pay periods, paid on the fifteenth and at the end of the month (EOM).

- Productivity is 20% of personal production.
  —Personal production is *everything* on an exam-room ticket.
  —Personal production for inpatient surgery is a 50% split.
  —Refills, over-the-counter sales, boarding, baths, etc. are credited to the hospital.

- The EOM payment is 20% of the *previous month's* production, less the mid-month base payment.
  —Next year, base pay will be 20% of this year's production divided over twenty-four pay periods (this is called "no-salary-ceiling" compensation).
  —The reception team controls the equitable-client-access scheduling.

THE SECOND YEAR

For the second year of a new graduate doctor, the last six months of the first year are taken into consideration. The personal production from that period is multiplied by two. Twenty percent of that number is computed as the second year's annual base compensation. Twice-a-month pay periods usually prove best for budget tracking, paid on the fifteenth and the last day of the month.

The rest of the story can be quite different, based on your performance. Compensation is based on client perceptions, staff perceptions, community perceptions, owners' perceptions, and fiscal success of the practice. Keep the following points in mind as you move into your second year:

- Since every practice wants to improve patient-client service, you need to ask the clients about their perceptions. A once-a-quarter survey on the quality of service would provide client feedback about each provider, as well as the practice system that supports the client access. Each quarter, it would set the criteria for the next three months.

- The individual veterinarian's involvement in community activities is important—to the practice and to her own quality of life. This community activity should be of your own choosing and be one that promotes community image, health, wellness, and your identity to community members.

- There is also a concern in most practices regarding your timely and satisfactory performance of all administrative and nonpatient-care responsibilities. This could be as simple as following a dress code or as complex as the training of outpatient nurses. These include one-time and recurring tasks that may be assigned from time to time by the practice leadership.

- An evaluation by the paraprofessional team of each doctor is important, addressing harmony, synergy, and quality of performance. This could be a simple survey, done quarterly, to establish the criteria for the next three months. Team members should be able to help form the team standards.

- Regardless of the individual effort, a program-based budget sets goals and objectives for the products and services being offered by the practice. All staff members should be working to attain or exceed the financial projections for the programs being offered. Projections should provide for a total annual growth of at least the inflation rate (Consumer Price Index, or CPI) plus 6% (projected need to support a benefit-plan investment program, debt retirement, and capital-expense procurement).

- Practice consultants indicate that they counsel employers to expect new associates to produce $400,000 to $500,000 per year. Associates should ask a potential employer if the practice can support at least $400,000 in gross production.

EMPLOYEE BENEFITS

Recent graduates looking for current information on employee benefits can get an idea of how meager the benefits packages offered to starting veterinary associates are by looking at the annual surveys published in *JAVMA*. The 2001 survey showed that:

- 35% of the employers covered by the study offered disability insurance

- 70% offered health benefits

- 25% offered a retirement plan

- Approximately 20% of the employers reflected in the *JAVMA* study granted no benefits at all.

This approach doesn't make much tax sense with respect to benefits such as medical, disability, and life insurance; professional dues; and licensing fees. Current tax laws allow the practice to deduct all or part of these as a business expense *and* the employee receives these benefits tax-free. By having the employer provide these types of benefits, you can save 25% to 40% of the value of the benefits in taxes depending upon your individual tax situation. Logic would imply that it is prudent to take advantage of such lucrative tax breaks.

The value of a particular employee benefit depends, of course, on your personal situation. For instance, if you have health problems, medical benefits may be more important than extra cash, whereas medical benefits have no value if you receive medical coverage through your spouse's employer. If you have young children, flexible hours may be the most important benefit.

Among the various employee benefits, you *cannot* afford to be without some form of health insurance, disability insurance, professional-liability insurance, and a retirement plan.

The following profile describes the typical benefits packages for full-time and part-time associates in small-animal practices, according to AAHA's *Compensation & Benefits*, Third Edition. If a benefit was offered 50% or more of the time, it is included in the package description below.

Full-Time Associate

- Thirty-six-hour workweek to achieve full-time status

- Six paid holidays per year

- Ten paid vacation days per year after one year of employment

- Five paid sick days per year

- Retirement plan

- $993 annual CE allowance plus travel expenses paid for by practice

- Five paid CE days

- Employee health insurance (89% of premium paid for by employer)

- Liability insurance

- License fees and professional association dues

- Employee pays practice's cost for services, pharmaceuticals, and over-the-counter products

- Four uniforms

Part-Time Associate

- Employee pays practice's cost for services, pharmaceuticals, and over-the-counter products

- Three uniforms

- Flexible work schedule

Health Insurance

Tax deductible to the employer and tax-free to the employee, it makes sense for the employer to provide health coverage, particularly since group plans are available through state and national veterinary associations, including the AVMA. Moreover, the actual cost per individual covered in employer-provided group plans is almost always considerably less than in an individual plan. Group-plan coverage is usually better than individual coverage and will frequently cover persons with preexisting health problems, whereas individual plans will not.

Disability Insurance

You have a much greater chance of contracting an illness or suffering an injury that will prevent you from working than dying. Your ability to earn a living is your greatest asset. Foregoing disability insurance is like playing Russian roulette with more than half the cylinders loaded. There is no adequate substitute for disability insurance. Social Security does provide some disability benefits, but eligibility is very strict. Workers' compensation covers only certain injuries, and benefit periods are short.

If the employer provides group disability coverage, the premiums are tax deductible to the practice and tax-free to the employee. Any benefits you receive if you become disabled will be taxable income to you as the employee. Associate veterinarians buying individual coverage cannot deduct the premiums, but benefits received are tax-free.

Professional Liability Insurance

This is another benefit that is tax deductible to employers and excluded from employees' taxable income. For reasons of self-defense, most practice owners will cover themselves and their associates, usually by purchasing a policy through the AVMA Professional Liability Insurance Trust. The only way to determine if a prospective employer's coverage is adequate is to study the policy. Key issues to investigate are the level of coverage, the cost of the premiums, the dollar amount of the coverage, and whether there are exclusions to the coverage.

Life Insurance

Approximately 30% of the employers in the *JAVMA* survey and 23% of employers in the AAHA study provided life insurance to their associate veterinarians. Life-insurance premiums

are relatively inexpensive, are tax-deductible to employers, and are either entirely or partially free to employees, depending on the policy amount. The benefits payable to the policy beneficiaries are also tax-free.

Life insurance is necessary only if you have dependents who cannot fend for themselves if you die. In most cases, this will only be if you have minor children or a spouse who cannot work.

To provide for dependents, term life insurance is generally sufficient. Beware of whole-life insurance in its myriad forms (whole life, universal life, variable universal life, and variable life). This type of insurance combines the death benefit with one or more tax-advantaged investment vehicles. Such insurance is quite expensive and is generally suitable only for high-income persons who wish to save for retirement and have already made the maximum permitted contributions to all other tax-advantaged retirement plans available to them (such as profit-sharing, 401(k) plans, and IRAs). Although permanent life insurance almost never makes financial sense for starting veterinary associates, insurance salespersons nevertheless love to aggressively push whole-life life insurance because of the high commissions and fees generated by these policies.

Retirement Benefits

Until the 1980s, most working Americans did not have to worry about saving for retirement. Employers would fund traditional pension plans, called "defined *benefit* plans," under which eligible employees would receive a fixed portion of their salary upon reaching retirement age.

To cut expenses and save costs, employers increasingly have switched to defined *contribution* plans under which the employees fund their own retirement out of their compensation. Thus, employers have transferred the burden and worries of retirement to their employees.

Relying on Social Security is risky. As everyone should know, unfavorable demographics make it unlikely that Social Security will provide future generations with the same level of benefits as early (i.e., at age sixty-five) as it does to current retirees. Remember—the payroll taxes collected on employees' salaries fund the retirement of *current* retirees, not the employees from whom the tax was deducted. Between 1990 and 2030, the number of Americans over age sixty-five will double, while the workforce will have grown only by 25%. By 2030, many people over age sixty-five will still be working because they cannot afford to retire.

> Relying on Social Security is risky. As everyone should know, unfavorable demographics make it unlikely that Social Security will provide future generations with the same level of benefits as early as it does to current retirees.

Retirement plans have varying features and are difficult to compare. Some general questions to ask include (although not all questions may be applicable to all plans):

- What type of plan is it?

- When are employees eligible to participate (e.g., after one year's employment)?

- For defined contribution plans, what is the maximum annual contribution limit, and will it be excluded from the employee's taxable income? Is the maximum the same for all participants?

- In which investment vehicle(s) are contributions invested, and how risky are they? *Beware of plans that invest exclusively or primarily in stock of the employer. If the employer goes bankrupt, you lose not only your job, but also the value of your retirement savings (because the stock will be worthless).*

- When do benefits vest (when are the funds considered 100% yours), and how are they taxed?

- How much money has the employer contributed to the plan in recent years?

- Are part-time employees excluded from the plan?

If the employer provides no retirement benefits, you must save on your own and should instead negotiate a higher salary. A sound way to start saving is through an individual retirement account (IRA). IRAs allow tax deductibility of contributions and tax-deferred growth of invested contributions.

Employees of mutual-fund organizations, such as the well-respected Vanguard or TIAA-CREF, and investment advisors will be happy to explain IRA mechanics to the uninitiated. As always, the slogan "buyer beware" applies, and you are encouraged to learn as much as possible before investing. The amount you can contribute tax-free to an IRA is rather small, though ($3,000 in 2004); if you limit your retirement savings to your IRA contributions, you will not save enough in most cases.

Time Off

VACATION

All veterinarians, including associates, need time off to prevent burnout and declines in productivity, particularly in practices where sixty-hour-or-more weeks are the norm. Nevertheless, about 25% of the employers reflected in the survey published by JAVMA offered *no* vacation leave, and another study found that the average paid vacation time among the surveyed contracts was a skimpy 9.3 days per year. Most practices increase vacation time, with seniority, up to fifteen days.

Calculation of daily vacation pay is easy if you are on a fixed salary; divide your annual salary by the days worked per year (about 240 for full-timers). If you are on a straight commission system (no base salary), vacation days may not be paid at all by the employer. If you are paid, calculating vacation-day value is more complicated because your compensation fluctuates. One recommended method is to use your average daily salary during the three months preceding the vacation. In hybrid systems, some practices value vacation days as if you were on a fixed salary; this penalizes good income earners. *Hybrid-system vacation days should be paid on the basis of the higher of base salary or the average daily salary during the three months preceding the vacation.*

Other vacation issues include:

- When starting veterinary associates first become eligible for vacation (e.g., after the first nine months of employment)

- How fast vacation time is accrued during the year

132

- Whether unused vacation time can be carried forward to the next year(s)

- How much advance notice the employer must receive regarding a proposed vacation

- How long an employee must be employed before vacation days are paid to her upon termination

OTHER LEAVES

Ask the same questions about the following types of leaves as for vacations (eligibility, accrual, carry-forwards, scheduling, etc.):

- **Holidays**—Many practices, although not required to do so, offer paid legal holidays, except possibly for President's Day, Martin Luther King Day, and Veteran's Day. About 40% of the employers reflected in the *JAVMA* survey offered paid legal holidays. AAHA's study shows that full-time associates receive an average of six paid holidays.

- **Personal leave**—According to AAHA, 93% of full-time associates and 23% of part-time associates are offered paid vacation days at one year of employment. The average number of paid days are 9.5 and 6.3, respectively, for associates who have been with the practice for one year.

- **Sick leave**—About 52% of the employers included in the *JAVMA* survey offered paid sick leave. The AAHA study, *Compensation & Benefits*, reports that 60% of full-time associates and 15% of part-time associates receive paid sick days. Employers offer an average of 5.4 and 3.3 days to full-time and part-time associates, respectively.

- **Continuing-education leave**—A majority of states mandate some form of continuing education. According to the *JAVMA* survey, about 62% of employers granted veterinary associates continuing-education leave. The AAHA study shows that an average of 4.7 days are offered to 81% of full-time associates. An average of 3.7 paid CE days are offered to 28% of part-time associates.

Continuing-Education Expenses

More than 75% of the employers in the *JAVMA*

survey and more than 90% of employers in the AAHA study reimbursed at least some continuing-education expenses for full-time associates. These expenses are tax-deductible to the employer and tax-free to the employee. AAHA reports an average $993 CE allowance for full-time associates and $595 for part-time associates. You would be well advised to ensure that your contract specifies a deadline for reimbursing your continuing-education expenses, since many practices are quite slow to do so. Seek continuing-education programs that help you to develop skills and increase your self-esteem.

Licensing and Drug Enforcement Agency (DEA) Fees

According to AAHA, about 63% of employers pay licensing fees for their full-time associates. State licensing fees range from about $100 to $450 per year. Recent graduates may consult the "Digest of Veterinary Practice Acts" section of the *AVMA Membership Directory and Resource Manual* for current information regarding state licensing fees. When the employment contract requires you to work exclusively for the practice, it is more fair for employers to pay licensing fees (which, in any event, are tax-deductible to employers and tax-free to the employee). When the employment contract allows you to work for any number of practices, it is more fair for you to pay such fees.

If you are acting as an agent of a veterinarian registered with the DEA, you may administer and dispense controlled substances but you *cannot* order or prescribe them. It is generally less costly and administratively burdensome if not all veterinary associates of a practice are registered with the DEA, as long as at least one DEA-registered veterinarian is available at all times to prescribe and order controlled substances. Prospective associates should discuss this matter with their employers.

Professional Association Dues

There are many advantages to membership in national and state professional associations. These organizations also defend the political and legislative interests of veterinarians—a crucial function in today's society. It is in the best interests of all veterinarians that national and state associations be as financially strong as possible. Approximately 60% of the employers reflected in the *JAVMA* survey paid the professional association dues of veterinary associates. AAHA reports that 65% of employers pay dues for full-time associates, and 27% pay dues for part-time associates. Such payments are tax-deductible to the employer and do not count as income to the employee. In practices with numerous employee veterinarians, paying 100% of the dues of all associates may be cost-prohibitive. In this case, the dues might be split between the employer and employee.

Other Employee Benefits

The sky is the limit when it comes to employee benefits. Other benefits you may encounter include:

- **Automobile expense reimbursement**—To the extent you are required to use your vehicles for the business of the practice (e.g., to respond to emergency and house calls), you should be reimbursed for a portion of the insurance, general maintenance, registration and inspection fees, fuel, repairs, depreciation, and lost-opportunity cost (based pro-rata on the miles driven on practice business).

- **Child care**—Child-care benefits are almost unheard of, but as more women join the profession, benefits in the form of on-site child care, arrangements with local child-care organizations (i.e., employer-funded discounts), and/or flexible spending accounts may become more common. Flexible spending accounts allow parents to pay a limited amount of child-care expenses with pretax dollars, subject to certain IRS rules. This means you save taxes on money paid for child care.

- **Loans**—You may be forced to reject what would otherwise be your dream job because your student debts are too large for the compensation being offered, or you can't afford to move to the job. A short-term loan by the employer may make all the difference.

- **Housing allowances**—If you are looking for cheaper housing, be aware that under certain circumstances, practice owners can save on payroll taxes by providing on-site housing to their employees.

- **Speaking engagements**—If you are paid to speak at a public function, keep your honorarium unless the employer pays your engagement expenses. If you are not paid, then you need to decide whether you or the employer should pay your expenses. An additional issue is whether the employer will provide paid or unpaid time off so that you can give the talk, or whether you must use vacation or personal leave.

- **Pet care**—Many practices offer discounts on veterinary services and supplies for their employees' pets. You will want to know the details of such plans, especially if you have a "Noah's Ark" full of pets. Pet health insurance can also be offered.

- **Work schedule**—A balanced and predictable work schedule can be worth a lot. This includes recurring three-day weekends.

- **Personal time**—This may include accumulating one hour of personal time (paid) for every twenty scheduled hours worked, plus eight hours per tenure year awarded as a thank-you.

- **Feeling of belonging**—It is important to feel that you are part of a caring healthcare-delivery team (pain management, humane care, patient advocacy, work harmony, etc.).

FRANK AND FULL DISCUSSION

When dealing with compensation and benefits, the "warm and fuzzy" approach often leads to misunderstandings, resentments, and separation. Most new graduates leave their first job within a year, and many of those who do stay for a second season are plotting their next move for something

> **Full and frank discussion of compensation and employee-benefit issues increases the likelihood that the employment relationship will succeed.**

else. This high divorce rate in the employer-employee relationship suggests that few new associates and employers get it right the first time.

Full and frank discussion of compensation and employee-benefit issues increases the likelihood that the employment relationship will succeed. "Full" discussion reduces the possibility of misunderstandings and mismatched expectations. "Frank" discussion reveals whether the parties can tolerate a little tension without ruining their relationship—also a good test of whether their personalities can mesh.

You are well advised to consult what has become the veterinary employment relationship "bible": *Contracts, Benefits, and Practice Management for the Veterinary Profession,* written by James F. Wilson, DVM, JD; Jeffery D. Nemoy, DVM, JD; and Alan J. Fishman, CLU, CFP. Ignorance in this area can lead not only to a thinner wallet, but also to life-altering catastrophes if medical insurance, disability insurance, or retirement planning are overlooked, disregarded, or not accounted for.

SELECTING A LAWYER TO HELP YOU

Negotiating an employment contract can be long, painful, and complicated. It therefore makes as much sense to seek professional help in this endeavor as it does to take a pet to a qualified veterinarian when it is sick. Besides bringing technical expertise, your lawyer can be a useful buffer between you and your employer. There are only two real obstacles to involving a lawyer.

- Your lawyer may upset or scare off the employer. Lawyers always "complicate things" and "screw up deals" with all their nitpicking. There is some truth to these criticisms, but what escapes attention is that almost all of those deals shouldn't go through anyway. Moreover, you can rest assured that your prospective employer has some familiarity with lawyers and that his or her lawyer has prepared the employment contract your employer wants you to sign. Some employers, however, will be spooked no matter what. In that case, you can always leave your lawyer in the background.

- Lawyers are expensive. In dealing with lawyers' fees, the first rule is to try to obtain a flat rate (rather than billing by the hour). This way your maximum cost is fixed. Most important of all is to make sure you understand how you will be charged. Here, you must be blunt. Do not hire a lawyer without being absolutely clear about his or her fees. (And yes, it should be in writing.) Many lawyers are also willing to provide recent graduates with discounts or credit. Lawyers know that you are broke and are (or should be) less interested in the fees generated in reviewing (and perhaps negotiating) your employment agreement than in starting a long-term relationship with a promising veterinarian. A smart lawyer wants you to think of him or her whenever you have a problem, or want to buy into a practice, not gouge you right off the bat.

When selecting a lawyer, trust your instincts. If you don't feel comfortable with him or her, get another one. There are plenty around. You find a good lawyer the same way you find a good doctor—by word of mouth.

Your lawyer should be at least as smart as you are. Do *not* hire a "dumb" lawyer. Check out potential candidates just like you would when selecting a mechanic to work on your classic collector sports car. It is a relationship in which many times you must direct the activity.

COMPARING JOB OFFERS

Before you make any final decisions, it is wise to compare salaries and benefits offered by practices in different areas of the country. See Table 9-1 for a way to make these comparisons. An interactive template is also available on the CD that accompanies this book.

In Table 9-1, you'll see that our fictitious associate has written her definition of the ideal practice. We've covered many aspects of the job here, including type of practice, compensation method, base salary, many different benefits, ownership potential, availability of mentors, geographic region, and emergency call. You may want to add to or subtract from this list of characteristics, but

Table 9-1
COMPARING JOB OFFERS
A fill-in-the-blank version of this table is available on the companion CD.

	MY IDEAL JOB OFFER	OPPORTUNITY DURANGO, COLORADO	OPPORTUNITY DUBLIN, OHIO	OPPORTUNITY PHILADELPHIA, PENNSYLVANIA
CASH COMPENSATION				
1. **Base**	$45,000	(-) $39,000	(-) $43,000	(+) $51,000
2. **Production Potential** (based on $200,000 gross production over base)	20% over base; potential value $40,000	(-) 12% over base; potential value $24,000	(-) 16% over base; potential value $32,000	(-) 18% over base; potential value $36,000
BENEFITS				
1. **Vacation**	2 weeks paid (included in base pay)	(+) 2 weeks paid (included in base pay)	(+) 2 weeks paid (included in base pay)	(+) 16 days paid (included in base pay)
2. **Continuing Education**	$1,000/year allowance; freedom to pick what convention	(-) 1 meeting registration; value $300	(-) 1 meeting registration, hotel; value $500	(+) 1 national meeting registration, hotel, transportation; value $1,000
3. **Sick Days/ Personal Time**	1 per month paid; value $2,077/yr	(+) 1.5 per month paid; value $2,700/yr	(-) 6 per year paid; value $992/yr	(+) Up to 14/yr; carry over; value $2,746/yr
4. **Flexibility in Work Schedule** (can modify work hours for personal needs)	Yes	(+) Yes	(+) Yes	(-) No
5. **Medical Insurance**	Employer pays 100%; value $3,000/yr	(-) Employer pays 1/3; value $1,000/yr	(-) Employer pays half; value $1,500/yr	(-) Employer pays 2/3; value $2,000/yr
6. **Dental Insurance**	Employer pays 100%; value $1,200/yr	(-) Not offered	(-) Employer offers in plan; employee pays	(-) Not offered
7. **Vision/Rx Insurance**	Employer pays 100%; value $400/yr	(-) Not offered	(-) At employee expense	(-) Part of flex pre-tax option up to $650; value $182 in tax savings
8. **Life Insurance**	$150,000 death benefit; premiums paid by employer; value $375/yr	(-) Available but at employee expense	(-) Employer pays half of premiums for $300,000 death benefit; value $250/yr	(+) Employer pays 100% premiums for $200,000 death benefit; value $425/yr
9. **Liability Insurance**	Employer provides; value $385/yr	(-) Pays in clinic name	(-) Pays in clinic name	(-) Pays in clinic name
10. **Short-Term Disability Income Insurance**	Employer pays private policy; value $3,300/yr	(-) Private policy, employer pays $167/mo; value $2,004/yr	(-) Not offered	(-) Not offered

Table 9-1 (continued)
COMPARING JOB OFFERS

	MY IDEAL JOB OFFER	OPPORTUNITY DURANGO, COLORADO	OPPORTUNITY DUBLIN, OHIO	OPPORTUNITY PHILADELPHIA, PENNSYLVANIA
BENEFITS (CONT'D)				
11. 401(k)/Retirement	Employer matches first 3% of salary dollar for dollar; value $1,350/yr	(-) No, but historically pays $2,500 bonus	(-) Investment program offered; employer pays mutual fund management fees ($120/yr); no match	(-) Employer matches first 3% at 50 cents per dollar; value $765/yr
12. Sabbatical	Available at 5 yrs; value 6 month's pay, $22,500	(-) Not offered	(-) Not offered	(-) Yes, at half pay; value $12,750
13. Veterinary Licensing and DEA Fees	Employer pays; value $500/yr	(-) Employee must pay for own veterinary license and DEA fees	(-) DEA license in clinic name; employee must pay for own veterinary licensing fees	(+) Employer pays licensing up to $600/yr
14. Association Memberships	Employer pays AAHA, AVMA, and one state VMA; value $600/yr	(-) State only; up to $200/yr	(-) State or AVMA; up to $275/yr	(+) State, local, AAHA, and AVMA; up to $700/yr
15. Child Care Fees	Employer provides $5,760/yr	(-) Not offered	(-) Not offered	(-) Discount at local day care of $2/hr ($16/day) as part of flex account; up to $3,000/yr pre-tax; value $840/yr in tax savings
16. Vehicle Provided	Yes; value $4,800/yr	(+) Yes; value $6,000/yr	(-) Not offered	(-) Not offered
EQUITY				
1. Partnership (Stock)	Available	(-) Not in employment agreement	(-) Not it employment agreement	(-) Not in employment agreement
2. Buy-In Agreement	Available	(-) Not in employment agreement	(-) Orally stated but not in employment agreement	(+) Available
3. Ownership	Available	(-) Not offered	(-) Orally stated but not in employment agreement	(+) Available

Table 9-1 (continued)
COMPARING JOB OFFERS

	MY IDEAL JOB OFFER	OPPORTUNITY DURANGO, COLORADO	OPPORTUNITY DUBLIN, OHIO	OPPORTUNITY PHILADELPHIA, PENNSYLVANIA
MENTORSHIP				
1. Formalized Mentoring Program	Available	(-) Not in employment agreement	(-) Not in employment agreement	(-) Not in employment agreement
2. # DVMs in Practice	At least 2 full-time besides me	(-) 1 full-time	(+) 2 full-time	(+) 3 full-time
3. Network of DVMs	Yes	(-) Fairly isolated community	(+) Near university and specialty practices in Columbus	(+) Near university and multi-doctor specialty practices
4. Special Interests of DVMs in Practice	Yes, different focuses for different practitioners	(-) No, only general practice	(+) One practitioner likes cats	(+) One practitioner is boarded in internal medicine, one is oriented to dentistry, and one likes exotics
5. Proximity to University Teaching Hospital or Specialty Practice	Yes	(+) Colorado State University is 4-1/2 hrs away; no specialty practice nearby	(+) Near Ohio State University (20 min away)	(+) Near University of Pennsylvania (35 min away)
OTHER				
1. Housing Availability Within Easy Commute	Yes	(+) Yes	(+) Yes	(-) Difficult
2. Practice's Gross Last Year	$1M	(-) $546,000	(-) $897,000	(+) $1.8M
3. Accredited by AAHA	Yes	(-) No	(-) Not yet, but working on it	(+) Yes
4. Type of Practice	Companion animal	(-) Mixed, mostly companion animal	(+) Companion animal	(+) Companion animal
5. Career Path Potential	Yes, helps meet requirements for specialty board	(-) No	(-) No	(+) Yes Internal medicine, dentistry, exotic medicine
6. Geographic Mobility	Area of country where I want to live or access to preferred lifestyle	(+) Yes	(+) Yes	(-) No
7. Emergency Call	No	(-) Yes, must take rotation; can earn extra $60/call;	(-) Yes, must take rotation; can earn 40% of charges/call;	(+) No

Table 9-1 (continued)
COMPARING JOB OFFERS

	MY IDEAL JOB OFFER	OPPORTUNITY DURANGO, COLORADO	OPPORTUNITY DUBLIN, OHIO	OPPORTUNITY PHILADELPHIA, PENNSYLVANIA
OTHER (CONT'D)				
8. Moving Expenses	Yes; value $7,500	(+) Yes; up to $8,000 with 2-yr work contract	(-) Not offered	(-) Yes; $2,500 limit
TOTAL POTENTIAL VALUE OF OFFER	$117,096 Without equity consideration or sabbatical; no emergency work	$94,004 (Plus bonus potential; however, not in offer) Without equity consideration or sabbatical; emergency work included in figure	$92,987 Without equity consideration or sabbatical; emergency work included in figure	$98,758 Without equity consideration or sabbatical; no emergency work
RATIO of (+) to (-)		8/25	9/24	17/16
YOUR RANKING AS OF		**#3**	**#2**	**#1**
5/8/05				

Adapted from Dr. Kerri Marshall

we've erred on the side of completeness to make your job evaluation task easier.

For each job offer, you'll write the specifics of each particular aspect of the job, along with a plus or minus. A plus indicates that it meets or exceeds your definition of the ideal. A minus sign indicates that it does not meet your definition of the ideal job. At the end of the list, you'll see a ratio of pluses to minuses, which will allow you to easily rank your job offers. The spreadsheet included on the accompanying CD has room for you to add additional jobs and characteristics if needed.

GOLDEN HANDCUFFS

The term "golden handcuffs" refers to the concept of making it too costly for an associate to leave an established position. While most associates start at a base salary (calculated at less than 20% of their personal production), a practice owner may remove the salary cap for you if he wants to keep you around. This practice owner will give a one-half percent increase in productivity pay each year that your personal production goes up. For example, let's say your base salary is $40,000, and you earn 20% of the service revenue that you generate. Your personal production increased this year, so next year, you'll earn your base salary plus 20.5% of the service revenue that you generate.

Once you reach 22.5%, though, you should start negotiating for ownership equity because most companion-animal practices cannot afford to pay you more than 23% of your production without capping your total compensation. In "ownership-track" situations, the practice owner may choose to substitute a pay raise with an ownership share of the practice. In that case, you may forfeit your ownership shares if you leave the practice, plus your noncompete clause will kick in immediately. Be sure you understand what the consequences are if you have this kind of agreement, and get it in writing.

RESOURCES

Books

*Beyond the Successful Veterinary Practice: Succession Planning & Other Legal Issues.*by T. Catanzaro, R. Deegan, E. Guiducci.

Compensation Alternatives and Methodologies by T. Catanzaro.

Compensation & Benefits by AAHA Press.

Contracts, Benefits and Practice Management for the Veterinary Profession by J. Wilson, J. Nemoy, and A. Fishman. Available through AAHA.

Economic Report on Veterinarians & Veterinary Practices by the American Veterinary Medical Association.

The Equine Veterinarian: A Complete Profile by E. Blach (editor).

Veterinary Compensation in New England: A Descriptive Study by T. Lynch.

Magazine Articles

"Employment, starting salaries and educational indebtedness of year–2001 graduates of US veterinary medical colleges." JAVMA, Vol. 220, No. 2 (2002).

"Employment of male and female graduates of US veterinary medical colleges." JAVMA, Vol. 220, No. 5 (2002).

Websites

Veterinary Practice Consultants
www.v-p-c.com
A consulting firm providing veterinary practices with team building, leadership, and management assistance.

Vetsuite 2003
www.vetsuite.com
Vetsuite 2003 brings together three powerful educational tools for the veterinary clinic with the goal of "Improving Revenues Through Education." A subscription to Vetsuite 2003 includes both online access to the Vetsuite Medical Center, Vetsuite Website Builder, and Novartis Support Center, as well as offline access to Vetsuite for Windows.

CHAPTER TEN

Mastering Negotiation

Samuel M. Fassig, DVM, MA

IN THIS CHAPTER, YOU'LL LEARN:

- **Common negotiation mistakes**
- **The six steps in the negotiation process**
- **How to ace your next argument**
- **How to prepare for high-risk negotiation**

NEGOTIATION AS AN ART

Whether or not you know it, you're a negotiator. The things you negotiate range from what restaurant to have dinner at or what movie to see, to buying a house or getting a loan.

You negotiate by arguing, and it takes practice. You might think of argument as a negative process, filled with screaming or fear of retaliation. But arguing can take many forms, and when you do it right, it can be a positive experience.

Arguing, or negotiation, should not be confused with intimidation. Being at odds with someone else, merely to be contrary or difficult, is not negotiating or arguing. It is not winning. It's just being disagreeable.

Learning *when* to argue is as important to winning as learning *how* to argue. If you are a good observer, you'll learn that you can win an argument without really arguing. Winning is getting what you want. It often includes assisting others in getting what they want or letting the other person talk himself out of his own arguments.

In the employer-employee relationship, you, as the employee, have considerable power. Winning may mean you get the salary and benefits you need, and the employer gets a worker who may contribute more than what the employer could ever force an employee to do.

In today's world, if you argue for more money or are in negotiation for a job, you must always demonstrate that the dollars you will receive will create more revenue and more profit for the employer. You cannot win one of these arguments by lamenting that Sarah and Jessie are hungry, or Jimmie needs new shoes, or you cannot pay your student loans. You must put forth an argument that is directed toward generating more profit for the business. Here are a couple of valid arguments:

- My average transaction charge has been consistently 20% higher than other associates because I have superior client communication skills.

• I am asking for this salary because of my added skill as a journeyman-level farrier. And I bring to the practice considerable experience with equine foot-lameness issues. This can draw a considerable number of new clients to the practice and increase what we do for your current clients. I look forward to being on a percentage-of-production basis in the future. Until then, I will enhance the scope of what this clinic will accomplish for clients, in part due to the use of my special tools and farrier ability.

> In today's world, if you argue for more money or are in negotiation for a job, you must always demonstrate that the dollars you receive will create more revenue and more profit for the employer.

• I have interned at three different facilities in the last year, which means I bring you already developed time management and surgery skills. This will translate into less training time for you, which means you and I will both be earning revenue sooner.

In his book *How To Argue and Win Every Time*, noted trial attorney Gerry Spence claims that "Everyone is capable of making the winning argument." He also frames the process as "Winning is getting what we want, which also means helping others get what they want."

Negotiation Rules and Principles

Before negotiating the terms of your new job or that next pay raise, use these rules to give you a head start in the process.

• Negotiations are voluntary events. Either side can walk away at any time.

• Negotiations happen because at least one of the parties wants to change a part of what is in existence, believing a mutually satisfactory arrangement/agreement can be obtained.

• Both parties have power. If one of the parties had the power position and could mandate a solution, there would be no negotiations.

• A successful outcome of negotiation is that both sides get at least part of what they want.

• The timing of negotiation can be a significant factor. Timing sets the tone and influences the overall climate for a successful outcome. If a negotiation is approached too soon, one side may become defensive or end the dialog. If applied too late, the opportunity may be lost.

• In any negotiation, the personal values, perceptions, attitudes, people skills, and emotions which surface during the process will influence the progress and ultimately the results.

• Successful negotiations are not created through verbal wars, escalation of conflicts, fighting, or heavy-handed tactics. In fact, between trained negotiators, encounters hardly ever result in overt conflict.

• To be successful in negotiations, you must observe and listen to determine the best means of persuasion, and then put that persuasive approach into play at the appropriate time.

• You cannot negotiate if:
    – You are not in a position to bargain.
    – You do not have sufficient time to effectively prepare.
    – Your demand is unreasonable, and you already know it.
    – Your long-term objectives may be compromised if you negotiate now.
    – You are not aware of where you are in the negotiation process at all times. Making concessions in the opening phase may be premature and get in the way of reaching the target goal.

Common Negotiation Mistakes

Even skilled negotiators make mistakes. In his book *Deal-Breakers and Breakthroughs*, John Illich highlights some of the common critical mistakes made during the negotiation process.

• Entering a negotiation with preset mental mindsets and assumptions

- Not knowing who has the final negotiation authority

- Entering a negotiation with only a generalized goal as a final outcome of the negotiation

- Failing to advance arguments and positions of substance

- Losing control over seemingly unimportant factors

- Failing to let the other side make the first offer

- Ignoring time and location as a negotiation tool

- Giving up if there seems to be a deadlock

- Not knowing the right time to close

Here are some simple ways to avoid common negotiations mistakes.

- Be an active listener. Do not interrupt. Talk less.

- Build understanding by asking open-ended questions.

- Paraphrase, show a sense of humor, and make positive comments. Summarize often.

- Ask for a break if things seem to be "off the agenda," which helps maintain control.

- Set clear, specific, detailed, realistic goals for yourself before entering a meeting.

- List one or two good reasons for your claim or position rather than seven or eight weak ones.

- Look for the "common ground."

- Avoid weak language (*I hope, I prefer, I would like*) and avoid emotional outbursts, blaming, personal attacks, or sarcasm. Words like "unfair" and "unreasonable" are irritators, which can provoke a defensive or aggressive posture by the other party.

THE GIVE AND TAKE OF NEGOTIATING

The negotiation process can be compared to weaving. Its product is a solution that is stronger than the individuals' positions, just as a woven cloth is stronger than the individual threads. While the parties may have different levels of power or strength when they enter the negotiation, the agreement can create a solution with greater durability and strength than either can create alone.

Steven P. Cohen, in *The Negotiation Skills Company Newsletter* of July 2000, commented about the importance of paying attention to the other party's interests during negotiation. "To achieve optimum results from negotiations, we need to pay attention to interests of the parties and their constituents . . . A fair negotiation process aims at addressing those interests so that the parties can create an agreement that will be fulfilled according to the promises each party has made."

There are many interests at stake in negotiations, including satisfying your ego, saving face, humoring the boss, getting a good price, or achieving a goal. Sometimes it is easy to reach agreement, and other times it is more difficult.

Positional Versus Interest Bargaining

Positional bargaining usually involves someone wanting to win it all, or at least the biggest pieces. This type of bargaining is usually inefficient. The agreement could have been stronger because each party did not know what the other really wanted.

Positional bargaining often leads to one party gaining more short-term profit or advantage over the other party or hard feelings after the negotiations are over. Interest-based bargaining is integrative and value added. In a negotiation, it is important to be able to distinguish between positions and interests—both yours and those of the person with whom you are negotiating. The choice of focus will affect your negotiation style and influence the outcomes.

Example

Positional Approach

Potential employee: *"I need a salary level of $350 a month more than you are offering."*

Employer: *"I cannot go that high. It would not be fair to the other associates and it would create an inequity in the work force."*

Interest Approach

Potential employee: *"I need a salary level of $350 a month more than you are offering in order to cover moving costs."*

143

Employer: *"I cannot go that high. It would not be fair to the other associates and it would create an inequity. However, we have an arrangement with Sunshine Movers, which provides a 25% discount to my employees."*

With an understanding of why you want a greater salary, the potential employer informed you about the discount. In this case, if you did not give your reasons why you needed a higher compensation level, the result may have been less than satisfactory for both sides.

It is always good to ask yourself *why you want what you want.* This helps you get a better understanding of what your real goals are. It may be the key to opening up better deals for you in the long run.

Bargaining From a Position of Power

What kind of power does someone have in today's work world to really negotiate salaries, benefits, or working conditions? Remember—you have power and you need to negotiate from a position of power. It is preferable that you do not discuss salary or compensation details until after you have been offered a position. If salary is an issue brought up by the employer during the interview, phrase your response along these lines: "What range did you have in mind for this position?" Or, "I have a range in mind. However, I need to know the bigger picture before I can make my decision based on salary. Tell me more about the practice. I would especially like to know . . ."

Before you start discussing compensation, you need to understand how badly they need you and what you have they need and can really use. The only way you can learn that is by asking questions and doing homework regarding that practice. Doing so gives you a measure of the relative balance of power. Understanding the balance of power gives you leeway in negotiations. If during the process you continue to highlight what you bring that fits what they need, the higher your value may become in their

eyes, regardless of where they started from regarding compensation expectations.

When preparing for negotiation, or after it has begun, don't just ask yourself, "What do they want?" It is also important to ask, "Why do they want it?"

It is equally important—and often more difficult—to ask the same questions about your own views. Many champion negotiators find they will be more successful if they focus on understanding their interests as they enter discussions. If they haven't started out with a perfect package and closed mind, the ideas others present may actually improve their final result. Weave the cloth to meet your needs and those of your employer.

SIX STEPS IN THE NEGOTIATION PROCESS

In essence, the negotiation process has these six steps:

1. Preparing

2. Developing a strategy

3. Getting started

4. Building understanding and common ground

5. Bargaining

6. Closing with agreement

> Before you start discussing compensation, you need to understand how badly they need you and what you have that they need and can really use.

Preparing

To prepare for negotiations, you need to identify the issues and objectives for the discussion:

- Setting your objectives
  Examples are:
  —Top line objective (first thing asked for): flexible work schedule
  —Target objective (goal): ability to work four ten-hour days instead of five eight-hour days
  —Bottom-line objective (minimum you can accept): a forty-hour work week

- Assessing the other side's case
  Examples are:

—Flexible schedules have never been done before, and we cannot break the custom. If everyone wanted to do that, we would have to hire more people.

—If our hourly staff needed to support this plan, we would have to pay overtime—it would cost too much.

- Assessing strengths and weaknesses
  Examples are:
  As you listen, you hear that the employer:
  —Is afraid of change and wants things just as they are
  —Makes assumptions without testing them
  —Has the power to implement or defeat the proposal
  —Is out of touch with services that clients are asking for and the times they want access to the healthcare provider team (i.e., until 7 P.M.) because of commuting patterns in the employer service area
  —Does not like to interview and hire new help, especially lay help
  —Does not have the time or patience to train new people

  You know that you:
  —Are able to bring energy into the workplace
  —Can help with the interviews and training of new hires
  —Will be happier on the job and have higher productivity and more community involvement to help grow the business if you have a flexible schedule

Developing a Strategy

Your strategy is based on the manner in which you and the other party approach negotiations and the desired outcome. Be careful not to make hard and fast elaborate plans beforehand. Remain flexible but focused. Based on your assessment of the situation as it unfolds, your understanding of the style you tend to use under stress, and what you see as the style being employed by the other side, you

will need to plan what style of negotiation you will use during the meeting.

WHAT NEGOTIATION STYLE TO USE

Kenneth Thomas and Ralph Kilmann identified five distinct categories of approaches people take (style) based on their character, their strategic intent, and their value orientation.

The following conflict management styles are based on the Thomas-Kilmann Conflict Mode Instrument (TKI).

> Collaboration works by mutually exploring alternatives that meet or exceed parties' needs and expectations. It can be characterized as, "Not my way, not your way, but another way."

- **Collaborating**—Manages conflict by maintaining interpersonal relationships and ensuring that both parties achieve their personal goals. Enables people to work together so everyone can win. Collaboration works by mutually exploring alternatives that meet or exceed parties' needs and expectations. It can be characterized as: "Not my way, not your way, but another way." The strategic intent is to resolve conflict or interpersonal difficulty to the mutual satisfaction of all the parties, both in terms of the issues and the relationship. The process of collaboration typically involves relationship-building, full problem definition, exploration of alternatives, and joint decision-making.

- **Compromising**—This approach assumes a full win-win is not possible. The negotiating stance involves a little bit of winning and a little bit of losing. People choose a compromising style when it is important for them to satisfy some of their interests, but not all of them. People who compromise are likely to say: "let's split the difference" or "something is better than nothing." The objective is to find some expedient, mutually acceptable solution.

- **Accommodating**—To the accommodator, managing conflict involves maintaining the interpersonal relationship at all costs, with little or no concern for the personal goals of the parties involved. Giving in, appeasing, and avoiding conflict are viewed as ways of protecting the relationship. People who choose an accommodating style put their interests last and let others have what they want. They believe that keeping a good friendship is more important than anything else. The strategic intent is to settle conflict by satisfying the concerns of the other.

- **Controlling**—This is a power-oriented approach. It is the method used whenever the use of force (power and leverage) is applied to defend a position, because you believe it is correct or you simply just want to win. It is a competing style in which the person puts his/her interest before anyone else's interests no matter what the cost to the relationship. The strategic intent is domination or winning at the expense of the other.

- **Avoiding**—An avoider views conflict as something to be shunned at all costs. This style is evasiveness. A person choosing the avoiding style might say, "You decide and leave me out of this." This approach often leads to a high degree of frustration for all parties involved. Personal goals are often unmet, and the interpersonal relationship fails. This style might take the form of diplomatically deflecting an issue, postponing an issue until a better time, or simply withdrawing from what is perceived as a threatening situation.

HOW AND WHEN TO USE EACH STYLE

1. Collaborating

- *Tactics:* Noncoercive, legitimate, open, persuasive, exploratory, and creative

- *Your stance:* You assert your self-interests and fully cooperate with the other by attempting to reach mutual understanding and a mutual agreeable settlement.

- *How you feel toward the other:* You are cooperative. You perceive all parties as equals or colleagues who share the problem and the responsibility for achieving a mutually satisfying resolution. You treat the other in a caring and respectful manner.

- *Collaboration style is best when:*
  —The issues are too important to be compromised
  —When the objective is to integrate different points of view
  —You need a commitment from the other to make the agreement work

—The relationship with the other person is important and you wish to build and maintain it

2. Compromising

- *Tactics:* Expedient, 50/50 split, and concessionary

- *Your stance:* You are moderately assertive. The objective is to achieve a fair exchange and distribution of the gains.

- *How you feel toward the other:* You are cooperative, whereas the other person is seen as someone opposed to an equal sharing of the problem or to accepting responsibility for solving the problem.

- *Compromising style is best when:*
  —The issues are important to you but you cannot afford to be too controlling
  —The relationship is important; however, you cannot afford to accommodate
  —Opponents of equal power are committed to mutually exclusive goals
  —You need to find temporary solutions to complex issues
  —You need to find an expedient solution in as short amount of time as possible
  —It is the only alternative to no solution

3. Accommodating

- *Tactics:* Reactive by the accommodator, coercive by the other

- *Your stance:* You are unassertive because the issue is less important than the other's concerns. If not in an equal power position, you may tend to be more submissive. If you have a power position, you may be assertive.

- *Your stance toward the other:* Cooperation and affiliation with the other is the key. Submissive accommodation is external but not internal. Assertive accommodation mirrors a mutual strategy.

- *Accommodating style is best when:*
  —You find out you are wrong, your assumptions were faulty, or your perceptions were incorrect
  —You wish to be seen as practical, sensible, and reasonable

146

—The issues are more important to the other party

—You want to build "credits" for future issues

—You want to minimize loss when you are in a weak position

—Harmony and stability of the relationship with the other person are more important to you

4. Controlling

- *Tactics:* Coercive, below the belt, full of pressure, deceptive, dehumanizing, physically intimidating, high tension

- *Your stance:* You are aggressive or highly assertive. You want to win at all costs despite resistance.

- *Your stance toward the other:* You are noncooperative. The other is the enemy and is in your way, or there is an emergency.

- *Controlling style is best when:*
  —Quick, decisive action is critical (for instance, in an emergency)
  —The action needed to resolve the situation is an unpopular choice
  – Indisputably, you know you are right
  – The other party would take advantage of any cooperative approach

5. Avoiding

- *Tactics:* Defensive in nature. Characterized by rationalizations, denial, pseudo agreement, escape

- *Your stance:* You are nonassertive. The issue and the relationship are not valued or seen as important enough to make an effort. You may be fearful or arrogant depending on your perception of your power position.

- *Your stance toward the other:* You choose *not* to cooperate by refusing to engage in conflict.

- *Avoiding style is best when:*
  —The issues are not important to you
  —There are more pressing concerns which need your attention
  —There is no chance of meeting or achieving your objectives

—There are minimal benefits for you; the aggravation of negotiating outweighs any benefit

—People involved in the negotiation process need to cool down to regain perspective

—You need time to gather more information, do additional research, and adjust to the flow of the process

—Someone else could resolve the conflict more effectively

Getting Started

While preparing for the first meeting, decide what tactics you will use initially, where you will negotiate, when you will negotiate, and what the meeting will look like.

When you are negotiating for employment, the use of a neutral location may be desirable. Otherwise, there is the element of home-court advantage for the employer. This may result in you not having equal footing or your position of power may be reduced. If on the employer's home court, such as the clinic, your negotiations may also be subject to interruptions, thus breaking your train of thought and reducing your focus.

Timing is important. You need to have your facts together, be adequately prepared for the conversations to follow, and have practiced your delivery and style. Avoid starting any negotiations on the spur of the moment.

HOW TO START THE FIRST MEETING

Your careful attention to how the first meeting is conducted is an important preparatory tactic. What are your goals and objectives for the first meeting? They may well shape the climate and outcome of the negotiation process. Do not expect that one meeting will result in an agreement. This is a process. Sometimes it is a short one, and sometimes parties need time to think about it and come back to discuss and negotiate further. Try not to be in a hurry.

- **Reintroduce yourself**—You may have made an impression during the interview, but a lot will have been forgotten. Take the time to get reacquainted.

- **Cover the process issues**—State why you are meeting, emphasize the importance of getting agreement together from the beginning, and state how long the meeting is to last.

- **Have an opening statement and seek one from the other party**— An opening statement conveys information about a party's attitudes, aspirations, intentions, and perceptions of the other party and the issues in dispute.

Example

148

You: *"Dr. Creighton I am very excited about your offer of employment and because of my background in canine reproduction I can help grow that aspect of your business. Your hospital is progressive and well equipped, and your staff is well trained. I know I will enjoy the environment you have created. I am here to see how we can get to an agreement regarding the rewards for working in your practice, especially regarding how my productivity payments will be determined. I am a dedicated worker and see myself helping you grow your practice. I need some clarity so we can agree how that productivity will be rewarded."*

Dr. Creighton: *"Well Dr. _____, I think you are a bright young veterinarian, and my staff and I think you have potential. Let me share what I am offering . . ."*

As soon as you have acknowledged the other party in some manner and set the parameters of the meeting, let the other person do the talking. This will help you adjust in case you have made some miscalculation. The other person's style may be more collaborative or more competitive than you expected.

As you listen to the other person and get a picture of his or her position, you can adjust your pitch about your position.

The convention is that you always demand more than you expect to get and offer less than you expect to give. Therefore, your opening position should be far from where you hope to settle. This gives you time and space to negotiate for your target settlement.

There is also consistent evidence to show that the more you ask for, the more you get. Remember

there may be adverse consequences resulting from any extreme position. The use of specific facts and figures to support your position may be timely, but do not drown the other side, especially in the beginning. This negotiation is between you and the other party, not the average or mean of all veterinary graduates or what anyone else is getting. Listen as the other person tells you what is important. Respond in those terms.

It is also typical to reject the first and perhaps other early offers. The general rule is never to accept the first offer, however attractive it may seem. In the same way, never make your best offer first, as the other may reject that and use it as a starting place for his or her negotiations, causing you to get less out of the deal.

In general, your opening position regarding specifics should open the doors to gaining more information from the other person, establish a starting place, and allow you to probe into the other person's way of thinking.

Building Understanding and Common Ground

This phase of negotiation has three components:

- Getting information

- Testing assumptions, arguments, and positions

- Using timing and adjournments

GETTING INFORMATION
In negotiation, information is power. The more information you can get from the other side, the better it is for you. The quality of that information depends on the questions you ask.

- Open questions:

 —"Tell me about…."
 —"Please describe what you think are the…."
 —"Could you share a little more about…?"

- Probing questions:

 —"What do you mean by…?"
 —"Could you tell me more about…?"

- Closed questions: These questions establish specific points of fact with "yes" and "no" answers.

—"What is the patient load…?"

—"Do you board dogs?"

- Hypothetical questions: These questions encourage the other party to explore his or her ideas or feelings about a particular subject.

  —"Say I was a client and brought in a … for…. How would you handle that at your hospital?"

TESTING ASSUMPTIONS, ARGUMENTS, AND POSITIONS

- Do not interrupt the responses of the other person. Let him or her talk.

- Be sensitive to body language—yours and the other person's.

- Say only what is needed. Do not volunteer more information than asked for.

- End each statement you make with a direct question to the other person.

- Avoid being sidetracked. Stick to addressing the issues and your position.

- Regularly summarize what has been said.

USING TIMING AND ADJOURNMENTS

The timing of questioning is a technique used in the negotiation process to:

- Focus attention to an area—"Can I ask a question regarding what you are proposing?"

- Get more specific information—use the questions with who, what, when, where, and how.

- Give information—"Can you help me solve this problem? Here's what's happening . . . ."

- Get the other party to move—"Is this your final offer?" or "Can you get back to me with a revised proposal for our next meeting?"

- Bring a party's thinking to a conclusion— "Would you please summarize those last points for me?" or "How about we adjourn and meet tomorrow to continue?"

Bargaining

Bargaining has three characteristic parts:

- Receiving and giving concessions

- Breaking through deadlocks

- Moving toward agreement

RECEIVING AND GIVING CONCESSIONS

A concession is a modification of a previous position you held and defended. Concessions are expected in the negotiation process; yet, you try to move as little as possible. You need to know exactly where you intend to stop conceding. Help the other party save face by providing a rationale for him or her to make a concession. When the concession is made, repeat the offer out loud. Use hypothetical questions, like, "What would you say if I were to…?"

Any concessions you make may have long-term consequences. Think them through carefully. If you make a concession, state your reasoning first, then the concession.

Here are some important points to remember about concessions:

- Enter into a negotiation with possible concessions in mind.

- The best concessions are usually small ones.

- When concessions are offered, they should apply pressure toward reaching the objective and an agreement.

- You need to promote the other's willingness to make concessions.

- Know how to deal with concessions offered in packages.

BREAKING THROUGH DEADLOCKS

Deadlocks happen when both parties hold opposing views and objectives, and one party refuses to make concessions to keep negotiations alive. Sometimes deadlocks are used as a deliberate tactic to force the other person to reconsider his or her position and make concessions.

To break a deadlock you can try the following:

- Ask more questions to gather information.

- Attempt to find the barriers blocking progress. Ask something like, "Can you tell me why we are having so much trouble finding an acceptable solution?"

- For the time being, agree not to agree on the sticking point. Take time to reflect and resume negotiations on that issue later.

- State the consequences to the other party if there is a failure to reach a negotiated agreement.

- See if the party is willing to try a proposed solution for a period of time.

- Call in an outside party to act as a mediator, go-between, or arbitrator.

MOVING TOWARD AGREEMENT

The purpose of negotiation is to reach agreement. The closer you are to reaching an agreement, the more sensitive you must be to the discussion. Paying attention to the nonverbal aspects is critical.

To facilitate movement toward agreement, provide explanations as to why you want the person to take certain actions. Let the other party know what kinds of things you value and are likely to appreciate in the future. Use humor to reduce tension and to create a bond between yourself and the other person. Describe to the other party the emotional content of what he or she is saying in a concerned and nonjudgmental way.

Closing With Agreement

To reach an agreement, the other party needs to be convinced that he or she cannot push you any further. To effectively project this, the nature of your concessions should become minimal and given less and less frequently. Your previous willingness to move has evaporated despite pressure being applied. You reinforce this as your final offer and suggest that the other person talk it over with others in power.

To ensure you achieve credibility for any statement about your position as being final, *how* you make such a statement may be as important as *what* you say. Your final offer of agreement needs to be timed to coincide with a period of constructive discussion, not during a combative phase.

Before declaring the agreement is done, do the following:

- Clarify the terms of the agreement. Remove ambiguous words or phrases. Ensure that there is a full understanding by both sides.

- Ensure that there will be implementation and compliance, and that everyone knows who is responsible for what.

- Ask: "Who gets how much, of what, when?"

- Try to get the agreement in writing when the agreement is made.

- If the agreement is oral, send a written letter of understanding as soon as possible to the other party listing the points of agreement, disagreement, interpretation, and clarification.

Additional Hints for Successful Negotiating

SEPARATING THE PEOPLE FROM THE PROBLEM

You may have heard the phrase: "Hate the sin, not the sinner." If you choose to view the problem as one that needs to be resolved, rather than viewing someone who holds a contrary viewpoint as a person needing to be defeated, the odds of a successful collaboration increase. Try modifying the seating arrangement so you are not facing each other across a barrier. Seek an environment that makes it feel like it is "we" versus the problem, not "you" versus another.

USING SILENCE AS A TOOL

Silence is a terrific tool. This is true for two reasons:

- If one party is highly opinionated or emotional, if his approach is threatening or extremely demanding, keeping quiet after he finishes speaking can be quite unsettling to him. It is like jujitsu; you allow him to be tripped up by his own forcefulness. Most people are troubled by silence in the midst of heated discussion.

- Sometimes silence is viewed as disapproval, but since no specific disapproval has been voiced, it cannot be treated as an attack. When met with silence, people tend to modify their previous statements to make them more palatable.

USING ACTIVE LISTENING

Silence is an important element in the crucial tool called active listening. The discipline of active listening requires that you focus on what another person is saying. Don't spend your time shaping a stinging response or thinking of some witty remark to satisfy your ego. The job of a good negotiator is to listen to and understand what others are saying. You cannot make an intelligent response to an opinion you do not understand. If you lose focus, you will lose ground. Remember—your goal is to get what you want as a professional, not to be cute or witty.

Active listening produces results, sometimes dramatic ones. The listener may actually be able to get a clearer picture of the other party's ideas. If the listener's response shows just how good a job he or she has done listening, it can shock the other party making that person think, "Good grief, she actually paid attention to me!"

One other terrific result of active listening is that focusing on other opinions can also give you the chance to reflect on the process and strategy. Stepping aside and taking a dispassionate view of what is going on can make you much more effective as a negotiator. If you're in a negotiation, it is a cardinal rule to listen actively. Pay as much attention to what *is* said as to what is *not* said.

ASKING QUESTIONS

When issues occur to you that another party may be failing to address, ask questions. Don't be afraid to continue asking questions until you are genuinely sure that you have understood what the other party really means. Even when you think you understand, ask, "Am I correct in my understanding that you said 'xyz'?" There is no such thing as a stupid question.

PAYING ATTENTION TO DETAILS

In the negotiation process, it is also essential to pay constant attention to how the ultimate agreement will be fulfilled by the parties once the hands are shaken or the contract has been signed. Paying attention to the small details protects you from surprises once the agreement has been reached and it is time for the parties to deliver on their promises.

The "small print" is seemingly inconsequential details thrown into agreements that can turn into monsters later on. If you are dealing with people you don't know very well or with people who are more sophisticated than you are in this particular aspect of business, it is even more important to question the details. An even wiser move is to try

to learn about this employer's reputation, talking to other people with whom the employer has reached similar deals and employees who left. Also, find out how often this position is open. If it seems to be open every nine months or so, it may be a clue that this employer has a problem retaining staff. Find out why.

GETTING LEGAL ADVICE

It is good business practice, even if everything seems okay—you really like the employer and the staff—to exercise a moment of caution. Before you sign the agreement, have it reviewed by a reputable attorney who will look after your interests. It may cost you a couple of hours of his or her time but may save you considerable misery later. It is always good to have someone who is knowledgeable review any work-agreement document you sign. Ask your attorney any and every question that comes to mind, because you are the one who will have to fulfill the terms of the signed document. A good employer will be glad to give you a few days to review it.

Based on what you learn from your attorney, you may have to go back to the table to renegotiate or clarify something in the document. Keep an open mind, because the employer may not have realized that something contained in the document was worded unclearly or that the attorney had inadvertently left out something you and the employer had agreed to. Not all employers are out to cheat you.

It is not realistic to think you can anticipate all the possible problems that may arise during the term of an agreement. Thus, it is important to negotiate fairly and with civility so that if questions need to be raised during the life of the contract, the relationship among the parties won't stand in the way of dealing with what comes up later on.

PURSUING FAIRNESS

If all the participants view the process as fair, they are more likely to take it seriously and buy into its result. This can have an important impact on the substantive result. If the negotiating parties can agree on standards against which elements of the agreement can be measured, it can give each a face-saving reason for agreeing. Refer to published salary surveys by associations such as AVMA or AAHA.

To be considered successful, an agreement must be durable. Parties who walk away from the table grumbling may regret their commitment and only grudgingly honor it. They may also find ways to sabotage it, saying it was the other side's fault.

IMPORTANCE OF HONESTY

Honesty is always the best policy. Tell the potential new employer that everything about their job offer is attractive, but the pay, the holidays, and other benefits are below the standard you are currently enjoying. Instead of getting in the person's face and asking: "Will you pay me $X per month?" which is a closed question and demands a "yes" or "no" answer, try asking: "What incentives can you offer me that will give me reason to come to work for you?" Make it clear that your financial interest is paramount.

It is worth finding out from the new employer whether paying you more will cause the business any particular problems. For example, will other employees expect to be paid more or will adding extra holidays cost money when other employees are included. Ask the hiring person what issues determine his or her capacity to determine the compensation package. You may hear things in what they say that give you an opportunity to come up with a creative solution.

Once again, this reflects back to the importance of thinking about your employer and his or her needs. Remember to be honest and to keep both your needs and those of your employer at the forefront.

BEFORE YOU AGREE TO ACCEPT A JOB

Imagine that you are ready to accept your first position, and you really need a job. Dr. Albert A. Johnson, owner of Feel Good Rx Animal Hospital in Ossipee, New Hampshire (*yes, there is such a place*), has just made you a straight-salary offer at the end of your interview. It is the first offer you have received. You applied for six open positions and had three interviews in as many weeks. After years as a student, someone seems to want you. It

> **Remember to be honest and to keep both your needs and those of your employer at the forefront.**

does feel good. Of course, sometimes any offer sounds too good to pass up, depending on your level of anxiety and need. Before you leap, consider some basic issues:

1. **Geographic location.** Do you like this part of the world? Can you walk or bike to work, or will you be spending a good part of your day commuting? Prior to accepting a position, consider the costs, both financial and personal, to a practice's location. How will you pay for relocation? Do you think you'll enjoy the commute? While an hour's train ride may be relaxing after a long day, consider the same journey on weekends and late at night before you decide, especially if emergency duty is required. Did you evaluate the practice? Would working there meet your goals? Can you afford the type of housing you want? Does the area afford a life and the lifestyle you seek outside of the practice? (See Chapters 9 and 12 for help when comparing practices and locations.)

2. **Don't say "yes" on the spot, no matter how good the offer.** You get what you negotiate; yet to do so, you need to be in a position of power. It is always wise to wait twenty-four hours before committing. Think of it as buying a car. Those twenty-four hours provide considerable time to do a little more research, evaluate the situation without the adrenalin surge, and be sure there will not be buyer's remorse tomorrow. For example, if you're considering a job offer and you are not living near the area, another trip back might be a good idea if you have any reservations. Sometimes your remembrance of an area on first impression is clouded by what you were doing at the time.

3. **Money can't buy happiness, but it can make misery more comfortable.** Don't settle for less than you believe you're worth. On the other hand, few new graduates should hold out for a six-figure starting salary or expect a large signing bonus. Do your homework. Ask other recent graduates about what to expect, and check out what is being paid in the market you

are considering. You can always make a counteroffer or set a formal date to reevaluate after a probationary period.

4. **Find out what kind of commitment is required before you get too excited about a position.** How many hours will you be required to work? Are you expected to work evenings and weekends? Will you work emergencies? Will you be on call? Are there any management duties with this position?

5. **Do you feel like you have no room to negotiate?** Take a moment. Rethink and revisit all you have heard during the interviews and conversations. *If the situation isn't right, be prepared to walk away.* However, before you do, make sure you have faced your demons. Try to fully understand what's in it for you to decline the deal. Sometimes a cooling-off period makes both sides more flexible. Talk it over with someone you trust. Give yourself credit for looking it over diligently and in detail and for being willing to come back with a counteroffer. Be confident in making choices you deem right and in your best interest. You decide when to argue and when not to argue.

6. **Words are often weapons, which can generate conflict.** After listening to your opponent, choose your words wisely. An assault is not an argument or a line of reasoning.

I Want the Job, But the Pay Is Below Market

Question: Dr. Johnson has indicated that he has decided to hire me but needs to meet with me again. I really want this job. It offers the opportunity for me to get started as a veterinarian, and I am familiar with the county the practice is in. The trouble is, I have discovered that they are considering wages between $30,000 to $36,000. The benefits package is worth about $2,800 per year. After extensive research about what is being paid to other associates locally, I find that the median is $40,000 for those who have less than one year of experience. I really want the job. How can I get him to pay the wages that I deserve and need?

Response: If you have said you'll take the job—knowing what the numbers are—then you have to enter into your face-to-face process indicating that you have had second thoughts—entirely because of the pay.

The important question is not how much you want or need them, but how much they want you. In your meeting(s) with Dr. Johnson's business manager, you should mention that no one has asked how much pay would be a sufficient incentive for you to join them. Then you should indicate that you've been thinking in the range of the "high forties", which means you're looking for at least $45,000.

You do want to ask questions like, "As I understand it, people with less than my experience are getting paid more than $40,000 per year. What is there in your offer that reflects my experience and offers me good reasons for wanting to work for you?"

Focusing on your own interests is more important than simply beating up the company. For example, if the location, working conditions, speed of salary increases, or other elements of the job are extremely attractive, then you have to measure the value of those issues against sheer cash. People take pay cuts to improve their quality of life—reduced commute, more flexible hours, and other benefits not measurable in dollars.

Before sitting down to negotiate, think about what is important to you. Evaluate how the various elements of the job impact those issues. Then, you can make a wise decision on what approach to take when you negotiate. See Chapter 9 for a job comparison worksheet.

Should I Take It or Leave It?

Question: I am about to be made a job offer from a doctor who has a reputation for making a "take-it-or-leave-it" offer. What should I do?

Response: Ask yourself a number of questions. Do I want this job? What kinds of elements of a compensation package would be appropriate for me—salary, retirement plan, paid vacation time, insurance benefits, company car, office with a window, company-supplied laptop computer, flexible hours, ability to work from home, daycare for a

153

young child, frequent salary review, etc.? Is this the only likely employer I can find in the geographic area I want to be in? Perhaps another acceptable alternative can be found. If you are fortunate enough, you might identify an alternative option ahead of time that gives you more bargaining power.

In addition, you need to find a way to communicate to your future employer that you are concerned about negotiation styles. For example, if she has a "take-it-or-leave-it" approach toward employees, does she take this same approach with clients or suppliers? And, if she does, is this the right business approach for you—and for her? Can you live with that business culture?

Rather than simply opening yourself to an offer that appears to require a flat "yes" or "no," you could choose to approach the conversation as an opportunity to learn more about the job and the employer. Ask as many open-ended questions as you can. Even if she says, "Here's the salary we offer; you can accept this offer or forget about working here," you can ask, "How would you advise me to sell the offer you have presented to my spouse, my friends, or even myself?" If they simply say, "That's your problem," it may be a really good time to give more serious thought to a possible alternative. Unfortunately, if people take advantage of you at the start of negotiations, it is likely to get worse in the future.

High-Risk Negotiations

If you find yourself headed toward a *tense* "high-risk" negotiation situation, take your power back by building your own "power envelope." Here is a quick exercise to regain your composure and power. Just before you are about to enter a negotiation, try these five steps:

1. Find a place to sit and close your eyes. Think about being surrounded by a pink or white light. Focus on your breathing for a moment. Take a deep breath in, then let it out slowly. Repeat this a few times. Then, sift back through your favorite memories (anything from when you were a kid to last week).

2. Imagine a time or a moment when you did a fantastic job at something—a little-league homerun, the time you reached the top of the mountain or did the flip off the diving board and won the meet for the swim team, the best PowerPoint presentation you ever gave, or the difficult case you treated with huge success.

3. Now, how did you feel? When did it happen? Who said what to you? What was it about the victory, achievement, or accomplishment that made it so special? Remember the moment when you knew in your gut that you really did it. Hear the cheers. Feel the joy and exhilaration.

4. Enjoy those warm vibrations all over again. Revel in the experience like it just happened. Bask in the moment and vow to take all those warm sensations with you.

5. Open your eyes. Get up and go for it! Your brain is now programmed for you to meet the challenge with "winning." Take the winning feeling, spirit, and attitude into the negotiations, rather than having "worried" messages choreograph your performance. As psychologists have said and proven in studies over and over again, "what you expect is what you get."

RESOURCES

Books

Cultures and Organizations by G. Hofstede.
Deal-Breakers and Breakthroughs by J. Illich.
Developing Interpersonal Skills Through Tutored Practice by D. Taylor and P. Wright.
Developing Management Skills by D. Whetten and K. Cameron.
The Essence of Negotiation by J. Hiltrop and S. Udall.
Getting to Yes; Negotiating Agreement Without Giving In by R. Fisher, W. Ury, and B. Patton.
How To Argue and Win Every Time by G. Spence.
Negotiating Terms of Employment by C. Buppert.
Pocket Guide: The Fine Art of Negotiating by S. Cohen.
Pocket Negotiator by G. Kennedy.
Social Conflict: Escalation, Stalemate and Settlement by D. Pruitt and J. Rubin.

Websites

Career/LifeSkills Resources Inc.
www.career-lifeskills.com
This company offers the test developed by Kenneth Thomas and Ralph Kilmann (discussed in this chapter) as well as other professional development assessment tools.

► CHAPTER ELEVEN ◄

Basics of the Employment Contract

Charlotte A. Lacroix, DVM, JD

IN THIS CHAPTER, YOU'LL LEARN:

- **The elements of an enforceable contract**
- **What you should include in an employment contract**
- **How to terminate an employment contract**

Many veterinary-school graduates and associate veterinarians accept employment positions without ever having signed or fully negotiated the terms of an employment agreement. This is probably because written employment contracts are not yet the norm in the veterinary field. The eagerness with which you seek to fulfill your dream of practicing veterinary medicine may cause you to overlook the importance of defining the employment relationship. Additionally, many veterinary schools do not provide students with sufficient training with respect to selecting, negotiating, or accepting their first jobs.

The importance of understanding the working relationship cannot be overemphasized. Too often, disputes and misunderstandings arise because the owner and associate failed to articulate their interests, desires, and expectations. A written employment contract sets out and defines the terms of employment and helps to ensure that both you and your boss honor your sides of the bargain.

WHAT IS AN EMPLOYMENT CONTRACT?

Generally, a contract consists of a set of bargained-for promises between two or more people, where one party promises to do something in exchange for another party's promise to do something else.

In the context of veterinary employment, the contract sets out the terms whereby you promise to provide veterinary services in exchange for the employer's promise to provide compensation and benefits.

A contract can be oral or written. However, contracts that exceed one year in duration must be in writing to be enforceable under the statute of frauds. Since employment contracts for most associates are for a term of one year or less, oral agreements are enforceable. Written employment contracts are, nonetheless, preferable to oral agreements, because the details of the terms of oral contracts are often not clearly articulated, which subjects their meaning to each party's interpretation and recollection of the communication. Additionally, well-conceived employment contracts entail more terms and promises than the average person can remember.

THE ELEMENTS OF A CONTRACT

Dr. James F. Wilson, in an article for *Veterinary Economics*, listed the key elements of a contract to make it enforceable. These include:

- **The offer**—This usually starts as a written job description. It could be an advertisement in a professional journal, posted on a bulletin board, or mailed to applicants. What usually happens is that associates ask for clarity and make counteroffers. Employers counter those, and before long, all parties are confused or, maybe, they reach an agreement. If the final offer is not written down, memory lapses will create additional squabbles.

- **The acceptance**—Again, it is best for all parties if this is written down. If a contract is accepted orally, it is usually by an "I accept" statement. However, there can be what are termed "actions in reliance." Actions by new associates, such as breaking existing leases and scheduling moves, searching for apartments near the employer's place of business, and informing other employers that they no longer are job applicants, all constitute acceptance—if employers know of or should have been aware of such actions. Likewise, actions by employers, such as withdrawing all job advertisements from journals and placement services, informing candidates that jobs are filled, or buying new equipment or hiring new staff in preparation for an associate's arrival, all constitute actions in reliance.

- **Meeting of the minds**—Unless some type of written document exists, it is very difficult to determine what the contracting parties originally intended. These documents can be very informal, such as the infamous cocktail napkin, complex written masterpieces, or something in between. The key is that a written record is required, especially to understand the terms of the deal at some future point in time.

- **Consideration**—Consideration means conferring a legal benefit to each party in conjunction with the incurrence of a legal detriment by each person. For example, Dr. Newgrad will receive a salary of $45,875 plus employee benefits (this compensation is the legal benefit) in return for working fifty hours per week and agreeing not to compete within three miles of Dr. Oldguy's small-animal practice for two years after the termination of employment (this is the detriment). Meanwhile, Dr. Oldguy receives the brain power, energy, time, and a promise not to compete from Dr. Newgrad (the benefit) in return for a duty to pay Dr. Newgrad's salary and benefits and to provide training and education (the detriment). This part of contract law can be complex, difficult to interpret, and challenging to enforce.

- **Contract terms**—The "terms" are the minute nuts and bolts of the understanding. They often contain the moral, ethical, and legal issues that can be minor parts of a deal.

BE PREPARED TO NEGOTIATE

A difficult challenge for many associates seeking their first veterinary position is the thought of having to discuss the terms of the employment relationship with their potential employers. This feeling of discomfort stems from the fact that first-year associates are generally nonconfrontational and willingly accept what they are offered. They have little or no experience in negotiating contracts, and few really know what they want or need in their first job.

By becoming an effective negotiator, you can overcome this uneasiness as well as bargain for terms of employment that are in your best interests. See Chapter 10, Mastering Negotiation, for tips and advice.

In approaching any negotiation, remember two lessons. First, no one is born a negotiator; it takes practice and planning. Those who engage in negotiations with a "fly-by-the-seat-of-the-pants" approach usually don't achieve optimum results because they fail to set clear and prioritized objectives or form convincing arguments. Second, the art of negotiation is the ability to frame your goals in the interests of the other. The key here is for employees to recognize and acknowledge the needs of the employers and subsequently persuade employers that their interests are interdependent. For example, some employers request that their employees agree to work fifty to sixty hours a week, yet are unwilling to provide more than one week of paid vacation. The challenge here is for you to get your employer to realize that an overworked and overtired employee is less effective and less enthusiastic and that it is in your employer's best interest to provide at least two weeks of vacation.

> Those who engage in negotiations with a "fly-by-the-seat-of-the-pants" approach usually don't achieve optimum results because they fail to set clear and prioritized objectives or form convincing arguments.

What You Need to Negotiate in Your Contract

In preparing your negotiation strategy, generate a list of issues you would like addressed in the employment agreement. Some of the more important terms and related questions include the following:

- **Term of employment**—Is there a period of employment, or is it "at will"? At-will employment means you or the employer can terminate the relationship at any time for any reason (except those reasons prohibited by law). Is the employment period for one year? Less than one year? Does the term automatically renew itself on the day of expiration? Does the contract provide for a time when the terms of the contract can be renegotiated for the subsequent year of employment? Is there a probationary period, whereby either party can terminate the relationship without further obligation?

- **Work schedule**—How many scheduled hours per week will you be expected to cover? How many additional nonscheduled hours are you likely to spend phoning clients, performing diagnostics, interpreting laboratory work, overseeing patient care, and performing miscellaneous management tasks? How many weekends per month will you be expected to work? How often will you

be expected to take emergency calls? Is the call schedule equitably distributed among the employed veterinarians?

- **Duties**—What will your responsibilities be? Will your time be equally apportioned between surgical and medical cases? Will you be expected to undertake management responsibilities? If so, will additional compensation or compensatory time off be provided for such efforts? Will you be expected to perform procedures you deem ethically wrong?

- **Performance evaluation**—Will the employer provide you with written and oral performance evaluations? If so, how often? Are these used in any way to determine salary increases? If so, how? Do you have the opportunity for written rebuttal and comments on the evaluation form?

- **Compensation**—Is the yearly salary fixed, or is it based on the revenue you generate? What percentage of which categories of income will you earn? What happens if someone takes over your case—do you get paid for generating that revenue? Is there an opportunity to get a bonus? If so, upon what is it based? Will you be compensated for emergency calls above and beyond your fixed salary? Can you work extra hours for additional compensation?

- **Salary range**—Does the salary and/or the amount you would earn from bonuses and production-based pay fall within the average range as reported in the *Journal of the American Veterinary Medical Association* or AAHA's *Compensation & Benefits*? What is the average salary offered to other associates in the same or similar geographic area? Significant variations exist between Southern California, New York City, and medium-sized cities near veterinary schools. Does the salary offered allow you to meet your budgetary needs?

- **Other benefits**—In addition to direct monetary consideration, what else does the employer offer? Carefully review the "average" package

157

offered to associates in *Compensation & Benefits*, consider what you need (see Table 9-1), and compare that with the employer's offer. Make sure benefits are addressed in the written contract:

—*Vacation.* Do you earn one week per year? Two weeks? More? Is there a limitation as to when it can be taken and how many consecutive days can be taken? How far in advance must you inform your employer of your desire to take vacation days? If vacation days are not used, can they be carried over and used in the subsequent year of employment, or are they lost?

—*Holidays.* Will you be expected to take emergencies or manage cases during holidays? If so, how often and on which holidays? Are you paid for holidays even if you don't work? Which ones?

—*Sick leave and disability.* Does the employer offer any paid time off for sick leave? Disability leave? How long can you be disabled before being terminated? If sick leave is offered but not used, can it be used in a subsequent year? Can you receive extra pay for not having used your sick days?

—*Continuing education.* How many days per year are you permitted to take off work to attend continuing-education seminars? Do you continue to receive your salary during those days? Does the employer provide a stipend for the costs of registration, travel, lodging, and meals? If so, how much? Do you choose the conference you'll attend or does the employer?

—*Association dues.* Does the employer provide a stipend for national, state, and local veterinary organization membership fees? How much?

—*Professional liability, health, and disability insurance.* Does the employer pay the premiums on your professional liability insurance? Does the employer have a health-insurance plan or pay for your health-insurance premiums? What percentage? Are your spouse and children covered? Does the employer pay for your disability insurance?

—*Veterinary license fees and DEA registration.* Does the employer pay these costs? Is a DEA license necessary?

—*Pet-care coverage.* Does the employer provide any discounts for the care of your family pets? If so, what kind of discounts will be provided? Do you receive discounts on pet foods? Pet products? Veterinary services? Is pet health insurance provided instead?

—*Retirement plans.* Does the employer have a retirement plan for you? When do you become "vested" or eligible? How much can you contribute?

—*Relocation (moving) expenses.* Most corporate (including veterinary HMOs) and government employers provide some form of moving expense reimbursement. If the private practice owner/employer does not offer this, it may be worthwhile to ask. Perhaps a "signing bonus" can be arranged to help cover these costs.

—*Temporary housing allowance.* This is another option to help cover some of your relocation expenses, especially if you are not able to bring the family until school is out, or until the moving van comes, or until you can find a place to live.

—*Short-term loan.* Because of debt load, many new graduates could use help during the transition to the new place of employment and to settle in. Employers may consider a promissory note with salary paybacks monthly from your wages of "bonus" earnings, even though you are unproven.

—*Vehicle allowance or mileage payments.* This may become important if the employer has more than one facility and you are expected to go from one to another. It may also apply if you are expected to make house calls regularly. It is essential to ask, especially if the costs of vehicle operation and insurance will be an issue for you.

—*Health-club memberships.* You may have different values than Dr. Oldguy does, because often you are more eager to maintain balance in your life. Dr. Oldguy may also consider this a motivational perk for you.

—*Profit sharing.* This is quite a value for you and something to negotiate when you are considering a long-term relationship with the employer. You may have to prove yourself first before you get this one.

—*Tax-free medical expense and dependent-care plans.* These plans are known as flexible spending, cafeteria plans, and section 125 plans. This benefit may be of value if you have children or expect large medical expenses.

• **Restrictive covenant**—Many employers require you to sign restrictive covenants that prohibit you from competing with the employer for a certain period of time within a set geographic area when you cease to be employed. Find out whether noncompete agreements are enforceable in the state where you are to be employed and, if so, whether the restriction seems reasonable.

• **Termination**—Can either party terminate the employment relationship? Must notice be given? If so, how much? Can the employer terminate you for cause without providing notice?

After considering these issues, your multiple options, and the employer's interests, you are well on your way to being prepared to negotiate your first employment contract. Once the terms of the employment contract have been discussed and agreed upon, it is advisable to have the contract reviewed by an attorney to ensure the agreement states the intent of the parties and complies with state law. Negotiation techniques are discussed in detail in Chapter 10.

GETTING OUT OF AN EMPLOYMENT CONTRACT

It is not uncommon for an associate to work with several different employers during the first few years of employment. In fact, you may decide to move on after being employed for only a few

months, long before your term of employment has expired. This may be a result of changes in your personal life, such as marriage, the birth of a child, illness, or the death of a family member. What is more common is that an associate becomes dissatisfied with the employment conditions. Shortly after being hired, you may decide you can find more suitable work elsewhere. This is often the case when the terms of employment are vague with respect to your duties and emergency schedules and when your employer fails to provide promised benefits. If you follow the advice in this book, though, the chance of finding the right employment relationship the first time around is much better.

> Leaving behind a disgruntled employer can have long-lasting negative repercussions if that employer has many contacts in the industry.

Irrespective of why you give your notice of termination before the term of employment has expired, you should carefully consider the consequences of such actions. Your early departure is often distressing and frustrating to an employer who has invested significant time and resources recruiting you, drafting and negotiating an employment agreement for you, and training you. For this reason, an employer may resent your early departure; this may be reflected in an unfavorable reference. Even if a reference is not requested, your reputation can be easily tarnished through casual conversation among colleagues. It is important to realize that the veterinary industry is very small, which means that word travels fast. Leaving behind a disgruntled employer can have long-lasting negative repercussions if that employer has many contacts in the industry.

In addition, if you have signed an employment contract and have agreed to work for a given period, consider whether your early departure constitutes a breach of contract, in which case your employer may be entitled to monetary damages. In the event of a breach, the damages reflect the costs to place an employer in a position he or she would have been in had you not prematurely terminated the employment relationship. Therefore, you may be required to compensate your employer for expenses incurred in locating another associate, as well as the amount of salary, if any, that must be paid to employ the new associate that exceeds the salary that would have been paid to you.

To determine whether an early departure would constitute a breach of contract, focus primarily on two provisions of your contract—the term and termination provisions. To start, determine whether the contract has a term, or whether the employment is "at will," in which case, either party can terminate the relationship at any time for any reason or for no reason. When contracts do not stipulate a term, the type of employment is deemed to be at will in most states. If the contract states a term of employment, however, you must then determine whether you can terminate the contract by providing your employer with advance notice of your intent to leave. The termination provision of the contract provides that information.

If there is no provision allowing for you to terminate your employment prior to the expiration of the contract period, it is likely you would be in breach of contract if you give your notice prior to the end of the employment period. In any case, before you terminate your employment, it is advisable to have the agreement reviewed by local counsel to ensure that your interpretation of the agreement is accurate.

THE BOTTOM LINE

While it is rare for you to find the "perfect" employment situation early in your career, you can enjoy the work environment and gain valuable experiences by ensuring that you have a "meeting of the minds" with your employer with respect to the employment relationship. The use of employ-

ment contracts facilitates the process by which the employee and employer arrive at a meeting of the minds, and it is usually recommended that you sign a contract prior to beginning work.

In the event you are dissatisfied with your employment and you wish to terminate your employment prior to its expiration, carefully consider the consequences of such an action, because it may negatively impact your career as a veterinary practitioner.

Refer to the contract template provided on the CD that accompanies this book for a veterinary-specific boilerplate that covers the points in this chapter and more.

RESOURCES

Books

Compensation & Benefits by the American Animal Hospital Association.

Contracts, Benefits, and Practice Management for the Veterinary Profession by J. Wilson, J. Nemoy, and A. Fishman. Available through AAHA.

The Employment Contract by W. Freedman.

Websites

LawDepot.com™
www.lawdepot.com
This site has boilerplate language for employment contracts. You fill in the blanks, and a contract is written for you. Buy a one-time license to use the material for $15 or a multiple-use license for $45. Templates are also available for purchase on *www.urgentbusinessforms.com* and *www.uslegalforms.com*.

▶ CHAPTER TWELVE ◀

Making the Move

Samuel M. Fassig, DVM, MA

IN THIS CHAPTER, YOU'LL LEARN:

- **What to expect when planning a move**
- **How much it costs to move yourself vs. hiring a commercial mover**
- **How to cut costs**

IS RELOCATION WORTH IT?

You have found a job you think you want and you have evaluated the practice and community. So far, you like what you see. But before you pack the first box, research the cost of living in the area where the practice is located. If you move to an area with higher living costs, you could end up with a lower standard of living—even if you are making more money. On the other hand, a lower-cost location can help you live like you're rich—even if you aren't. Consider the following hypothetical examples.

Example A

As a veterinary student at Texas A&M, Kraig was spending $375 a month to rent a small, two-bedroom apartment. His utilities were low (swamp cooler for summer, baseboard heat for winter). Basically, if he was frugal he could manage on $1,000 a month for living expenses, including payments on a three-year-old pickup truck and stall space for his horse (not including school expenditures,

clothing, and entertainment). After graduation, he considered taking a position at the racetrack near Arlington, Illinois. He discovered that the cheapest one-bedroom apartment he could find was $885 per month, and it would put him eight miles from the track, in the approach flight path of O'Hare International Airport. Anything closer to the racetrack cost $1,100 to $1,400 per month. He could not afford the $10,000 down payment for a townhouse with monthly payments of $1,675. Utilities reportedly averaged $327 per month in the winter and $228 in the summer. The insurance for his truck would be six times more than what it was in Texas, and he was looking at $142 a month for highway tolls. Boarding his horse fifteen miles away would cost $650 per month. If he lived in Wisconsin, housing and horse care would be less expensive, but the commute could be an hour and a half each way, further increasing his truck insurance, plus his annual mileage and toll charges would double.

Example B

Dr. Catherine Metz and her husband, Marty, were recent graduates—Catherine from Cornell University's College of Veterinary Medicine and Marty with an MBA from Columbia University. They took positions near Tulsa, Oklahoma. They moved "laterally" from a tiny, older house with no garage and in need of work that cost $298,000 to a three-year-old house that cost $295,000. However, in Tulsa they picked up 50% more living space, a couple of extra bedrooms, a three-car garage, a second fireplace, new appliances, a swimming pool, and two acres of nicely landscaped property. Property taxes in Tulsa are $1,230 per year, whereas in New York, they had been paying $4,100. Utilities were about the same.

These are the kinds of things you will need to take into consideration as you analyze a move to another area (see Chapter 9 for information on comparing job offers).

How Much Will Your Lifestyle Cost There?

Use Worksheet 12-1 to identify the differences in cost of living between your current and proposed locations. To obtain this information in the new community:

* Contact at least three real-estate or rental agents. The Internet is an easy way to find these contacts. Ask them for information on homes, schools, and preferred communities, as well as commuting distances. Most have these packets already made. Because they want your business, most will provide them free of charge.

* Contact a relocation company, especially if your employer is helping you with the costs of the move. Ask their staff to provide you with similar information. It is part of the service.

* Get in touch with the Better Business Bureau and chamber of commerce for the area. Ask for informational packets and guides to businesses.

Shari Steiner, in her book *Steiner's Complete How-To-Move Handbook*, suggests subscribing to your new town's newspaper for a month or two so that you can check out grocery promotions, car ads, housing and employment classified ads, and local news.

Many realtors and relocation firms have moving calculators that can also be used to compare expenses (see Resources section at the end of this chapter). If you have not held a job where you currently live, consider using AAHA or AVMA figures for the mean starting salary. This will help you decide if you should negotiate a higher salary in order for you to enjoy a lifestyle similar to what would be available if you stayed in the location you live in now.

COSTS OF MOVING

You have compared the cost of living and calculated how much it will take to make a living in your new location. Now, assume you have decided to take the job in the new town. How do you go about getting there, and what costs are involved? If your new employer is paying for all or part of your move, you are lucky. If not, you will need to be diligent and take every possible opportunity to save money.

The American Moving and Storage Association gives a number of suggestions. Visit their website at *www.amconf.org* or call 703/683-7410.

John Simon of Atlas Van Lines in Arlington, Illinois, indicates that peak moving dates are the weeks of Labor Day and Memorial Day. The number of moves for his company may rise from 1,500 per week to 5,000 to 6,000 during those two peak weeks. The rate of moving is also higher at the end of the month than in the middle of the month.

Evaluating the Costs for "Self-Haul" Moves

According to Simon, many graduating students move themselves because they have only a one- or two-bedroom move that would normally take up only about 10% of a fifty-foot commercial van. Before you sign an agreement for a truck rental, especially for an interstate move, ask questions. There are often hidden costs. It will also help you to compare a commercial estimate from a moving and storage company to determine which might be the most cost-effective method in terms of

162

WORKSHEET 12-1
Categories to Use for Location Cost Comparison
This worksheet is also available on the companion CD.

Expense Category	Current Location	New Location
Housing	$ _____	$ _____
Utilities Gas Water Sewer Electric	 $ _____ $ _____ $ _____ $ _____	 $ _____ $ _____ $ _____ $ _____
Home Phone Service	$ _____	$ _____
TV/Cable Service	$ _____	$ _____
Internet Service	$ _____	$ _____
Wireless Phone Service	$ _____	$ _____
Groceries[1]	$ _____	$ _____
Sundries[2]	$ _____	$ _____
Fuel for Vehicles	$ _____	$ _____
Property Taxes	$ _____	$ _____
Sales Taxes	$ _____	$ _____
Vehicle Taxes, Plates	$ _____	$ _____

[1] Price 10–15 basic items such as milk, bread, meat, soup, coffee, and produce, and compare them over a few weeks.

[2] Follow same steps as for groceries, except track things like shampoo, makeup, and toothpaste.

WORKSHEET 12-1 (continued)
Categories to Use for Location Cost Comparison

Expense Category	Current Location	New Location
Insurance		
Homeowner	$ _____	$ _____
Personal Property	$ _____	$ _____
Vehicle	$ _____	$ _____
Liability	$ _____	$ _____
Medical	$ _____	$ _____
Vehicle Maintenance		
Tires	$ _____	$ _____
Repairs	$ _____	$ _____
Oil Changes	$ _____	$ _____
Transportation Costs		
Public Transportation	$ _____	$ _____
Tolls, Fees	$ _____	$ _____
Parking	$ _____	$ _____
Free-Time Activities		
Green Fees	$ _____	$ _____
Gym Membership	$ _____	$ _____
Outdoor Activities	$ _____	$ _____
Spectator Sports	$ _____	$ _____
Movies	$ _____	$ _____
Dining Out	$ _____	$ _____
Clothing	$ _____	$ _____
TOTAL	$ _____	$ _____

Chapter 12: Making the Move

price, damage, and security control, and your personal time investment (including time lost from work if you are injured). If you throw your back out because you are moving, medical expenses may not be covered by your employer or be considered eligible for workers' compensation or disability. Check your insurance policy.

TRUCK RENTAL CHARGES

You must provide the origin, destination cities, month, day, and year of the move to the truck-rental company for them to determine if equipment is available. In certain locations, prices may vary. The peak season is May through September, which is likely when you will be charged higher rates. Most people move at the beginning or end of a month, which may also mean equipment is unavailable for your move.

The rental charge you are quoted includes a damage deposit that may or may not be refunded. It all depends on the condition of the vehicle when you return it; therefore, it is important that any dents or defects are noted on the rental slip at the time of possession.

> Make sure you rent the correct size of truck. Efficient truck loading is an art—not a science. You do not want to find out after a day of packing that you have run out of truck space.

You are usually entitled to a certain number of free miles (approximately 10% greater than the estimated map distance). If you go over that, there is a fee (about forty cents per mile). Estimates do not include state taxes or additional fees.

You will need a day to pack and a day to unpack; therefore, be sure to quote two extra days in addition to driving days.

Make sure you rent the correct size of truck. Efficient truck loading is an art—not a science. You do not want to find out after a day of packing that you have run out of truck space.

AUTOMOBILES

Are you going to drive your car(s) or tow one or more? Trailer rental packages are available from rental companies at additional costs of about $200 plus insurance (approximately $50) and are tied into the truck rental and length of the rental agreement. A full trailer may be preferable to a front-wheel dolly for hauling a personal vehicle.

This is for safety reasons, because the rental dollies do not usually have anti-sway devices to keep the vehicle in tow from swaying side to side behind the pulling truck. Car dollies do not protect wheel bearings on your car from side-to-side wear either—a problem that may surface after the move. Depending on the type of vehicle you are towing, other precautions may need to be taken to protect the drive train. Also, it is harder to see a vehicle on a dolly from the driver's mirrors than on a full-size trailer.

If you drive a vehicle, figure that the IRS considers mileage wear and tear at 36.5 cents per mile (in 2002). Compare that cost to trailer rent.

INSURANCE CHARGES

Rental-truck insurance may cost an extra $10 to $14 per day. The daily charge includes vehicle damage and medical and life insurance if the vehicle is involved in an accident. There may still be a deductible. The daily charge also includes reimbursement for cargo damage up to a stated dollar amount.

Theft may be a concern, especially if you leave a fully loaded truck unattended while you spend the night at a motel or in an unpatrolled rest area. Strongly consider buying theft insurance, especially if your auto insurance will not cover you. Also, check with your auto insurance company to see if your policy will pay for vehicle damage if your car is being towed or is on a trailer. If you do not have comprehensive coverage, you may need supplemental insurance depending on the replacement value of your automobile.

OTHER EQUIPMENT RENTALS

Furniture pads cost ten dollars per dozen to rent. An appliance dolly or furniture dolly may cost an additional five to ten dollars to rent.

PACKING AND LOADING

Although you may be able to collect boxes from local merchants, you might consider purchasing specialized boxes like wardrobes, dish packs, or mattress containers to help secure your cargo in transit. The cost of packing materials varies from state to state and from company to company. *UHaul.com* estimates that packing materials cost about $500 for a one-to-two-bedroom house and $140 for each additional bedroom. Some appliances and electronic equipment (copiers, audio equipment, and computer drives) need special attention before being moved. If you have to hire that out, it will also increase your moving expense.

FUEL

The truck is full of fuel when you pick it up. You must return it full of fuel or you will be charged a premium if the rental company has to fill the tank (two to three times higher per gallon). How much will it cost to operate a truck? In general, a twenty-six-foot, manual, fully loaded diesel truck will average nine to ten miles per gallon. If you travel 1,600 miles, you will consume about 160 to 178 gallons. At a price of $1.689 per gallon, your estimated fuel cost will be between $270 and $300. Also keep in mind that fuel prices peak during the summer.

PER-MOVE VALUE OF TIME

Who is going to pack, unpack, and pick up, drive, and return the truck? Figure out your hourly wage, then multiply that times the estimated number of hours for yourself, your spouse, and your family to pack, pick up the truck, load, drive, unload, unpack, and return the truck. In addition, figure out what the hotel/motel charges might be along the way and at your destination.

DESTINATION CHARGES

If your house or apartment is not available when you arrive, you must consider:

- Where will you store your possessions?

- If you are renting a mini-storage unit, what is the security level? Are you insured for actual replacement costs from perils such as fire, flood, theft, smoke, and other losses?

- Will you have to rent another truck to move the goods in storage to your new house or apartment?

- Will you have to pay for help in loading and unloading the truck again?

OTHER COSTS IN A SELF-MOVE

- Food costs money—for friends during packing and unpacking, and on the road.

- Trash—do you need a dumpster for rubbish as you clear out your current residence? If so, how big of a dumpster do you need, and how much does it cost? Who will call the trash company to come and remove it?

- Childcare expenses

- Will lifting and unloading cause old injuries to resurface?

- Security of the load while the truck is moving (cargo damage) and when you have stopped to sleep (theft/vandalism), especially if the trip takes more than one day

- Bridge and highway tolls, as well as bridge and tunnel clearances en route—most commercial rental trucks will fit under interstate bridges. However, if you are sightseeing, make sure you know how high and wide the truck is before you enter narrow roads and get stuck or cause damage to the truck and cargo.

- You may run into schedule problems due to detours, construction delays, equipment failure, and driver fatigue, forcing an earlier stop to rest.

- Do you have the emergency road-service numbers with you to call in case there is a mechanical or tire failure or an accident?

- Before taking possession of the truck, do your own safety inspection for tire wear and inflation levels. Make certain that all the lights are operating. If you are using a trailer, be sure that all connections are safe and operating properly and that all mirrors and windows are intact and operational. Be sure you understand from the rental agent how everything works on the truck and trailer, and ask if you must stop at any state weigh stations along the route. In some states, all trucks over 10,000 pounds gross vehicle weight must stop, and all trucks pulling trailers must stop at scale and weigh-safety stations. If you do need to stop, make sure you have the rental papers and a copy of the truck registration materials. Failure to have them may cause delays.

- If for any reason you are thinking about taking the truck out of the country (i.e., Canada or Mexico) as part of your travels, become familiar with United States customs procedures and import/export regulations and those of the country through which you will be passing, even if it is just for sightseeing. Also, see if the rental company will allow it. As a veterinarian, you know there are drugs, drug-delivery systems, and substances that are legal for you, as a licensed veterinarian, to have in your possession in the United States. However, they may be forbidden in other countries, even if you think it is an "open border." If you have them in your possession or on your person, you run the risk of being detained and having everything in the truck unloaded and inspected. These items can be confiscated, and you could be assessed fines, have your vehicle impounded, and, for some offenses, be detained or arrested and have to pay any associated legal fees.

- Personal trailers—most truck-rental companies will not allow you to pull anything but their equipment behind their rental trucks. Doing so without telling them may subject you to additional fees or void insurance protection coverage if you are in an accident with the rental truck. In addition, your own insurance carrier may take a dim view of attaching your equipment to a rental vehicle without permission clearly stated in the rental agreement.

Moving With Plants and Pets

Plants are subject to shock when changes in temperature, light, and moisture conditions occur. Trucks can get hot, cold, and dark. The vibration may loosen potting soil, causing root damage. Plants may also tip over or get crushed. Consult your nursery for information about your particular plants.

When you move across state lines, you will likely need to have a completed health certificate for your animals—dogs and horses especially. If you leave the state in which you are licensed, and you are not licensed in the state where you are stopped, it is too late for you to write your own. In the event of quarantine violations, you may be putting your license in jeopardy or be subject to disciplinary action by the state boards of veterinary medicine in which you are licensed.

All but four states require proof of rabies vaccination for dogs, and many require it for cats. A few states have border inspections of all animals being transported; others have random inspections. Inspections can occur at weigh stations or where "port of entry" signs appear.

If you move or are transporting animals across state lines, call or write the state veterinarian, and check with the Animal Plant Health Inspection Service (APHIS) or other appropriate authority for any restrictions or rules. Although in the past many states have been lax on checking health certificates during automobile transport, being in a truck may subject you to more scrutiny due to increased security related to biohazards. It is not really worth your career to circumvent regulations that you as a veterinarian are expected to uphold.

Using Commercial Movers

If you are planning to use a commercial mover, you will need to select a carrier company and schedule the move well in advance—six to eight weeks before the moving date. Four weeks is the absolute minimum. With short time frames, expect difficulties.

Moving companies provide various services for a considerable range of fees. Ask around for the names of and contact information for moving companies from friends, neighbors, your university human-resources department, relocation companies, your new employer, or the Better Business Bureau, which has information about the number of complaints against a carrier and the success of the resolution of the claims. The AVMA also offers a moving program as a benefit of membership.

Referrals may be tricky. Someone telling you that their movers did a great job may not be enough. Most companies are independently owned and operated, and although some are affiliated with a big national name, that does not guarantee any level of service. The best buy could be a small mom-and-pop outfit. A key point to remember is that interstate moves are regulated, while local moves are not.

167

The Federal Highway Administration (*www.fhwa.dot.gov/*), formerly the Interstate Commerce Commission, requires that if you are moving interstate, the mover must provide you with a consumer booklet entitled *Your Rights and Responsibilities When You Move* and information regarding the mover's participation in a dispute-settlement program. Get it and read it.

When you choose a moving company, be sure you know all of the following:

- All the rates and charges that will apply (Ask, ask again, then ask once more.)

- The mover's liability for your belongings (damage, breakage, loss, repair)

- Details of how the pickup (packing) and delivery (unloading, unpacking) will work

- What insurance protection you will have (from the mover) or if you need to get additional insurance (perhaps on your own or with the moving company) to protect your cargo

- Which items might be better off traveling with you (e.g., computer, furs, jewelry, firearms, stamp and coin collections, family photos, veterinary drugs, high-value equipment)

- If your load is being combined with someone else's to make a full truck. If so, and if all your possessions do not arrive, how do you get your stuff? If the shipment does not arrive as scheduled due to dropping a partial load, are you compensated? How can you get just your belongings on the truck and no one else's?

- If, on arrival in the region, the truck is going to be unloaded in a warehouse, with your belongings stored and then loaded onto a local truck for delivery to you, how are you protected from loss, damage from the elements, and damage to your possessions due to the additional handling? Are you compensated for or protected against pests and insect infestation of your cargo? (This can be a significant problem if you are moving to southern states or in the summer and your shipment is offloaded if you are moving.) If not, you may want to consider hiring a commercial pest controller to come in and treat the new residence within a week after your move-in. Roaches, fleas, spiders, and other critters are very adaptable and set up housekeeping in a hurry.

WAYS TO CUT COSTS

- **The discount**—Most long-distance moving companies determine charges based on the American Moving and Storage Association's book, *Tariff 400*. It states what the charge should be for hauling a certain number of pounds of cargo a given number of miles. To stay competitive, movers will then discount the tariff as much as 40 to 60% to get your business. Ask the moving company's representative or sales agent how much the discount is and try to negotiate a lower rate. Get at least three estimates to give you leverage. If possible, include a company in the destination city for an estimate as well. You might get a deal if he needs to get a truck back and can pick up your load to offset returning an empty truck.

- **Flexibility on moving dates**—As with self-haul rental trucks, movers are very busy from mid-May to mid-September. They usually are looking for work in January and February. Discounts during high moving periods, such as June and July, will probably not be as deep as in December through March, which could yield you an additional 5% to 12% discount. In addition to the month, if you give the movers some leeway on pickup and delivery dates (three to five days on pickup and the same for delivery), you might also be able to negotiate a better deal.

- **Packing**—You can save money by packing some items yourself, especially the nonbreakable things like books, VCR tapes, clothing, and general office supplies. In most cases, let the movers pack the high-value and breakable items such as china and dishes. In general, you can buy boxes and packing materials from companies like Ryder or U-Haul less expensively than from the mover, who will also sell you boxes, tape, and packing paper. Grocery-store boxes are okay if they are in good shape, but if they were previously used for produce, they may attract bugs. Ask for boxes at an office-supply store. They usually cut up boxes but might save some for you. They also sell boxes and may give you a special rate if you are buying in large quantities. Laura Bruce, in her article for *Bankrate.com*, "Quick Take on Moving: Estimates of Moving Costs," lists common packing-carton sizes (in cubic feet) and common suggested uses. Table

12-1 summarizes these figures, along with suggestions from the author. Tuff Crates are especially good because you can see what is in them, they stack, they are tough, and they are fairly watertight with duct tape on the center of the lid (available at Home Depot, Wal-Mart, and Lowe's).

- **Reducing the weight of the load**—Moving is a great time to clean house. If you have not worn or used something for a year or so, consider selling it, giving it away, or throwing it away.

- **Tax deductions**—Keep all receipts, including those for tape, boxes, and other miscellaneous materials. You will be able to deduct allowable expenses on your income tax return.

> Keep all receipts, including those for tape, boxes, and other miscellaneous materials. You will be able to deduct allowable expenses on your income tax return.

COSTS YOU MAY NOT BE ABLE TO REDUCE

- **Additional transportation charges**—These are charges that compensate the mover for services performed in high-labor-rate areas, such as major metropolitan areas. These charges can range from $1 to $3 per 100 pounds or higher in cities like New York, Los Angeles, San Francisco, and Chicago. Moving companies hire locals to load and unload the truck and are at the mercy of the local labor market.

- **Special services**—When the mover needs to hire a specialist to perform certain tasks, like disconnecting gas appliances or disassembling a piano or pool table, you will be charged an extra service charge. It is very common, and

169

Table 12-1
PACKING-CARTON SIZES AND USES

Carton Size (cubic feet)	Carton Size (inches)	Uses
1.5 cubic feet	16⅜ x 12⅝ x 12⅝ inches	Books, records, tapes, canned goods, shoes, silverware
3.0 cubic feet	18⅛ x 18 x 16 inches	Small kitchen appliances, lamp bases, small outdoor tools, pots and pans, electronic gadgets, small bathroom items, hand-held horse-grooming equipment and supplies
4.5 cubic feet	24 x 18 x 18 inches	Nonhanging clothes, larger lamps, lamp shades, linens, bedding, nonbreakable kitchen products (e.g., muffin tins, Tupperware, baking pans)
6.0 cubic feet	24 x 18 x 24 inches	Stuffed toys, blankets, pillows, area rugs, winter coats
12-gallon polyethylene Tuff Crate (side-hinged folding lid, clear bottom)	21¾ x 15¼ × 12 inches	Files, magazines, professional journals, books, notebooks

many moving companies hire third-party companies that provide this type of service.

- **Bulky items**—Lawnmowers, boats, snowmobiles, and shop equipment (e.g., large table saws and compressors) may cost extra to move. It will also cost extra for the movers to drain and neutralize fuel tanks. The mover may refuse to move some of these items altogether due to safety reasons.

- **Access service charges**—You will be charged extra if it is difficult to access your residence. If the mover has to walk more than seventy-five feet from the truck to the door, you pay extra. If there are stairs or an elevator to reach your apartment, you will pay more. The cost is usually between $1.50 and $2.00 per hundred pounds.

- **Shuttle fee**—If the mover cannot get your belongings on or off the truck due to narrow streets, low branches, electric wires, or restrictions, and your belongings must first be placed on a smaller truck, then taken to the larger van, you will be charged a shuttle fee. Depending on the size of your shipment, this can be a most unpleasant surprise for you. The moving-company sales representative at the origin end will include such a charge in the initial price quote. However, because he or she cannot see the destination location, this fee may be tacked onto the end of the move.

- **Payment on delivery**—Unless other arrangements have been made in advance (such as your employer paying for your move), the mover will demand that you pay for the move when the goods are delivered and before they are taken off the truck. If you do not have the certified check or payment the mover requires, your belongings may be put into storage until you pay. You will be charged extra for the storage and possibly for handling.

THE MOVING ESTIMATE

The fee for an interstate move is based on the weight of the load, the distance it is shipped, how much packing the mover must do, and other services required from the mover. Movers will give you an estimate of the cost. To help them with this process, show them everything to be moved. Do not forget the attic, the cellar, the storage shed, or anywhere else you store items that must be moved. Reach a clear understanding of who packs what, and how much packing the mover will need to do. Anything omitted from the estimate but later added to the shipment will add to the cost.

A good sales representative will go room to room, basement to attic, and garage to shed and will write down everything he or she sees. Unfortunately, inexperienced representatives take the customer's word on items that need to be moved. For example, he or she might ask the customer, "Is there anything in the basement that goes?" The customer replies, "No, just the washer and dryer and the folding table." The inexperienced representative comes up with a low-ball estimate. The more experienced person goes down into the basement and may come out with 2,000 pounds more. The customer says, "Oh, I completely forgot the metal shelves, the Christmas decorations, and the kid's train set."

When an estimator goes through the house, he or she is completing a table of estimates called the "cube sheet," which helps calculate the cubic footage. This determines the amount of room needed on the truck. This is where there can be big differences between moving companies on the estimate, depending how thorough and seasoned the sales representative is.

Most movers offer two types of estimates—binding and nonbinding. A binding estimate is a written agreement that guarantees the cost of the move. It is based on the items to be moved and the services listed on the mover's sheet. Anything added later will cost extra and may delay the move.

Whenever possible, especially with large loads, get a binding estimate with everything spelled out. Movers are allowed to charge you for making a binding estimate. If you get a binding estimate and you are being charged for it, you may want to ask for a "not-to-exceed" estimate.

A nonbinding estimate is not guaranteed—it is just an approximation. Final charges will be determined once the load is weighed. It does not bind the mover to any costs, and there is no guarantee that the final cost will be what the estimate indicates. Movers cannot charge you for making a nonbinding estimate. A smart consumer will say, "I would like to have a binding estimate, and then I would like to have the truck weighed, figure that cost, and pay the lower of the two." A good mover will do that automatically, but it is always good to ask.

At the time you get the estimate, also discuss payment arrangements. Most movers will accept cash, a certified check, or a money order. Most do not accept personal checks. Only some will accept a credit card. Ask first and get it in writing. Always get a receipt when you pay.

Once you have three or four estimates, find the one with the most weight, the longest carrying distance, and all the extras. Call the others back and ask them to revise their estimates based on the exact same categories. The time to ask for the deep discount is when they all get on the same playing field.

The discount reflects the quality of service you will receive. By the time you have dealt with three or four companies and gotten referral and background information on each carrier, you will know which company you really want to move your belongings. The cheapest in price may provide the lowest quality of service.

Example

Say you are going to move from Davis, California, to New York City. You have a two-bedroom townhouse (1,000 to 1,200 pounds per room). There are no extraordinary items, and nothing requires special crating (such as antiques or large paintings). Your total load is 6,000 pounds. You are moving 2,836 miles with four appliances (washer, dryer, refrigerator, freezer). Only the washer needs servicing. There is one flight of stairs in your new home. You do not need any additional insurance coverage, and there are no unusual services, such as crating or hoisting. An average discount (42%) is given because you are planning to move on June 15. Tables 12-2, 12-3, and 12-4 summarize the costs for this move.

MOVER'S LIABILITY FOR LOSS OR DAMAGE

All interstate carriers must assume some liability for the value of the cargo that they transport. There are different levels of liability and charges for each option. Most movers offer four levels of liability coverage.

- **Released value**—This is a no-additional-cost option that provides minimal protection. The mover assumes liability for no more than sixty cents per pound per article. Loss or damage claims are settled at sixty cents per pound. Say, for example, a ten-pound stereo speaker valued at $1,000 is lost or destroyed. The mover is

Table 12-2
TRANSPORTATION-RELATED MOVING CHARGES

Transportation Charges	Weight/Size/Mileage	Cost
Transit charges	6,000 pounds for 2,836 miles	$8,996
ATC (Davis)	6,000 pounds × 2.25 cwt	$135
ATC (NYC)	6,000 pounds × 3.80 cwt	$228
Appliance services		$37
Appliance reservicing		$25
Stair carry	6,000 pounds × 2.00 cwt	$120
Total Transit-Related Charges		**$9,541**

Table 12-3
PACKING CHARGES

Containers	Number Required	Price per Container	Total Container Cost	Packing Cost per Container	Total Packing Cost	Unpacking Cost per Container	Total Unpacking Cost
Dish Pack	7	$25.20	$176.40	$43.05	$301.35	$17.20	$120.40
1.5 Cu. Ft. Carton	15	$5.35	$80.25	$11.10	$166.50	$4.40	$66.00
3.0 Cu. Ft. Carton	14	$7.70	$107.80	$17.25	$241.50	$6.95	$97.30
4.5 Cu. Ft. Carton	10	$9.25	$92.50	$21.15	$211.50	$8.50	$85.00
6.0 Cu. Ft. Carton	2	$10.65	$21.30	$24.15	$48.30	$9.70	$19.40
Wardrobe	4	$19.75	$79.00	$12.60	$50.40	$3.15	$12.60
Dbl. Mattress	4	$16.15	$64.60	$12.25	$49.00	$4.85	$19.40
Mirror	6	$20.30	$121.80	$39.30	$235.80	$15.75	$94.50
Total Packing Charges			**$734.65**		**$1,304.35**		**$514.60**

172

Table 12-4
ESTIMATE OF TOTAL CHARGES FOR THE MOVE

Total	Charges
Transportation-related charges	$9,541
Cartons	$735
Packing	$1,304
Unpacking	$515
Total before discount	$12,095
42% discount	($5,080)
TOTAL AFTER DISCOUNT	$7,015

liable for no more than $6. There is no extra charge for this coverage, but you must sign a statement on the bill of lading agreeing to it.

- **Declared value**—The valuation of your entire shipment is based on the total weight of the load times $1.25 per pound. As an example, a 6,000-pound shipment is valued at a maximum of $7,500. Any loss or damage claim under this option is settled based on the depreciated value of the lost or damaged item(s) up to the maximum liability value based on the entire weight of the shipment. A $1,000 speaker, then, is covered up to $1,000, based on depreciation. If the speaker is five years old, it could be depreciated at 10% per year and you would get $500. The mover is entitled to charge you $7 for each $1,000 of value.

- **Lump-sum value**—This is similar to the declared value. The lump-sum value is determined if the declared value of the shipment exceeds $1.25 per pound times the weight of the shipment, and you want to purchase additional liability coverage from the mover. If, for example, you declare the value of your 6,000-pound shipment to be $10,000, the mover will charge you $7 per each $1,000 of declared value. In this case, that amount would be $70. You must declare this on the bill of lading.

- **Full-value protection**—If you elect to purchase full-value protection, any item that is lost, damaged, or destroyed will either be repaired or replaced with like items, or a cash settlement will be made for the current replacement value, regardless of the age of the lost or damaged item. Depreciation is not a factor. The cost for this type of protection varies from mover to mover.

- **Extraordinary value**—Extraordinary value must be declared separately on the bill of lading and must exceed a value of $100 per pound. Movers are permitted to limit their liability for loss or damage to articles of extraordinary value under all four liability options cited above.

These optional levels of liability are not insurance agreements governed by state insurance laws. They are authorized release rate orders of the Surface Transportation Board of the U.S. Department of Transportation. Other insurance products may be available. Check with the mover or your own insurance company for products and rates.

HOW TO PLAN YOUR MOVE

Plan Ahead. Pick a moving date that is flexible and that offers you the best discount you can get. Carefully go through at least three estimates from different companies, comparing them to see which company best suits your needs and budget.

Packing. Schedule packing with the mover a day or two before the moving van is loaded. The services of a trained packer and the right packing materials will definitely make it a better move. While packing items yourself can save you some of the per-carton expense to pack and unpack, movers will usually not accept any liability for damage to items packed by owners.

Be present when your goods are packed. An inventory of your goods will be made, and it is important to resolve any disagreements prior to signing the inventory list. Have valuable items listed separately. Be sure boxes are marked with contents and the type of room they go to.

Moving Day

- Be available when the movers arrive.

- Make sure the delivery arrangements have been fully discussed with the mover and are clearly understood.

- Beds should be stripped and ready to be packed.

- Let the moving crew disassemble goods. However, make sure the boxes containing parts to reassemble are clearly marked or noted.

- Read the bill of lading closely before you sign it.

- Provide the mover with information as to how to contact you at the destination.

- When you are traveling, keep in touch with the mover's agent.

At the Destination When the Truck Arrives

- Check your goods for damage and any missing items. Note that the number of items on the inventory sheet did, in fact, arrive. Note the condition of every box. If a box is damaged, write it on the inventory sheet and have the

173

driver confirm it in writing. This will make any claims go much faster, with some being handled on the spot.

- Do not sign the inventory sheet until you have inspected your furniture and the exterior of all cartons.

- You have nine months to report any damage you notice after unpacking. It is to your advantage to report it early. The mover must acknowledge receipt of your claim within 30 days and must deny or make an offer within 120 days of receiving your claim.

- Remember—the mover's liability is limited to the level cited on the bill of lading at the time your belongings were loaded.

DEALING WITH THE STRESS OF RELOCATION ONCE YOU ARRIVE AT YOUR NEW HOME

Learn the Geography

Part of the stress from relocation is dealing with unfamiliar geography and the loss of places where you did business. "Where do I go now to get the car fixed?" "What about a bank and a grocery store?" "Where can I get my hair done, go to a gym to work out, and find affordable computer parts?" Scary or adventurous? It depends in part on your attitude and ability to adjust.

By exploring what the new area has to offer, you will open doors to meeting new people and networking with those in your new neighborhood. It will generate some excitement and energy as you get a sense of control back in your life. As you travel around the various parts of town looking for restaurants, shops, and places you could take people who come to visit, you will get to discover the "flavor" of the area. You do not have to actually wait until the car breaks down to go out and interview some garage owners.

Play tourist. This can help you break the ice when you are talking to clinic staff and clients; you can also invite these people to share their stories. It will most assuredly jump-start your ability to feel like a part of the community and be closer to those for whom you are now providing animal healthcare services.

Ask the local distributor and pharmaceutical representatives for advice on where to go, what to see, where to eat, etc. Most likely, they know every inch of town, or at least all of their service territory. Not only will this help you glean information about the area, but undoubtedly they will also share their perception of all the practices in town, give you their biased look at the competition, and let you know who and where the specialists are for patient referrals. (For you, this could also mean identifying a potential mentor.) Keep this relationship on a professional level. Maintaining a friendly professional position builds respect and a positive image. Let them know you have a specific interest in whatever part of veterinary medicine you are passionate about. Representatives will talk about you to others in their territory as the "new doctor at the clinic." The impression you make is important, even though you may not be in charge of buying. They can help build or tarnish your image in both the local and professional communities.

Social Support and Friendship

One of the most significant parts of relocation is the loss of familiar friends and social support. Psychologists indicate that when people get uprooted and are forced to move away from familiar people or places, they often get sick. They are ill more often and are absent from work at a higher rate than their coworkers.

In summing up the general protective nature of social ties, psychiatrist Robert Taylor said, "When people have close relationships, they feel less threatened, less alone, more confident, and more in control. Knowing you have people you can turn to in times of need can provide some very important feelings of security, optimism, and hope—all of which can be great antidotes to stress."

Studies in Michigan, North Carolina, Sweden, and Japan indicate that people who are socially isolated—the unmarried, divorced, widowed, people with few friends, and people who have few church or social contacts—are three times as likely to die of a wide variety of diseases than those who have happy, fulfilling social lives. Having good relationships seems to:

- Help you resist infection

- Protect you from disease

- Protect you from stress

- Make you healthier, both physically and mentally

- Help you live longer

It is important then, when you find yourself in new surroundings, to be outgoing instead of isolating yourself.

Barbara Powell, in her book *Good Relationships Are Good Medicine*, makes the point that a full and rewarding social life can nourish the mind, the emotions, and the spirit. Good physical health depends as much on these aspects as it does on a strong, well-functioning body. So make a point of building new friendships as soon as possible after you've settled in to your home.

RESOURCES

Books

Mind/Body Health: The Effects of Attitudes, Emotions, and Relationships, Second Edition by B. Hafen, K. Karren, K. Frandsen, and N. Smith.

Packing and Moving Tips That Could Save You a Fortune by J. Marc.

Smooth Moves by E. Carlisle.

Steiner's Complete How-To-Move Handbook by S. Steiner and C. Steiner.

Websites

Bankrate.com
www.bankrate.com
You can access two helpful articles on this site: "Quick Take On Moving: Estimates of Moving Costs" by L. Bruce.
"Moving Costs: How to Save Money" by L. Bruce.

monstermoving.com
www.monstermoving.com
You'll find school reports, city profiles, a mortgage calculator, and lots of other good moving information on this site.

Realtor.com
www.realtor.com
Click on the "Moving" tab for pre- and post-move checklists and a place to get bids on moving your belongings.

The Riley Guide
www.rileyguide.com/relocate.html
This site has many helpful links to moving-related sites and a salary calculator (what you'll need to make in the new location to compare to your salary now).

Special Acknowledgment
For providing information handouts and materials on relocation as resource information, giving permission to use them for reference, and taking the time to be interviewed.

Mr. John C. Simon, National Account Manager
NOFFS-Atlantic Relocation Systems
1735 E. Davis Street
Arlington Heights, Illinois 60005-2887
Phone: 847/870-3200 or 800/323-7791
www.atlanticrelocation.com

CHAPTER THIRTEEN ◄

When Private Practice Isn't Your Cup of Tea

Carin A. Smith, DVM

IN THIS CHAPTER, YOU'LL LEARN:

- **How to apply your degree outside of traditional practice**
- **Where to find out about other careers**

You did your research, accepted a job, and now, after working there for the past few months, something isn't right. Or maybe you haven't even started looking for that first job and don't even know where to start. What is your next step?

First, try to determine whether the lack of fit is between you and this particular practice, or if it's between you and private practice in general. Give yourself enough time to make adjustments in your life at home and at work. Don't be too quick to blame others for your problems–you may only find that the same problems arise again in the next job.

"I'd quit my job in a minute, but there are no other jobs here, and I'm not confident that I'd find work! I just feel stuck." Think again. There are a huge number of choices available to you. Only *you* create the limitations on what you can do, and only *you* can make the choices that are right for you. Life is a series of trade-offs. If you must live in a specific location, then don't expect to find your dream job there. If you must work in your dream job, realize that other aspects of your life must "give" to allow you that freedom. It is *your* choice.

Before you start looking at career alternatives, recognize that stereotypes could interfere with your decision-making. We all have stereotypes about

certain jobs that are based on influences from our teachers and families, or that may be based, in part, on our encounters with only a few people working in various fields. Try to start your search with a fresh outlook. Talk to people who are working in a wide variety of jobs. Join special-interest groups to meet more people in your field of interest. Most of these groups are listed in the *AVMA Directory* (see the Resources section at the end of this chapter) and most hold meetings in conjunction with national veterinary meetings.

"I really hesitate to move out of private practice, because then I'd be wasting my education!" One stumbling block is the common assumption that you are somehow "wasting" your veterinary schooling if you are not in private practice. Yet, can you imagine saying to someone in small-animal private practice, "Aren't you wasting your education? You never use the bovine medicine, the basic virology, or the histology that you learned!" *No one* uses everything they learned in school, and *everyone* needs to learn additional skills before they are comfortable in the jobs they choose. The only waste of your time is if you continue to work in a job you don't like while trying to prove that you are "using" your schooling.

Nonetheless, simply disliking your current job won't propel you into a better job. You must be driven by more than a desire to get away from something. Instead, define what it is you want to do. What attributes of a job are most important to you? What do you like most about your current work? Use that information to help guide you to a new position.

You will read and hear a lot about opportunities (or lack thereof) in various areas of veterinary medicine. Use that knowledge to assess your realistic chances of successfully finding work. However, realize that even in job niches with low numbers of veterinarians, there are *some* people doing that work. If it is the kind of work you love, don't let the statistics frighten you. You could be that one person who fills the niche.

WHAT ARE YOUR OPTIONS?

You have several options other than full-time private practice as a veterinarian. You may want to enter an internship and possibly a residency in order to become a board-certified specialist. You could work in a large-group or corporate setting, or in a small-town, one- to two-person practice. Additional choices include part-time or relief work, and housecall or mobile practice. Many of these choices transcend the boundaries of specialties and of small-animal, mixed, and large-animal practices.

Your decision about where you want to live has a large impact on your choices. Veterinarians who prefer to work in a group practice or corporate setting will be limited to locations where the population can support such a practice. Those who prefer small-town life will likely work in a small practice with one or two other veterinarians. Veterinarians in smaller practices often see their own emergencies and are more intimately involved with the day-to-day management of the practice.

Part-Time and Relief Work

Part-time work is becoming more plentiful. You could even work two part-time jobs, resulting in full-time work for yourself while filling a need for two different clinics. A part-time veterinarian must put a lot of effort into communicating with staff and other veterinarians in order to ensure continuity with staff communication and patient care.

Part-time veterinarians differ from relief veterinarians in several ways. Part-timers are employees who work consistently for one or more hospitals. They are expected to show up during designated hours on designated days. They are paid on a regular payday and should receive prorated benefits. They are also valued, long-term members of the hospital team. It is the regularity and control over your work that the hospital has—not the actual number of hours worked—that create the part-time employee designation.

Relief veterinarians run their own service businesses. They work a series of short-term, temporary jobs for many different hospitals. Relief veterinarians may work more than once for one hospital, but they do so on an intermittent basis. Relief veterinarians set their own fees and may accept or decline each job on its own merits.

Relief work requires enough experience that you are comfortable working as the only veterinarian, and with a variety of people, equipment, and supplies. It is not a good job for a new graduate. Relief work is sometimes thought of as a stepping-stone or a temporary way to earn money while you decide on a long-term position. However, many veterinarians do relief work on a full-time, permanent basis.

"I started doing relief work as a temporary thing while deciding what I'd really do. Now I've had a full-time relief business for four years! I control my schedule, and I'm appreciated wherever I work. I enjoy working with different people, and I learn a lot from every practice."

Housecall Practice

"I knew I wanted to stay in private practice, but I wanted a more personal relationship with my clients and to be able to set my own schedule. I still work as hard, or harder, than I did in a regular practice, but it's my decision." Housecall veterinarians are increasing in number throughout the United States, as

> **Housecall veterinarians are increasing in number throughout the United States, as seen by the growth of the American Association of Housecall Veterinarians.**

seen by the growth of the American Association of Housecall Veterinarians. Starting your own housecall practice can be a low-cost stepping-stone to opening a full-service clinic, or it can become a long-term, stand-alone service. As with relief work, housecall work requires enough experience that you are comfortable with performing procedures and making decisions on your own. Like relief veterinarians, housecall practitioners are small-business owners who must manage and run their own businesses.

Housecall veterinarians may work out of a standard automobile or may become mobile veterinarians, using a vehicle that provides a facility for surgery, radiology, and other procedures. The extent and type of work that housecall or mobile veterinarians are allowed to perform is governed by individual state laws. Check your state veterinary practice act for details.

Internships and Residencies

More and more graduating veterinarians are entering internships. Before you do so, define the outcome you want to achieve. New veterinarians may enter internships simply to better improve the medical or surgical skills they will need in private practice. However, some private-practice employers would prefer to hire those with more *people* skills—something obtained by working in private practice and not necessarily in an internship. Others say they are not willing to pay a higher salary to someone who completed an internship. The lesson—explore your expectations for the outcome before you enter an internship.

You may also pursue both an internship and a residency with the goal of board certification. Specialists can work in private practice, academia, industry, and government. Veterinary specialists in certain areas are in high demand. Your choice of specialty has an effect on where and how you can work. Small towns are unlikely to be able to support the work of a specialist. While some specialists are in high demand in cities (e.g., ophthalmologists, oncologists, and clinical pathologists), others may find there is a limited market

for their expertise (e.g., large-animal medicine). Choosing a specialty with a limited market means that you have less choice in where and how you work. Explore your expectations for the outcome of your advanced study before you begin.

Government

The number and type of job opportunities for veterinarians within government entities are vast. "Government" includes city, local, state, and federal positions. These positions include both those specifically labeled "DVM" and those for which veterinarians are qualified, but which don't specifically limit their qualifications to the DVM degree. Government jobs stand out with their great benefits. Be sure to include the value of these benefits when making salary comparisons.

"I had never thought of working for the government, but then I found out about the opportunities for advancement and additional education. I can do a lot of different things, but still work within the same structure. And the time off is really nice. I have no regrets about this decision. I love my work!" Cities and counties have public-health departments that may hire veterinarians to oversee food safety, monitor zoonotic disease, and help establish policy. Cities that run their own animal shelters may hire a full-time staff veterinarian. Cities and states may hire veterinarians for animal-care facility inspection; these veterinarians travel to breeding and research facilities to ensure that animals are properly cared for.

State governments have several career options for veterinarians. Many of these options focus on public health or control of food-animal or zoonotic diseases. Departments of public health hire a wide variety of scientists, including veterinarians. State departments of agriculture (sometimes called the livestock board) have several veterinarians on staff. Their work ranges from evaluating livestock to supervising meat inspection to other management and supervisory positions.

Veterinarians who work for the federal government report high job satisfaction and good pay and benefits. Yet the number of federal agencies that employ veterinarians, and the types of

> **Veterinarians who work for the federal government report high job satisfaction and good pay and benefits.**

179

jobs veterinarians can fill in the federal government, can be overwhelming. Adding to the confusion is the way you must apply for any federal job—with a generic form. Those who are able to make their way through the paperwork maze are rewarded with satisfying jobs that range from hands-on clinical work to fascinating, cutting-edge disease research.

Many federal employees give this advice: Apply for any civilian federal job, just to "get in the door." Subsequently, you will learn about many more job opportunities, and as an "insider," you will have a much easier time finding the specific work you desire. Yes, it's a leap of faith—but those who made the leap report they are glad they did.

Industry

If your stereotype of the "industrial veterinarian" is limited to pharmaceutical-company technical service, take another look. The category called "industry" is both large and small. It is large in that it includes a huge variety of jobs, with the potential for even more. It is small in that the total number of veterinarians working in these jobs is just a tiny percentage of all the veterinarians in the United States.

To get an idea of some of the choices within industry, spend some time in the exhibit hall at the next large veterinary meeting you attend. Choose a time when the hall is quiet and others are attending continuing-education sessions. Ask the veterinarians who work at the various exhibits about their work and about the work of their colleagues. You may be pleasantly surprised at the variety of work they do, and about how much these people love their jobs.

"I enjoy my job because I get to meet and talk with veterinarians all over the country. I enjoy the travel, the challenges, and the lack of a set routine. I even get to travel worldwide. It's a great career!" Some veterinarians in industry are in positions you never see unless you go out of your way to find them. They include veterinarians who work in companies such as Gore (makers of Gore-tex®), bio-medical-research firms, and computer-database firms. Joining the American Association of Industrial Veterinarians and attending their meetings can help you meet some of these people and find out more about their jobs.

No matter what company you work for, jobs in industry fall into several major categories. The best-known are the *technical service* jobs. Veterinarians in these positions learn the technical details about their company's products or services and work to educate other veterinarians about them. They may give seminars to veterinarians about the diseases or disorders for which their products or services may be used, they travel and work at the exhibit hall of major meetings, or they answer telephone inquiries from other veterinarians about their products.

Veterinarians may also work in *research and development* (R&D). Many of these jobs include hands-on work with animals. Veterinarians may do basic or applied clinical research, care for research animals, or manage research departments. Some of these positions require a PhD or board certification, whereas others simply require that you have some research experience.

Regulatory affairs and *product development* are other areas in which veterinarians work. Every company that makes a product (drugs or equipment) for veterinary use must meet the regulatory requirements for that product. The regulatory veterinarian becomes familiar with these regulations and assists the company with compliance. That means working with the research department to ensure that the appropriate studies are done, and then cooperating with the regulatory agency (e.g., FDA) in providing the needed data or studies. Veterinarians working in product development create new products and oversee the process, from basic research studies through clinical trials and approval.

Veterinarians can fill many other jobs within industry. Some may start their own companies, producing anything from software for veterinary clinics to wheeled carts for disabled dogs. Others may choose to work overseas. With enough experience, a veterinarian can become a self-employed consultant to industry.

UNLIMITED CHOICES

Other jobs include working with associations and organizations, teaching veterinary technicians, working for international-assistance groups, and working with wildlife rehabilitation centers or environmental groups. "Consultants" are veterinarians in *any* type of work who become experts in one area and then work to educate others about what they have learned. Some veterinarians have combined careers, such as law and veterinary medicine, to create their own specialty niche. If you have a special area of interest, follow it, and you may find that you create your own career.

RESOURCES

Associations

American Association of Housecall Veterinarians
225 E. 74th St.
New York, NY 10021
www.athomevet.org

American Association of Industrial Veterinarians
PO Box 488
Oskaloosa, KS 66066-0488

American Veterinary Medical Association
1931 N. Meacham Road, Suite 100
Schaumburg, IL 60173
847/925-8070
www.avma.org

Association of Veterinary Practice Management
Consultants and Advisors
511 N. Country Ridge Court
Lake Zurich, IL 60047
847/719-2477
www.avpmca.org

National Association of Federal Veterinarians
1101 Vermont Avenue NW, Suite 710
Washington, DC 20005-6308
202/289-6334
users.erols.com/nafv/

Books

AVMA *Membership Directory and Resource Manual.*
Career Choices for Veterinarians: Beyond Private Practice by C. Smith.
The Housecall Veterinarian's Manual by C. Smith.
The Relief Veterinarian's Manual (and Survival Guide) by C. Smith.

Websites

Federal government job applications
www.usajobs.opm.gov

VRS Inc.
www.vetrelief.com
This site is the interactive employment hub for relief veterinarians.

CHAPTER FOURTEEN

Mistakes Do Happen

Samuel M. Fassig, DVM, MA

IN THIS CHAPTER, YOU'LL LEARN:

- Why it's okay to make mistakes
- How to handle criticism
- How to be a leader when your team makes a mistake

No one does everything right the first time, every time, all the time. In today's workplace, if you don't fall on your face both regularly and painfully, you're probably not learning. The only people who don't make mistakes are the ones who aren't creative and don't take risks.

If your boss cannot accommodate, and even reward, failure, you will not advance at that practice. Why? Because doing things wrong is perhaps the best source of innovation. Innovation not only allows you to survive, it helps you grow. David Kelly, CEO of the design firm IDEO, says, "...enlightened trial and error beats the planning of flawless intellects... The reason is simple: The best solutions to most problems are rarely the most obvious." James Joyce said it poetically: "Mistakes are the portals of discovery." Think about it. What did you ever learn by doing something right the first time?

IBM's rumored motto regarding mistakes is legendary: Fail faster. World leaders, industry leaders, and scientists have a wonderful legacy of being wrong in a big way. Edison's tolerance for "mistakes" is renowned. The European "discovery" of America was a mistake. The invention of Ivory Pure Floating Soap, Teflon, and Post-it Notes were mistakes. GM's bizarre Gremlin was a substantial flop, but it paved the way for the ever-popular hatchback. The list of famous failed computers is long, including Apple's Lisa and the PalmPilot's predecessor, Zoomer. Obviously, in many instances, development failures bred innovation. Since the road to success is paved with failures, the faster you move through them, the faster you will find a way that works.

> When you make a mistake, get over it quickly, reflect on the experience, learn the most you can, and move on.

Not all business failures are so glorious. Small Business Administration statistics indicate that 65 out of 100 business start-ups vanish without a trace within five years, and 90% are gone within ten years. If you fly airplanes for a living, you probably shouldn't make mistakes, and it is also a good idea to minimize mistakes while you're in surgery. But sometimes doing things wrong is a prerequisite for doing things right. When you make a mistake, get over it quickly, reflect on the experience, learn the most you can, and move on.

SEEKING THE RIGHT CULTURE

Many companies say they encourage mistakes, yet they intimidate and punish the mistake-makers. As soon as that happens, a better-safe-than-sorry attitude is fostered. The problem with better-safe-than-sorry is that sometimes, when you err on the side of caution, you approach treatment without proper scientific protocol and do more harm than good.

A good mentor will train you to savor your mistakes and will understand the strange paths that lead you astray. By creating a safe place where you can take the risk to explore rather than ignore what happened or what went wrong, you get to process what you experienced. You are afforded the opportunity to analyze and amend, investigate and correct. It is the ideal environment to work in.

How would it feel to work for an employer who didn't penalize mistakes, but rather encouraged them? What if you got a bonus for the most brilliant (or most flagrant) mistake of the month, provided you had to share what you learned and what you would do differently if presented with the same scenario again? Wouldn't you feel empowered?

Obviously, there is a level of quality beyond which mistakes are not a viable economic or ethical alternative. If the outcome of your actions impacts life and death, the cost of "trial and error" to get to perfection is not justified. Mistakes happen. As a veterinarian, though, you have an obligation to be a life-long self-directed learner. You must try to be right, every time, especially where life is at stake. Seek a mentor who will help you learn from your mistakes. Take the risk. Share and learn.

Facing Criticism

Criticism can help you make positive changes. Imagine how difficult it would be to improve if no one ever gave you any feedback. But criticism is only one person's opinion. If you let that criticism mold the way you feel about yourself, you are letting your happiness depend on others. When you are being criticized, look objectively for something useful and positive in what is being said. Discard the rest.

Some people are anxious to complain and criticize just because they take a perverse pleasure in putting others down. If you are making a sincere effort to be the best that you can be and living in keeping with your values and sense of self, is it really that important what other people think? There are many people whom you will never please no matter what you do. That is their problem, not yours. Try to learn from your critics, then move forward with confidence and commitment.

BEING A LEADER WHEN DISASTER STRIKES

Rather than spending time deciding who did what wrong, pointing fingers, and placing blame when your team makes a mistake, restate where you want to go and what will get you back on track. This can be a group or individual effort.

Staff debriefings can be a very positive learning experience for everyone. When addressing mistakes, you need to ask:

- What worked?
- What didn't work?
- What was missing?
- What do we do next?

Consider this example: A progressive practice had scheduled an in-clinic presentation on vaccines and principles of immunology. On the day of the presentation, the staff was reeling from the unexpected death of a client's pet to whom they had all become attached. Recovery, which included rehabilitation therapy and extensive nursing care, had been going well for weeks. The patient's owner had become like one of the staff. Suddenly, the patient died. Every team member was second-guessing, wanting to place blame, and questioning his or her medical skills. Rather than sitting through the continuing education session on vaccines and immunology, the entire staff asked and answered the four questions listed above.

The process of answering the four questions put the staff back into the mode of "team" so that they were able to reflect without judgment and determine what they needed to do to grieve the loss, rededicate themselves to learning, and ascertain what each of them needed to do to move on. They also identified how they might better serve this client and apply the lessons from this event to other clients. A week later, they were a cohesive unit, motivated and looking forward to working together. The practice owner's wisdom and leadership allowed the team to learn from a negative experience.

> Use the mistakes you make as opportunities to improve your customer service, medical, and interpersonal skills.

If you are tempted to criticize a team member, ask yourself why you have that urge. Is the intention of your criticism to destroy or to support? If your intention is to support, why not try challenging rather than criticizing that person? For example, instead of saying, "Your skills are so weak, you will never get a promotion," say, "You know, I think you can get that promotion if you will develop your skills in this area." Both statements point out the weakness. Which statement would you respond to better? Which is the most helpful?

LEARNING FROM MISTAKES

Although the hallmark of progress is making mistakes and learning from them, repeating them—especially the same ones over and over—is definitely not a good thing! Use the mistakes you make as opportunities to improve your customer service, your medical skills, and your interpersonal skills. Because you have the title "Dr.," the staff will look to you to model the appropriate behavior.

REFERENCES

Nierenberg, G. *Doing It Right the First Time: A Short Guide to Learning From Your Most Memorable Errors, Mistakes, and Blunders.* John Wiley and Sons, 1996.

Ward, K. *Decisions Without Mistakes: Common Sense Decision-Making Strategies for Today's Managers and Leaders.* Writers Advantage, 2003.

CHAPTER FIFTEEN

The Mentor—Your Personal Guide to Success

Linda L. Black, EdD, LPC

> IN THIS CHAPTER, YOU'LL LEARN:
>
> - What a mentor is
> - How to find a good mentor
> - How to make the most of a mentoring relationship

WHAT IS A MENTOR?

The concept of mentoring is ancient. Homer described the archetypical mentor as the "wise and trusted counselor" whom Odysseus left in charge of his household during his travels. Athena, in the guise of Mentor, became the guardian and teacher of Odysseus's son Telemachus. In modern times, the concept of mentoring is applied in practically every learning environment. In academia, the term mentor is often synonymous with faculty adviser. There is a fundamental difference, though, between mentoring and advising. A mentoring relationship is personal as well as professional, whereas an advising relationship can be distant and one-sided, focusing on limited aspects of the student's performance.

Although an adviser can also be a mentor, the mentoring relationship is defined by its quality. A good mentoring relationship develops over an extended period, during which a student's needs and the nature of the relationship tend to change. A mentor tries to be cognizant of these changes and varies the degree and type of attention, help, advice, information, and encouragement provided.

A mentor is also someone who takes a special interest in helping you develop into a successful professional. An effective mentoring relationship is characterized by mutual respect, trust, understanding, and empathy. A good mentor is able to share life experiences, wisdom, and technical expertise. A profound listener, a careful observer, and a good problem-solver, a mentor will make an effort to know, accept, and respect your goals and interests. A mentor establishes an environment in which your accomplishment is limited only by the extent of your talent, imagination, and desire.

Characteristics of a Good Mentor

Effective mentoring need not always require large amounts of time. An experienced, perceptive mentor can provide a great deal of help in just a few minutes by making the right suggestion or asking the right question. A good mentor:

- Listens carefully.

- Keeps in touch—The amount of attention that a mentor gives you will vary widely. If you are doing well, you might require only "check-ins" or brief meetings. If you have continuing difficulties, you might need several formal meetings a week. An experienced mentor will keep you on his or her "radar screen" to anticipate problems before they become serious. Likewise, if you need help, ask for it. Do not assume your mentor knows everything that is going on in your life.

> A good mentor allows you to clearly see his or her attitude toward work, communicates feelings about his or her professional career, and shares frustrations as well as passions.

- Understands professional ethics—The earlier you are exposed to the notion of scientific integrity and ethical behavior, the better prepared you will be to deal with ethical questions. A good mentor will remember to explain ethical dilemmas that arise in his or her own work.

- Acts as a skills consultant—You must augment your veterinary-specific knowledge and experience with a variety of other skills if you are to make the best use of your talents. You will need to develop general communication skills, such as the ability to express yourself clearly and understand others' responses. A good mentor will help you develop these skills:
    - Planning and organizing—Many new associates have little experience in organizing tasks and making good use of time.
    - Writing—The ability to write clearly is essential to most careers, especially those with administration and management components.
    - Communicating verbally—Speaking is at least as important as writing. As an associate, you must be able to present ideas, diagnoses, test results, and other findings to colleagues, as well as to your clients and specialists in other fields. A good mentor will look for opportunities to include you in his or her network of social gatherings, professional groups, and community projects.
    - Teaching—Teaching is a skill that you can begin to develop by conducting staff-training sessions and client seminars. Developing the content with your mentor will build a stronger connection between the two of you. Another benefit is that you will become an "expert" in the eyes of the hospital staff.
    - Working as part of a team—Learning is often most effective when done within a community. Cooperative problem-solving skills can be developed through group exercises and objectives. A good mentor will help you look for ways to develop leadership skills and work on team-development activities.
    - Creative thinking—A productive veterinarian is one who approaches problems with an open mind. A mentor who gives you permission to move beyond timid or conventional solutions will challenge your thinking.

- Provides a role model—In a good mentoring relationship, the mentor, as the senior partner, is a role model through word and actions. A good mentor allows you to clearly see his or her attitude toward work, communicates feelings about his or her professional career, and shares frustrations as well as passions.

DECIDING IF YOU WANT A MENTOR

Mentoring is an interactive relationship, with formal and informal aspects, that develops over time. Willing and informed faculty and board-certified or seasoned veterinarians are critical to your successful mentoring relationship. Keep in mind that faculty members and practicing professionals balance teaching, research, seeing patients, and their personal lives with mentoring. If you find a mentor who is willing to take the necessary time to work with you, it usually means that mentoring is a part of that person's personal value system—it is part of the process of giving something back to the profession.

Before you set out to find a mentor, first ask yourself why you want a mentor. The answer to this question is critical. Mentoring is a multifaceted relationship that takes time and energy that some people simply cannot commit. Understanding your desires and expectations of the mentoring relationship will help you establish a good mentoring match. Ask yourself these questions:

- What do I want a mentor to do for me?

- Do I really feel I could benefit from a mentoring relationship?

- What qualities do I want in a mentor (e.g., advanced training, guidance, support, challenge, sponsorship)?

- What would I bring to a mentoring relationship?

- Do I have the time and energy to commit to a long-term relationship?

- Do I know the interests of potential mentors?

- If I find a likely candidate, am I willing to approach him or her and demonstrate my interest?

- What will I do if the potential mentor is not interested?

In academia, ask these questions to assess the likelihood of finding a good mentor in the faculty:

- How and to what degree are faculty and students involved with one another?

- What seems to be the nature of these relationships (e.g., primarily task-focused, or socially/ personally focused)?

- Do you hear other students discuss mentoring relationships they have with faculty or other professionals?

- Has anyone (e.g., faculty, advanced graduate students, clinicians) invited you to be involved in projects or activities beyond the normal scope of your schoolwork?

- Do you know whom to ask for help on any topic?

In private practice, ask these questions to assess the likelihood of finding a good mentor in one of the practice owners or even another associate veterinarian:

- How and to what degree are the practice owners and staff professionally involved with one another?

- What seems to be the nature of these relationships (e.g., primarily task-focused, or socially/ personally focused)?

- Do practice owners and staff or associate veterinarians currently have mentoring relationships?

- Do you hear other associate veterinarians discuss mentoring relationships they have with practice owners or other veterinarians?

- Has a practice owner or another associate veterinarian invited you to be involved in projects or activities beyond the normal scope of your work?

- Do you know whom to ask for help on any topic?

- Do other associate veterinarians speak of feeling valued and involved in their learning and professional development?

Most mentoring relationships begin in a structured and formal fashion and then progress to a less structured and more informal relationship. If you understand the nature, demands, and boundaries of a mentoring relationship, you are more likely to be an active and successful participant in the process.

Unfortunately, some mentoring relationships begin without clearly defined roles, expectations, and goals. In these situations, the student can feel bitter because her needs are not met. This is not meant to dissuade you from seeking a mentor; it is a reminder that it is important for you to have a clear understanding of what a mentoring relationship is and is not, and to communicate that to your potential mentor.

> **Most mentoring relationships begin in a structured and formal fashion and then progress to a less structured and more informal relationship.**

FINDING A MENTOR

The process of selecting a mentor is foreign to the average student and new graduate. Indeed, you are accustomed to looking to a faculty member or other trusted professional for instruction, guidance, and support. These relationships, while helpful, are typically formal and task-oriented. They place you in a one-way rather than an interactive relationship. You will still take on the role of student in a mentoring relationship, but now your classroom is the workplace and your status is that of a professional.

190

Rarely do mentors seek out students. Because you are initially in the role of learner, the responsibility for seeking and selecting a mentor is yours. Begin by investigating the match between a potential mentor's area of interest and your own. You can investigate the interests of the potential mentor through more formal methods (e.g., informational interview, professional and/or association meeting, discussion of referral cases, and, if you are a student, discussion of a professor's orientation toward the clinical sciences). The mentor's professional demeanor, the classes taught, the types of patients seen, articles or books published, the presentations given, and stated areas of research are factors to consider when assessing whether you have shared interests. Once you have this information, you can evaluate the benefits of selecting a particular mentor. If you decide that it would be a good fit, initiate a meeting to discuss an ongoing relationship.

Mentors may be professors you had in the past, people you have worked with, a current employer, or some other professional. Potential mentors should know you before they agree to become involved in a mentoring relationship. Volunteer for projects that will allow you to work together in a less formal environment.

You will need to clearly articulate to the potential mentor your expectations of the relationship. Because mentoring relationships are mutually beneficial, you should be prepared to discuss what you bring to the relationship, such as access to interesting cases or knowledge of a topic the mentor is interested in but doesn't know much about. The demonstration of mutual interest and the potential to contribute to the relationship signify to the mentor that you are willing to do more than just take.

You are responsible for extending an invitation to the mentor that the mentor can accept or refuse. You need to be prepared for the possibility that the mentor may refuse the mentoring opportunity for any number of reasons. While a mentor's acceptance of your invitation can be exhilarating, a denial might leave you feeling wounded. It is critical that you realize that some

mentors have the desire to mentor but lack institutional support or the time to do it. The denial of an invitation to be your mentor may or may not be related to you. Do not take a refusal personally. A mentor candidate may explain the reasons for turning down your request, but don't force the issue.

Mentoring Teams

Sometimes a mentoring team may work best for your situation. For example, you start a job as a new associate. The owner is talented in dentistry but has limited time to mentor you. You might be able to enlist a more seasoned associate to bring you up to speed on the basics. The owner will allow you to observe and assist with some procedures. The understanding, then, is that you will complete the activity with the junior associate, who is mentoring you with regard to basic dentistry techniques, and then, as questions arise, you will have access to the senior mentor.

No mentor can know everything you might need to learn in order to succeed. Everyone benefits from multiple mentors of diverse talents, ages, and personalities.

> No mentor can know everything you might need to learn in order to succeed. Everyone benefits from multiple mentors of diverse talents, ages, and personalities.

MAKING THE MOST OF THE RELATIONSHIP

There is no single formula for good mentoring. The nature of a mentoring relationship varies with the knowledge, skills, and activities of the student and the mentor. In general, both parties must share the common goal of advancing the personal growth of the student.

In a mentoring relationship, there should be mutual responsibility and accountability for the relationship. A mentoring relationship initially involves a power differential, with you in a subordinate position. Both you and your mentor should demonstrate and expect professional courtesy and ethical behavior from one another. Ideally, mentors are responsible for modeling professional and ethical behavior because they hold a position of power inherent in the mentoring relationship. Certainly, a mentoring relationship involves getting to know one another on a personal level, and both parties must be comfortable with some level of personal disclosure.

Mentoring can resemble a love relationship due to its intensity, informality, and mutuality. Occasionally it can be confused with romantic love, which results in chaos when other factors come into play. It is critical that you and your mentor have realistic expectations of the relationship. You should feel empowered throughout the mentoring relationship to voice any concerns you have regarding the nature of the relationship without fear of retribution. A mentor who asks anything less of a student is not mentoring.

The hallmarks of a thriving mentor–apprentice relationship are credibility, accountability, and professionalism. Both people understand that they can depend on one another to complete tasks and activities in a timely manner, honor the relationship, and display ethical behavior. Mentors seem to be attracted to protégés who demonstrate a sensitivity to the mentor's time demands; who do not abuse the relationship by boasting or bragging to others (a possible source of perceived favoritism); and who demonstrate initiative, dedication, a strong work ethic, and a self-directed learning orientation. No one benefits when a mentor or apprentice is too "possessive."

Formal interaction develops over time into a mutually beneficial relationship marked by trust, support, respect, and balance. The once hierarchical relationship becomes collegial, and the mentor and learner recognize and honor the gifts of a mentoring relationship. In fact, the best way to honor a mentoring relationship is to go on to mentor others.

REFERENCES

Angelini, D. 1995. "Mentoring in the Career Development of Hospital Staff Nurses: Models and Practices." *Journal of Professional Nursing* 11 (2): 89-97.

Association for Women in Science. 1993. "Mentoring Means Future Scientists." *Association for Women in Science.*

Bolles, R. The 1997 *What Color Is Your Parachute?* Ten Speed Press, 1997.

Brill, J. 1993. "The Debt That Cannot Be Repaid: Mentoring Helps Others While Bringing Satisfaction To the Mentor." *ABA Journal* 79: 100.

Committee on Science, Engineering, and Public Policy. 1995. "On Being a Scientist: Responsible Conduct in Research." National Academy Press.

Gerstein, M. 1985. "Mentoring: An Age Old Practice in a Knowledge-Based Society." *Journal of Counseling and Development* 64 (2): 156–157.

Gilley, J. and Boughton, N. *Stop Managing, Start Coaching.* McGraw Hill, 1996.

Hodgson, C. and Simoni, J. "Graduate Student Academic and Psychological Functioning." *Journal of College Student Development* 1992; 36(3): 244–253.

Kanigel, R. *Apprentice to Genius: The Making of a Scientific Dynasty.* Johns Hopkins University Press, 1986.

Lankard, B. *Trends and Issues Alerts: The Role of Mentoring In Career Education.* ERIC, 1996.

Miller, G. "Earnings, Feminization, and Consequences for the Future of Veterinary Medicine." *JAVMA* 1998; 3: 340–344.

Nielsen, N. "Is the Veterinary Profession Losing Its Way?" *Canadian Veterinary Journal* 41: 439–445.

Orpen, C. 1995. "The Effects of Mentoring On Employees' Career Success." *Journal of Social Psychology* 135 (5): 667–668.

Struthers, N. 1995. "Differences in Mentoring: A Function of Gender or Organizational Rank." *Journal of Social Behavior and Personality* 10 (6): 265–272.

Whitely, W., Dougherty, T., and Dreher, G. 1991. "Relationship of Career Mentoring and Socioeconomic Origin to Managers' and Professionals' Early Career Progress." *Academy of Management Journal* 34 (2): 331–351.

Wollman-Bonilla, J. 1997. "Mentoring As a Two-Way Street." *Journal of Staff Development* 18: 50–52.

Zelditch, M. "Mentor Roles." Proceedings of the 32nd Annual Meeting of the Western Association of Graduate Schools, 1990.

RESOURCES

Associations

American Association for the Advancement of Science (AAAS)
www.nextwave.org
AAAS publishes an online magazine as a career development resource for scientists.

Association for Women in Science (AWIS)
www.awis.org

Books

Connecting: The Mentoring Relationships You Need to Succeed by R. Clinton and P. Stanley.

Mentoring: Creating Connected, Empowered Relationships by V. Schwiebert.

Magazine Articles

"The Role of Mentors in the Career Development of Young Professionals" by C. Wright and S. Wright in *Family Relations: Journal of Applied Family and Child Studies*, 1987.

Websites

Inc.com
www.inc.com/guides/growth/24509.html
Links to articles and resources for finding a mentor.

Management Assistance Program for Nonprofits
www.mapnp.org/library/guiding/mentrng/mentrng.htm
Links to articles about mentoring.

CHAPTER SIXTEEN

Building Self-Confidence and Gaining Respect

Carin A. Smith, DVM

IN THIS CHAPTER, YOU'LL LEARN HOW TO:

- **Create a great first impression**
- **Get clients to stop asking for the other doctor**
- **Gain respect from clients, staff, and your boss**
- **Confidently communicate with your boss**

You've successfully completed years of college and graduate school. You've even found a job as a practicing veterinarian. But you may not feel as confident as you'd like. Perhaps you look very young and are concerned that clients do not respect you. You may love doing surgery, but you want someone available to help you, just in case. You may chafe against your boss's restrictions on what you are allowed to do, but at the same time you worry that you don't know enough to handle some things on your own.

How can you get your boss, the staff, and your clients to give you more respect? How can you take on more responsibility while still having access to the help you need? How can you project confidence when you don't feel confident?

It's normal to feel nervous when you lack experience. But the first few years after graduation from veterinary school is when your medical and surgical skills and knowledge are the most up-to-date. How are you communicating that you have that knowledge and those skills? Why is there a difference

between how you see yourself and how you are perceived by your boss? Certainly, the practice owner has more experience to draw upon, but even experienced veterinarians encounter situations where they are unsure. How does the practice owner act when she is uncertain? How does that differ from the way you behave? What can you learn from watching others?

CREATE A GREAT FIRST IMPRESSION

Like it or not, people develop an instant first impression when they meet you. This impression is based on many different factors—how you dress, your eye contact, your posture, your tone of voice, and what you say. If something about any of those factors distracts clients, their ability to hear your message is impaired. In turn, that could interfere with your ability to help the pet.

Most people have a preconception of how a veterinarian should look and behave. Research shows that people expect doctors to look professional and behave confidently; they expect veterinarians to be kind to their pets and to communicate medical terms in a way they understand. You don't *have* to look or behave a certain way, but the more you deviate from what clients expect, the harder it will be for them to focus on your recommendations.

You may know veterinarians who "get by" wearing any kind of clothing, but as a young person who is worried about showing confidence, you need all the help you can get. Wearing a spotless white doctor's coat is one thing that will improve your appearance of professionalism. If you need to, have three or more coats available that you can rotate through as they get dirty. Keep a lint brush handy at all times.

If you think you look young, ask an experienced colleague for help. Specifically, do your hairstyle and clothing reflect your age? If you want to look older, you may want to make changes. No one should feel forced to create a "look" that does not fit her personality, yet you can make small adjustments in order to improve your appearance, generate confidence, and increase the respect you receive.

Your voice tone and pitch also affect how you are perceived. Do you speak very quietly and hesitantly? Does your voice go up at the end of each sentence, even when you are not asking a question? No matter what your intentions, such vocal delivery reduces clients' and staff's confidence in you. Eye contact and posture go hand-in-hand with vocal tone. The person who does not feel confident has hunched shoulders, avoids eye contact, and speaks softly.

The first step in changing these patterns of behavior is to notice them. Then ask your friends, the practice owner, or staff to help you set up role-playing situations so that you can practice your new way of presenting yourself.

One great way to gain more confidence in speaking is to join a Toastmasters group. These clubs help working professionals develop more confidence when speaking to individuals and groups. Specific exercises focus on "thinking on

> The person who does not feel confident has hunched shoulders, avoids eye contact, and speaks softly.

your feet"—teaching you how to formulate what you want to say in the midst of action. There are Toastmaster Clubs in nearly every city; visit *www.toastmasters.org* or look in your newspaper's activities section for information.

GET MORE RESPECT FROM CLIENTS

You may believe in the common myth that the "good" veterinarian somehow "knows" the diagnosis before she does any diagnostic work. Because of this assumption, you feel stupid standing in front of a client and saying, "I don't know what's wrong with your pet."

Do you know that experienced veterinarians face that problem many times each day? The difference is that they realize they should not be expected to just "know" what is wrong, and they don't make the client expect that, either. Both a new graduate and an experienced veterinarian may feel the same frustration when faced with a difficult diagnosis. Watch, however, the differences in what they say to the client:

New graduate: "I'm not sure what's wrong. We should probably do some tests. . ."

Experienced veterinarian: "We need to find out what is wrong with Fluffy so we can help her. The first step is to take some blood for laboratory tests. These will help us see what's going on inside Fluffy and find out what's wrong. Then we can choose the best treatment to make her feel better."

Note that neither veterinarian knows what is wrong. In the first scenario, the veterinarian focuses on herself and on the uncertainty. In the second scenario, the veterinarian takes charge of the situation, telling the client specifically what she *can* do to help Fluffy—focusing on the positive, on what to do, and on the pet's well-being. The veterinarian uses "we" to create a partnership with the client. *The client will focus on the same thing that you focus on.*

If you think that you get too little respect from clients and staff, what are you focusing on?

- What you don't know
- What you can't do
- How young you are
- How little you know
- YOU

There will always be some things you don't know, situations that are difficult, and diagnoses that evade you. There is little point in giving the client a list of what you don't know or can't do. To project confidence, focus on the things that you *do* know. Discuss the actions you *can* take.

When you think about people who project confidence and are well-respected, what comes to mind? Usually, it is how *others feel* when they are around this person. The focus is not on the confident person; it is on what that person is doing or saying to make others feel better. Sure, you notice that the person is confident, but *because* they are confident, you have no need to "pick them apart," noticing every wart or wondering what they don't know.

To avoid sending loud signals of "I'm no good!" stop focusing on yourself and instead *focus on the clients*. They would not be in front of you if they did not think you could help them. They *expect* you to help them.

> To project confidence, focus on the things that you *do* know. Discuss the actions you *can* take.

How Can I Get Clients to Stop Asking for the Other Doctor?

You may feel clients don't respect you because they specifically ask for the other doctor instead of seeing you. What can you do to keep that from happening? You can *reduce* the number of client requests for the other doctor, but you can't eliminate them. Self-confident veterinarians know that all people, including pet owners, have preferences and styles that differ from their own. Some clients may prefer one doctor to another. That's life. On the other hand, if the requests for the other doctor are still frequent, you should consider making some changes. Talk to the practice owner, the staff, and individual clients.

Talk to the Practice Owner

Has the practice owner introduced you to the clients, either in a clinic newsletter or when the clients come to the clinic? If not, ask her to do so. The practice owner could send a press release to the local paper, announcing your addition to the staff and relating positive information about you. She could write the same information in the clinic newsletter and post it in the reception area.

And, as the opportunity arises, your boss can introduce you in person to clients you haven't met.

Talk to the Staff

Have the staff members, particularly the receptionist, been coached about how to talk to clients about the new veterinarian (you)? If not, ask the practice manager to discuss this during the next staff meeting. The way the receptionist reacts to client inquiries will have a big effect on how you are perceived.

Hello, Mr. Goldberg. It's nice to see you and Max again! Say, before you go in to see Dr. Oldstuff, I want to let you know about our new doctor, Mary Newgrad. Dr. Oldstuff spent a lot of time looking for someone who would fit into this practice, and I think he's done a great job.

The receptionist can also smooth the way for you when clients make appointments by phone.

Thanks for calling, Ms. Grant. It sounds like Fred needs to be seen today. Today is Dr. Oldstuff's day off, but Dr. Newgrad is here, and we'd really like you to meet her. I think you may have read her profile in our last newsletter. We can fit you in at 2:00; would that work for you?

Talk to the Client

If the client hesitates when the receptionist tries to schedule an appointment with you, you can do your part by getting on the phone yourself.

Ms. Grant? Julie tells me that you aren't sure if you need to bring in Fred today, or if it can wait until Dr. Oldstuff gets back tomorrow. Can you tell me more about what is happening with Fred?

Notice that in the above conversation, you don't focus on why the client is reluctant to see you. Instead, you focus on the pet and what is best for the pet's well-being. Drawing out the client in conversation often works to ease the hesitation she may have about seeing you instead of the regular doctor. (The client discovers that you are a nice human being after all!) You can also ascertain whether waiting for the other doctor would harm the pet, and, if so, convey that concern to the client.

Finally, you can help by talking directly to clients when they are at the hospital. When time permits, make it a point to look around the waiting area and introduce yourself to waiting clients you've not met.

Mr. Hedden? While you're waiting for Dr. Oldstuff, I'd like to introduce myself. I'm Dr. Mary Newgrad, the new veterinarian here. How are you and Blackie doing today?

In the exam room, you may find that honestly discussing awkward feelings helps to dissipate them. Saying that you work with the other veterinarian lets the client know you are a team working for her pet's benefit. You can convey this without having it sound like you are inexperienced and need someone's help—instead, you are a professional member of a team that always discusses cases together.

Ms. Kane, I know you're used to seeing Dr. Oldstuff. You can rest assured that I will take the same care of you and Buster as he does. Dr. Oldstuff has gone over Buster's history with me, and we work together to ensure the best care for every patient—especially for Buster, since he's one of our best patients! Once we get the blood test results back, I'll review them with Dr. Oldstuff and then discuss with you the next step to take for Buster.

CAN'T GET RESPECT FROM THE STAFF?

Does this lament sound familiar?

I wish I could get along better with Julie, our technician. But she just ignores me when I ask her to do something for me! Then she bends over backward whenever the practice owner asks her to do something, or when she's watching her work with me. I wish she'd give me more respect!

Getting respect from staff members can be a challenge. Sometimes they have worked at the practice for years, and then you walk in, the new veterinarian, with the gall to try to tell them what to do!

Give Them Respect

To get more respect from your staff, you must first give *them* respect. That doesn't mean that you let them walk all over you, but that you acknowledge their experience. Ask them for advice when appropriate, and treat them as team members. You may need to focus on politeness, using words like "please" and "thank you" more often than you feel is necessary. If it makes your work easier, though, maybe it is necessary. People have more respect for others when they feel appreciated and respected themselves. Set aside a time to talk, and say something like this:

Julie, I know it's been a tough transition to have me start work here, especially after you've spent so much time with just one veterinarian. I hope that we can talk about any situations that are uncomfortable for you. I may do things differently than Dr. Black does, and I want to learn her methods. But I'd also like to show you the way I do things. I'm willing to listen to your suggestions, but I'd also appreciate it if you would have the flexibility to learn my approaches, too. Can we agree on that?

> To get more respect from your staff, you must first give *them* respect.

Clarify Roles

Sometimes you may need to talk to the practice owner or practice manager about the chain of command. Who is in charge of ensuring that people do their designated jobs? What is the procedure (if one is outlined at all) for dispute resolution within the practice? Be sure that your boss isn't undermining your authority (either unconsciously or consciously) by what she says to the other staff members. Set aside a time to talk. Ask for clarification of any chain of command.

Dr. Black, I am having trouble getting Julie to help me out during surgery. She seems to disappear to help you and the other doctors in the exam rooms just when I need her most. I am confused about her job. What should her first priority be? Can you help to define the roles of each staff member so that Julie can feel comfortable staying in back to help me while the other staff members help you in the exam rooms?

Stop the Complainers

Do you feel like a "dumping ground" for staff gripes? Unless you have the responsibility and authority to change what they're griping about, you probably feel frustrated. Yet, you want to "be nice," and so you listen and nod, or perhaps you gently defend the practice owner or the target of the staff members' gripes. It won't take long for you to get tired of being a garbage can, though. How can you "be nice" and stop this situation? Focus only on what you can control—whether or not people complain to you. Don't take on the position of negotiator or allow yourself to be used as a go-between for two bickering coworkers.

Julie, I understand that you are frustrated. However, I am not in a position to make any changes. It just makes me uncomfortable and frustrated, since I can't do anything to help you, and I feel caught in the middle. I suggest that you go to the practice manager to discuss your concerns. It's your decision whether you do that, but in the meantime, please don't bring these complaints to me.

Distinguish Between Friend and Employee

You may find that you are working with older staff members, or with people the same age as yourself, who have more years of experience but less education. That can create an awkward situation for you. How do you give direction to someone who is older than you? How can you maintain a friendly relationship with someone who is your age, but over whom you have authority? What happens if they show resentment for your position? Can you be friends with staff members?

No matter how much *you* would like to "just be friends" with the staff, and no matter how much you can forget that they earn less than you, *they* will not forget. They usually cannot ignore the fact that you have some control over their jobs and their paychecks. For many people, a certain amount of distance is necessary for them to be comfortable interacting with you at work. It takes a staff member of strong inner character to maintain a friendship with someone who occupies a superior position at work. So, don't be offended if staff members rebuff your attempts at "being friendly."

Only you can decide how "close" you want to be with the staff. Keep in mind that you may have to discipline staff members or discuss their performance. Be ready to do so within the framework of the relationships that you create. Think about how well you can separate your friendship outside of work and your working relationship at the hospital. If you can do that, but they can't, then do them the favor of taking the high road and putting the work relationship first.

Remember the main goal of the practice—to have everyone work as a team to help clients and their pets. To achieve that goal, maintain a respectful attitude toward everyone, and set boundaries on friendships and work relationships when necessary.

GET MORE RESPECT FROM YOUR BOSS

As a new graduate from veterinary school or a new employee at the practice, you are sometimes in an awkward position. You want to try out all the things you learned, but you aren't always sure of what to do. Sometimes, you feel as if the practice owner is hovering over you too much. You may feel uncertain about doing some kinds of surgery, but you want to try. You want the practice owner to have enough confidence in you that she will let you do some interesting surgical procedures, but you also want help if needed.

Ask for More Responsibility

How can you earn enough respect from your boss so that she will allow you to try new things, and yet give the help you need, when you need it? It's a balancing act, and the balance point that seems comfortable to you may be different than the one that's comfortable for your boss.

One way to approach the problem is to discuss it out loud. Why ignore the situation? You are both thinking about it, anyway. So just come out with it:

Dr. Smart, I have noticed that you are comfortable with my surgical skills for doing spays and neuters, but you still haven't scheduled any other surgeries for me. I know that I don't have much experience and that you hesitate to have me jump in over my head. I also don't want to be set adrift! Still, I would like to come up with a plan that would allow me to learn more and take on more surgery, without making you uncomfortable. What about allowing me to do some of the more complex procedures if and when they are scheduled on a day that's not very busy, so that we will have time to work together?

Don't "Discuss" Every Case

Are you sending out "I'm unsure" signals that you aren't aware of? Many young veterinarians fall into the habit of thinking, "I'll just run this plan by the practice owner before I start the treatment." Others all too frequently say, "Doc, while you're here, could you please take a look at this radiograph?"

Of course, good colleagues and team members do discuss difficult cases. But confident adults do not discuss every case, nor do they need the owner's approval for every decision they make. If you are "discussing" a lot of your cases with the boss, the message she may be hearing is, "I don't know what I'm doing." As a result, you may be treated as if you don't.

COME TO TERMS WITH THE CULTURE OF THE PRACTICE

Your confidence depends partially on your comfort level. Do you feel that you fit in at the practice where you work? Are you comfortable with the practice's goals, vision, and mission statement? (Does the practice owner discuss these with you?) How do your goals and vision mesh with those of the practice?

Earlier in this book, you learned how to create a mission statement for yourself. Sometimes the key to finding the reasons for feeling like a "misfit" in a particular practice may be in comparing your mission statements and visions.

Part of my vision includes helping the poor, but this practice does not help clients who love their pets but can't afford the bill. We don't have a special fund set aside for clients in need. If I knew that the hospital had a policy to care for those in need, I'd feel better about charging fairly for those clients who truly can afford our services. But all my boss can see is that I'm "giving away" services. He'd rather put an animal to sleep than set up a payment plan.

Or

My vision includes balancing my work life, family life, and time for myself. But my boss thinks that my request for job-sharing means that I don't care about my work! I'm as dedicated as I can be to this practice and to our clients. I'm willing to work extra hard to ensure continuity and communication between myself and the staff and clients, and to be paid in proportion to the work that I do. But I can't neglect the rest of my life just to please my boss.

Or

My vision includes working as part of a team, with everyone pitching in and contributing. But in this practice, with pay based only on production, I feel like we're all competing! I don't feel like I'm a part of a team at all.

If your vision appears to conflict with that of your practice, don't just give up hope or try to "endure" the situation. It is rare to find the "perfect" practice, with an owner whose vision is identical to yours. Still, you can work together with the practice owner and staff to see that everyone's needs are met.

Start by asking the practice manager to put a discussion of the practice mission and vision on the agenda for the next staff meeting. Try to find out all that you can about your practice owner's needs and goals. Then, phrase *your* needs in terms of what she will gain. Perhaps you can get what you want, if you also give your boss what she wants. Compare these two discussions:

> Dr. Black, I really can't finish what I have to do in a ten-minute time frame for an exam! I am just running myself ragged, and I can't get my work done. I am behind all the time. Could we please go to fifteen-minute exams?

The above statements focus on you and your needs, and your position seems to be that of asking your boss to fix the problem for you. But she has enough to think about already. Your boss is thinking:

> Why can't she just learn to be more efficient? I'm sure she is just in there gabbing with the clients, and I know she can get more efficient if we just make her do it. Taking up more time only costs us money! I haven't got time to bother with this.

You could address the needs of the owners and still meet your own goals with a different approach:

> Dr. Black, could we discuss the scheduling for exams? I know that sometimes I take longer than the allotted ten minutes for exams. I understand that I should be productive, but some clients and patients need more time than others. I have a possible solution—we could create different exam types, each with a different length of time allotted. For instance, we could break up our exams into five-minute blocks, with a vaccination booster or suture removal taking up only one block, an annual exam taking two or three blocks, and a sick-pet or multiple-pet exam taking four to six blocks. We'd actually save time on the shorter exams, where we really don't need fifteen minutes at all.
>
> I can help the receptionist set this up, using our current scheduling software. She has a pretty good idea of how long we take with different types of exams, and she can ask clients questions when they make appointments to determine how much time to allot to each. Would you be willing to try that?

> **If your vision appears to conflict with that of your practice, don't just give up hope or try to "endure" the situation.**

Notice that you came to the practice owner with, first, an acknowledgement of your contribution to the current problem. Then you presented a possible solution to the problem. You haven't negated your boss's perception that you take too long—she may be right, at least some of the time. You also have held your ground in stating that sometimes the allotted time is too short. Finally, you haven't just dumped the problem on your boss, you came up with a solution—not only what to do, but how to carry it out. And you volunteered to take the first step.

Try creating your own "presentation to the practice owner" for the following problematic situations. Include in your discussion:

- Your contribution to the problem
- What you think needs to change
- The advantages of this change to the practice (clients, practice owner, staff, *and* practice bottom line)

199

- What you will do to help make the change

Imagine you are the veterinarian whose vision it is to help the poor.

- How could the practice and its clients benefit from having a special fund set up for needy clients and special situations?
- Where will the money come from?
- What can you do to show that you will focus on charging fairly for your work once the fund is established?
- How would you express this to the practice owner?
- What could you offer to do to get the program started?

Imagine your vision is to job share or work part time.

- What information can you present about the benefits of job sharing and part-time work?
- What protocols can you suggest to the practice owner that will ensure good communication to clients and between staff who work different shifts?
- What kind of staff training will ensure that clients are told, in a positive way, about the part-time veterinarians' schedules?
- What are you willing to do to set up staff meetings and rounds to ensure communication lines stay open?

Imagine you want to be a team player rather than an individual competitor.

- What alternatives are there to working purely on production or being paid a straight salary?
- What information can you gather about the pros and cons of different types of salary structures?
- What information can you gather about the practice owner's reasons for paying on production?
- Can her needs be met in another way?

200

- What can you do to improve teamwork?

Know When to Stop

How do you know when the fit just isn't there? It's tough to know when to pull out of a bad situation. Some people give up too soon, losing out on the opportunity for learning and growth that comes with facing difficult situations and working through problems with other people. Others stay too long, feeling as if they are "giving up" if they leave the practice. (If you're staying because you don't think you have any other choice, see Chapter 13, When Private Practice Isn't Your Cup of Tea.)

Only you know when you have done enough. If you have not had any open discussions with the practice owner or staff members, it is probably too soon to leave. (Be sure you have actually set aside a time to talk. If you've only said something in the course of your workday, as a reaction to a specific situation, don't expect to get results. You must set aside a time to talk calmly.)

If you've had those conversations and there is still a wide discrepancy between your vision and that of the practice, it may be best to find another place to work—both for your own benefit and that of the practice. Leave before you (or they) become too angry or bitter to forgive and while you still recognize that the problem is simply one of differences in style, approach, or vision. Veterinary medicine is a small world, and you don't want to burn bridges. Leaving on a positive note will help your career in the long run.

RESOURCES

Books

Client Satisfaction Pays: Quality Service for Practice Success by C. Smith.

How to Gain the Professional Edge: Achieve the Personal and Professional Image You Want by S. Morem.

How to Say It for Women: Communicating with Confidence and Power Using the Language of Success by P. Mindell.

The Ultimate Secrets of Total Self-Confidence by R. Anthony.

Continuing Education

The Art of Veterinary Practice: Success for Life. AAHA seminar that offers practical techniques to help you improve interpersonal relationships and play a more productive role in the success of your practice. Contact AAHA at 800/883-6301 for more information or visit *www.aahanet.org.*

Dale Carnegie Training®. Courses help individuals create goals, communicate more effectively, and move beyond their comfort zones. Visit *www.dalecarnegie.com* for more information.

Websites

Toastmasters International
www.toastmasters.org
Through its member clubs, Toastmasters helps men and women learn the art of speaking, listening, and thinking.

CHAPTER SEVENTEEN

Why Your Boss Does That

Erin Landeck, MS, CPA

> IN THIS CHAPTER, YOU'LL LEARN:
>
> - How to see the practice through the owner's eyes
> - What you can do and say to fit in at the practice
> - How to make a heck of an impression on your boss

Your employer's approach to veterinary medicine and practice management may delight you or annoy the heck out of you. Regardless of your opinion, it is your responsibility to understand your employer's philosophy so that you can do your best within its confines. This doesn't mean you compromise your beliefs and ideals—you have to stay true to yourself. But if you keep an open mind and try to understand the practice owner's point of view, you will be a happier person and a more valuable employee.

There are hundreds, if not thousands, of decisions a practice owner must make on a monthly basis to keep the practice running smoothly. To help you understand how your employer approaches medicine and business, we briefly discuss the types of decisions a practice owner must make. After you read this chapter, you will have a better understanding of the practice owner's daily trials and tribulations. In addition, you'll see how to make your life, and your boss's, a lot easier.

THE BIG PICTURE

Practice owners set the direction for the practice. They see the "big picture" in terms of economic and medical trends and how those trends will affect the practice.

Mission

A practice owner must set an overall direction for the practice and communicate that direction to the staff. Most veterinary practice owners' missions, if they have articulated them, are something along the lines of, "To provide high-quality care to our patients." In the simplest terms, though, a veterinary practice team's mission is, "To save pets' lives and make them healthier." A mission should be short, sweet, and to the point—it should enable you to get up in the morning with a purpose. Question: Why am I going to work today? Answer: Because I'm going to save pets' lives and make them healthier.

As an associate, you can't really create a mission for the practice, but you should definitely be clear what that mission is. If the answer is unclear, encourage the practice owner to clarify the mission so that you can keep that in the forefront of your mind as you go about your day-to-day activities. You can also take a leadership role by reinforcing the mission with the staff at every opportunity. When a team member grumbles about the cost of a procedure that "poor Mrs. Smith" has to pay, turn it into a teaching moment by saying, "Sara, we are making Fluffy healthier, which is why we're here."

Market Trends

Do people have less money to spend? More money to spend? The human-animal bond is getting stronger, and pet owners are getting more and more information from the Internet. How does all of that information affect the practice's direction and the products and services they provide? A practice owner must keep tabs on the local and national economy, along with consumer preferences, in order be competitive in the marketplace.

Though it is not your responsibility to be an expert on the economy, you can certainly do your part by keeping tabs on what's happening in the local community and on a macro level. If you have information that could help the practice serve its clients better, share it with your boss. For example, you may learn from a friend about a major layoff that's coming in your community—let your boss know. It may affect the demand for services for a few months, and it's wise to plan for that contingency.

> If you have information that could help the practice serve its clients better, share it with your boss.

Competitors

What products and services are other veterinary practices providing? What are their prices? How do other practices' level of service and quality of facilities compare to this one? How does the practice distinguish itself in the market? A practice owner has to take all of that into consideration as she determines where the practice fits in the grand scheme of things.

Help improve the practice by sharing what you know about the competitors. If you have learned, for example, that most practices are not charging for writing prescriptions for medications that clients are going to buy on the Internet but your practice is charging a hefty fee, bring it up with your boss. Remember not to question your boss in front of the staff or take him off guard. These kinds of discussions are best held in private unless your boss has made it clear that he wants you to bring them up at any time.

OPERATIONS MANAGEMENT

There is an overwhelming amount of work that has to be done to keep a veterinary practice running and in good repair. Operations management encompasses everything from scheduling appointments to repairing equipment to choosing practice management software. Many of the duties in this realm are delegated to staff. A practice owner has to understand what to delegate, though, and must put the systems in place to make sure everything happens the way it's supposed to once it's been delegated.

Quality Control

A practice owner ensures that there are quality control procedures in place for all areas of the hospital. Each employee should be able to reference written processes and procedures that dictate how each situation is to be handled. Otherwise, it's a fly-by-the-seat-of-your-pants operation. Do you know the answers to these questions: How do we discipline an employee who is habitually late? How does the receptionist perform telephone triage? What is the standard procedure for treating an ear ablation? What is the answer when a client asks about the efficacy of FIV vaccine? Under what circumstances does the practice allow a client to pay her bill in installments? How often does each piece of lab equipment get serviced?

When trying to fit in at the practice, it's important not to tell the staff or the practice owner, "This is what you should be doing." So if they don't have written procedures, ask each question as it arises, and write down the answer so that you can refer to it in the future. Make sure that there is agreement about how a situation should be handled—the owner might want to handle it one way, but the receptionists have worked out a different system. If you run into that situation, make an observation to the owner— "When I asked the receptionists about scheduling geriatric exams, they told me it varies by doctor, but you said that each doctor should be scheduled for 20 minutes. I just want to be clear about it so that I budget the appropriate amount of time." You are not trying to get the receptionists in trouble, you are clarifying a policy to ensure that you are doing it the way you're supposed to.

> You also need to understand that if the practice has written procedures, the practice owner or even another associate may question your treatment plan.

You also need to understand that if the practice has written procedures, the practice owner or even another associate may question your treatment plan. Don't take it personally; just figure out where you departed from the procedure and make a note of it for the future. If you think that a particular procedure should change, bring it up with your boss in a nonthreatening way.

Safety, Security, Laws, and Regulations

The details of insurance coverage, OSHA regulations, ergonomic issues, and workplace safety would likely bore you to tears, so we'll be brief. Suffice it to say that the regulations are overwhelming in number, and they change every month. The practice owner has to keep on eye on all of these potential problem areas, even if she delegates the detail work to others.

You can do your part by always following the rules. If you don't know what they are, ask. Take the time to check Material Safety Data Sheets (MSDSs) before you handle an unfamiliar substance. Don't slouch over your keyboard and then complain that your neck and back hurt. If the practice has a dress code, follow it. (Many elements of a hospital dress code are there for your

and the staff's safety.) Label bottles with secondary container warning labels, no matter how innocuous the substance. Not only will you be protecting yourself, you will set a shining example for the rest of the staff.

Maintenance and Repairs

Not only does the practice owner have to worry about upkeep on the building, landscape, and parking lot, she has to ensure that all equipment is maintained properly. If you own a house, you know what a pain it is (and how expensive it is!) to get a building painted, replace the furnace, or arrange to have a clogged drain fixed on short notice. Imagine what it's like to keep the practice and all of its equipment running and in tip-top shape on top of caring for patients and running the business.

Here, too, you can make yourself valuable. First, make sure you clean up after yourself so that you don't contribute to wear and tear on the building or the equipment. Second, bring it to the owner's or practice manager's attention when you notice something needs to be repaired or replaced—don't assume someone else will do it.

Hardware and Software

The boss has to keep hardware and software up to date. This means upgrades, updates, and new equipment on a fairly frequent basis. From decisions about which practice management software to use to which kind of scanner will fit your needs, the boss has to be involved in the decision-making process at some level. Some practice owners spend lots of time on these issues; others would rather delegate most of it.

You know how you felt the last time your computer at school or home crashed for the third time in fifteen minutes, and you couldn't figure out why. Did you feel like throwing it out the window? So, think about how your boss feels when the fourth staff person in a row complains about the "slow" computer system, the inadequate accounting software, or the color inkjet printer that doesn't produce laser-quality images like the one at the last place she worked. You guessed it … you can help by *not* being one of these whiners. And if you have expertise in this area, you can bet your boss wants to make use of it. So the next time someone doesn't know how to fix the jammed printer or how to get out of a "hung" program, step in and lend a hand.

Appointment Scheduling

Some practices have been scheduling appointments the same way for thirty years: twenty minutes for all appointments except well puppy or kitten visits, which are thirty minutes.

Be sure you work as efficiently as possible within the appointment system used in your practice. If you simply can't see patients and clients in the allotted time, ask your boss for guidance. Maybe he would be willing to shadow you in a few typical appointments in order to give you some pointers for how to do things differently. Or you could ask to shadow him. How is he getting things done so quickly? In the opposite situation, where you have plenty of time to spare, use the extra time to mentor technicians or complete your medical records. You may want to suggest that you be scheduled for more patients in a given time period, but be careful how you approach your boss. You don't want to look like a showoff—ask questions rather than make demands.

Inventory

Your boss most likely delegates the bulk of inventory management chores to an office manager, head technician, or several different people. You can be sure, though, that she is keeping a close eye on what's sitting on the shelves. Having too much inventory is like taking a wad of cash, putting it on the shelf, and watching it collect dust.

Too little inventory means cranky clients and possibly lost business. Major concerns are staff time, how often the inventory turns over (another way of saying how many times per year the practice sells a product or group of products), and profitability. How does the practice get the best deal on surgical supplies, pharmaceuticals, food, and over-the-counter products? Inventory management is an art and a science, with the results showing in the bottom line.

When it comes to inventory, there are several things you can do to make your life, and the lives of those you work with, easier. First, don't demand that the person who orders inventory order your favorite drugs when there is a perfectly good substitute available. If there really is an issue of efficacy or new information, talk it over with your boss, not the person who orders inventory. Second, if you notice any expired inventory, notify the person who is responsible for sending it back. Third, if you take the last or second to last of anything, tell the appropriate person. Don't assume that someone will magically find out that you're out (unless there is a paper record that shows she was already notified).

Equipment

You want all of the latest toys, right? Well, so does the practice owner, but the boss has to consider whether that machine will pay for itself. When should the practice buy new equipment? What about buying used versus new? When should the practice get rid of the old stuff? These are a few of the questions a practice owner must consider.

So what can you do to help make these decisions? If you know how to do a financial analysis to project the costs and revenue related to the new piece of equipment, or if you're willing to learn, do it! The owner certainly will be impressed, and you may just get that new ultrasound machine. (See *Focusing on Diagnostic Testing and Imaging*, published by AAHA, for a step-by-step guide for how to analyze the financial feasibility of a new piece

> Be sure you work as efficiently as possible within the appointment system used in your practice. If you simply can't see patients and clients in the allotted time, ask your boss for guidance.

of equipment.) Otherwise, keep complaints to a minimum. Discuss case work-ups in terms of how the boss would like you to diagnose (or refer) within the limitations of the equipment that's available.

Medical Records

A practice owner must ensure that medical records are top notch. This means setting an example and creating quality control procedures to make sure everyone else follows that example. What needs to be recorded? What should be recorded? How will records be audited? What forms will the practice use? What types of consent forms do clients have to sign? Medical records speak volumes about the quality of medicine the doctors practice, so it's imperative that they be as thorough and neat as possible.

Your job first and foremost is to be a role model for how the boss wants medical records completed, even if she doesn't practice what she preaches. Also, thank any staff person who does a great job completing her portion of the medical record.

FINANCIAL MANAGEMENT

Financial management is the bane of many practice owners' existence. You may share that aversion to the business aspect of veterinary medicine, but the boss can't really afford to ignore it. He has to pay attention to productivity, money out, and money in on a weekly, if not daily, basis.

Managing the money means more than the net income—it means making sure there is enough cash in the bank to make payroll and pay a fair salary to himself, budgeting for the next year, and worrying about the value of the practice. It's a big job and the owner's responsibility. Even with a practice administrator overseeing the bulk of the day-to-day finances, a practice owner has got to keep his mind on the money all of the time.

Bookkeeping and Financial Reporting

The actual recording of financial transactions and generation of financial statements is delegated to either an accountant, bookkeeper, or office manager in most cases. The practice owner must understand the information, though, to keep the practice running smoothly. Are transactions being recorded accurately? What does the information on the income statement and the balance sheet mean? How does the data compare to other practices? Financial statements are an important scorecard for the practice's success, and they force the practice owner to consider how to improve revenue and control expenses.

The practice owner will decide whether or not to share all or part of the financial statements with you and the staff. It's best not to push this issue— if the boss is overprotective of the information, it may be because he doesn't want anyone forming opinions about him or the practice based on the financial statements.

Some owners don't want to disclose how much or how little they're actually taking out of the practice. (The average, by the way, is 19.4% of the practice's gross income split among all owners.) In any case, it's not really any of your business unless part of your compensation or performance appraisal is based on the numbers.

If the boss does share the numbers with the staff and use them as a scorecard for the practice's performance, it's your job to role model appropriate "cheerleading" behavior—talk about how you and the rest of the staff can improve the numbers when they're down and shout "Yea team!" when they're up. Also, if you have ideas about how to increase revenue or control expenses, be sure to present them to your boss.

Budgeting, Cash Flow, and Tax Planning

It's not enough just to record the financial transactions and review the financial statements. The boss has to plan for the coming years. Cash flow, tax planning, capital expenditures (business and medical equipment), revenue, and expenses are all parts of the formula. Sound complicated? It is.

Unless you have expertise in these areas, you probably shouldn't be involved. Just do your best to understand that the purchase of that expensive piece of equipment you were lobbying for might not happen—not because the boss is a cheapskate, but because there isn't the money for it right now, or perhaps the boss has determined that the equipment won't pay for itself.

Pricing

On average, about 74% of the practice's gross revenue goes right back out to pay for drugs, staff and associate salaries, rent, benefits, supplies, and everything else it takes to run a practice. Though there are several issues that affect revenue, pricing is chief among them. How does a practice owner set prices, anyway?

There are several theories about how to set prices that approach the issue from very different perspectives. But in the end, prices somehow have to keep pace with inflation, and they have to allow for enough money to keep the practice running.

> On average, about 74% of the practice's gross revenue goes right back out to pay for drugs, staff and associate salaries, rent, benefits, supplies, and everything else it takes to run a practice.

The best way you can support the practice is never to question pricing (unless you think it's too low). Charge the fee, don't discount, and charge for all services performed. It is not your prerogative to discount or skip charges, so don't do it. When staff grumble about fees, politely but firmly let them know that running a veterinary practice is an expensive undertaking, and the prices are what's necessary to pay their wages and provide the clients and pets with the best service and care.

Payment and Collection Policies

Unfortunately, providing services to clients doesn't always equate to collecting payment for those services. A practice owner must create a credit policy. This means figuring out who can charge and when and how much. Also, what is the procedure for those times when the client doesn't pay? What if a Good Samaritan brings in an animal hit by a car? All of these situations must be considered in light of the practice owner's philosophy about money and business.

What else is there to say except, "Follow the policy—don't make exceptions"? Don't make it your job to judge clients' ability to pay. If there is no policy, strongly and persistently urge your boss to create one so that everyone knows how to deal with each of the common situations: "I didn't bring my wallet," "I don't have any money," "This dog just got hit by a car!" and "Just put him to sleep."

Internal Control

Cash and other assets, including drugs, pet food, over-the-counter products, and equipment, are the practice's bread and butter and deserve protection. It's the practice owner's responsibility to ensure that there are adequate internal control procedures in place that prevent, as much as possible, theft of or damage to the practice's assets.

The best thing you can do is to *always* follow protocol, no matter how inconvenient. Set an example. Let's say that even the boss doesn't always follow the rules—maybe he takes a five-dollar bill out of the cash register every now and then without signing a receipt. This kind of example can lead to a free-for-all when it comes to ethical behavior. So, follow the rules—all of them—including how and when to account for controlled drugs, how to handle cash and credit card information, and how to sign materials out of inventory. If you see anyone breaking the rules, immediately tell the boss or follow the established protocol for communicating it to management. If there are no written protocols, just remember not to do anything you wouldn't want your employees to do if it were your practice.

HUMAN RESOURCES MANAGEMENT

"My job would be so easy if it weren't for all those darn *people* I have to work with." Have you ever caught yourself saying something like that? Human resource issues are among those most complained about and most dreaded by practice owners. In general, they ignore the issues when at all possible, delegate the ones they can't, and blunder through the rest.

208

Internal Communication

It is essential to keep every employee, from the most revered partner to the part-time high school kid that cleans cages, on the same page, or the practice may never achieve its true potential. The boss has to figure out not only what to say, but when and how to say it, including facilitating that next big argument between Susan and Margaret or making a "state of the union" speech at the next staff meeting. In any case, there has to be an official "party line" about everything staff-related that goes on at the practice, from the dress code to use of the phone to what to do if you catch someone doing something right. Internal communication should be frequent, consistent, and clear.

Your boss likely has had little to no training on how to deal with people issues, so cut her some slack when she messes up. What can you do to help? Ask questions so that you understand what the policies are (if they're not written), and then follow them. Also clarify what your boss sees as your role in staff communication.

Discipline and Firing

Disciplining and firing are two of the toughest tasks for any manager. The boss has to decide how to handle these issues and how you should handle them, too.

Often, an associate gets "stuck" with human resource management duties because the practice owner doesn't want to do it and doesn't want to delegate that kind of power to a nonveterinarian. Make it your job to understand how you should report performance issues to your boss and exactly what is expected of you with regard to human resource management.

> Make it your job to understand how you should report performance issues to your boss and exactly what is expected of you with regard to human resource management.

Hiring and Training

As easy as it may sound, hiring a new staff person requires tons of thought, time, and effort. First, there is the issue of defining the job and the required skills and knowledge needed for the job (there should be a job description for every position in the practice). Then, there is the matter of writing and placing the ad in the appropriate places and recruiting in other ways if necessary. Next, someone has to review the resumes and conduct phone and/or in-person interviews, test the candidates if applicable, check references, and offer the job. And it doesn't end when the new person walks in the door. There should be a protocol for "breaking in the new kid." Orientation and training are keys to a successful partnership between the practice and the new employee and should be intensive and thorough.

You may be called upon to be involved in any and all of these hiring and training tasks. And you may not know what you're doing. So ask questions about what the procedures are. If your boss or the practice administrator can't help you, ask for training. Don't just jump right in with both feet— not only could you be a poor ambassador of the practice, you could invite a lawsuit by asking inappropriate questions! When all else fails, ask to observe the process a few times before you become actively involved so that you can at least learn how things are done at that particular practice.

Benefits and Compensation

Unfortunately, pay in the veterinary field is low. Trained, educated technicians make an average of $13 an hour, which equates to an annual salary of $27,000. This is the pay for someone who can draw blood, run labs, and anesthetize an animal, among other things. Receptionists, who are the front-line ambassadors for the practice, make an average of $10 an hour. This is the pay for someone who can triage medical emergencies by phone, make or break the relationship with a new client, collect payment, reinforce the doctor's recommendations, and schedule that appointment for the dental cleaning before the client walks out the door. And it's not as if they make up for their low compensation in benefits. In fact, they work night and weekend hours, don't get great insurance coverage, and work in a stressful environment. So the boss has to decide how much of the pie to give to staff and how to divvy it up. Bonuses? Pay for production? If so, with what system? It's enough to give anyone the night terrors.

It's not really your job to decide on compensation and benefits issues, but you can offer new information if you have it. For example, if you go to a conference and listen to a great speaker talk about a new way to compensate employees and improve productivity, give the information to your boss and ask her to consider it.

As far as your pay goes, you should be up to date on the latest trends so that you are prepared with facts when you ask for a raise. The "I deserve it" motto is all too common among employees, and your boss has heard it dozens of times before. If you ask for more pay, either for yourself or the staff, make a logical case. Imagine what you would want an employee to say to you when asking for a raise. Would it be, "I just can't afford my rent because my husband left (or 'Jimmy needs new baseball equipment' or 'I took in another stray dog')"? Or would you like to hear, "Dr. X, let me tell you how I can make more money for you, provide better care for the patients, and provide better service to the clients"?

> Marketing to existing clients encompasses all of the communication the practice has with those clients, including every piece of paper given and every word spoken.

Performance Appraisals

Here's another issue that gives your boss a headache. How, when, and why should the boss review the employees' performance, including yours? Many practice owners just don't do it, or they do it infrequently, or when they do it, they botch it.

Again, this stems from lack of training. It may also stem from a lack of interest in doing it right. Veterinarians, though touchy-feely about animals, are scientists, and they are often not so touchy-feely about the people who work for them. It's not that they don't care, they just feel inept and lost when it comes to reviewing the performance of those who work for them.

If your boss doesn't schedule a performance appraisal for you at least once a year, ask for one. It's vital that you know how the boss thinks you're doing if you're going to fit in. The best thing you can do for a review is to be prepared. Review your goals from the prior year, along with the progress you've made toward those goals. Talk about your successes with clients, patients, and staff. Be able to summarize your accomplishments for the period and what you plan to change or improve in the next period.

Human Resource Laws

There are so many laws that relate to human resource issues, they can make your head spin. The practice owner either has to stay up to date on these laws or hire someone else to do it (i.e., a practice manager). There are laws that relate to sexual harassment, taking time off work, discrimination, payroll taxes, benefits, compensation, and practically any aspect of human resource management you can imagine.

You don't need to know these laws in detail, but you do need to have some understanding of those that apply to safety, discrimination, and sexual harassment. You need to keep yourself out of trouble and watch for any activity among the staff that could get you, them, or the practice owner in trouble. If you witness any improper activity, immediately bring it to the practice administrator's or owner's attention. Calmly state what happened, sticking to the facts and minimizing conjecture. As one of the "higher-ups" in the practice, you should be a role model in following HR laws and encouraging others to do the same.

MARKETING MANAGEMENT

When you think about "marketing," what comes to mind? You probably picture Yellow Pages ads and refrigerator magnets. In fact, marketing encompasses all of the communication the practice has with existing clients and potential clients. While much of the actual day-to-day details of marketing are delegated to various members of the team, it's the practice owner who must set the tone and oversee the process to ensure it is helping her achieve the practice's goals.

Existing Clients

Marketing to existing clients encompasses all of the communication the practice has with those clients, including every piece of paper given and every word spoken. The boss has to set the direction in terms of tone and quality. What kinds of printed pieces are given to the client? What do the handouts and brochures look like? Should the practice send a newsletter to clients, and what should it say? How are estimates presented? How do the receptionists answer the phone and greet clients? How should associates greet clients? Can the kennel person answer a question about fleas? What does the practice parking lot look like? How does the staff dress? All of these, and more, are questions to consider when marketing to external clients.

Knowing that your every move is being watched by clients and affecting their opinion of you and the practice can be a little scary, but you'll probably be a lot more careful about how you talk to them. Think about how you like to be treated when you go to your physician's office. Treat your clients as courteously as you wish your doctor treated you.

Potential Clients

Marketing to potential clients covers everything from how the receptionist answers the phone to visits to the local elementary school to the ad in the Yellow Pages. The practice owner has to coordinate marketing materials, set goals for each marketing campaign, and follow up to see what worked and what didn't.

The practice should have a marketing plan that details what kind of communication is sent to clients and when, but many practices don't. That's not to say that the practice doesn't offer a discount during Dental Health Month or try a bigger Yellow Pages ad, it's just that the message isn't necessarily consistent and it isn't necessarily used to meet the goals of the practice owner.

Though you may not have the skills and know-how (not to mention the authority) to write a comprehensive marketing plan for the practice, you can use your influence with the boss. If you have a good idea for a marketing campaign, explain how it will help achieve the practice owner's goals.

THE BOTTOM LINE

In this chapter, you've learned about the major decisions a practice owner has to make to keep the practice running smoothly. When you get upset, remember that the boss has a lot on her mind, so try to see things from her perspective. Do your best to fit in by setting an example and asking for clarification when necessary. This way, you can please your boss and make your life at work easier and happier.

RESOURCES

Books

Nasty Bosses: How to Deal with Them without Stooping to Their Level by J. Carter.
169 Ways to Score Points With Your Boss by A. Schonberg.

211

CHAPTER EIGHTEEN

Making a Connection With Your Clients

Carin A. Smith, DVM

IN THIS CHAPTER, YOU'LL LEARN:

- **How to successfully communicate with your clients**
- **How to deal with difficult clients**
- **How to talk about fees in a positive way**

Has this ever happened to you?

You thought you had done a good job with Max. You made an accurate diagnosis and prescribed the correct treatment, and the dog had done well, but the next time Ms. Goldberg came in to the clinic, she specifically asked for a different doctor. What went wrong?

Or this?

The last client of the day really got on your nerves. Of course he was upset that his dog was sick, but why didn't he listen when you told him what you were going to do? He kept repeating himself over and over and giving details about his pet that were irrelevant. Why couldn't he just shut up?

Client communication is one of the most difficult areas of practice. Unfortunately, clients won't go away. Once you learn to make the most of your client interactions, you'll start to enjoy them more, and the difficult clients won't be as difficult after all.

WHAT IS COMMUNICATION?

A better question might be, "What is successful communication?"

You may think that you have communicated successfully if you talk and the client nods in apparent agreement. What's missing here? It's a one-way street if only one person is talking. You have no idea what the client is thinking, what he or she has agreed to (if anything), or what his or her concerns or questions may be—*unless you ask.*

Successful communication starts when you send a message, but it requires that you then ensure that the message was received—and that it was the same one you intended to send. Furthermore, successful communication assumes that you, in turn, have received the message your client wanted to send to you. Your client's nodding may simply mean, "If I nod, I can get out of here and ask the technician what you are talking about," or, "I have no idea what that word meant, but you clearly assume that I do know, so I'm not going to embarrass myself by asking."

What you said: "Fluffy is very sick."

What the client heard: "Fluffy is going to die."

What you said: "We could do some blood tests or take X-rays to find out what's wrong."

What the client heard: "I have no idea what's wrong, nor am I sure what we should do to find out."

Communication includes more than just the words you say. In fact, the words you say are only a minor part of the message you send. Your body language, vocal tone, and eye contact all contribute to your message. The way you look and dress affects your message, too (if you don't look the way the client expects you to look, the client is distracted from hearing you). Be aware of *all* the messages you send.

TIME EFFICIENCY AND COMMUNICATION

You may think that successful communication takes a lot of time. You may even interrupt your clients in the interest of time and in the interest of "getting to the point." Yet, research shows that most people, if allowed to talk without interruption, will stop within two minutes. By allowing them to be heard, and by truly listening, you can get their full attention when you want them to listen to you. What's more, you may find out more about what's wrong with their pets.

After you have listened for a full two minutes (and only then), you may gently redirect the client to focus on the problem by using her name and by making statements or asking questions *about what she said*.

"Ms. Whitman, excuse me for interrupting, but I want to make sure I understand what has been happening with Fluffy. You said that Fluffy has not eaten since Monday and vomited twice yesterday. Can you tell me what the vomit looked like?"

Communicate in Many Ways

Do you like to read about how to do something new, or be shown how to do it? Would you prefer to learn by trying it yourself, or by watching someone else first? Just as you have learning and communication preferences, so do your clients. You don't necessarily need to analyze each person's learning style in order to meet his or her needs. You can ask clients what they prefer, but also make a habit of presenting information in many ways:

- Verbally
- In writing
- With video or audiotapes
- Through demonstration
- Through practice—having clients practice with your assistance
- Using models or pictures

"Ms. Townsend, my description of the surgery that Wilma needs may be a lot to absorb all at once. I have a written handout here that describes what we've discussed. I also have some pictures that show the surgery. Would you like to look at those? I can give you a few moments to review these materials. Then I'd be happy to answer your questions. Julie will also come in to show you how to give Wilma the medicine she'll need once she goes home."

Words That Help—or Hinder— Successful Communication

Certain words or phrases can interfere with successful communication. The first step in avoiding these words is to notice when you *do* use them. Then practice alternatives:

Instead of	You could say
No.	What we can do is… Your choices are…
We can't…	What we can do is…
I can't…	The practice manager (or Dr. Smith) can…
You have to…	Will you…? Would you mind…?

I don't know.	To find out, we can… (or I will…)
But	And

Watch Your Language

You may have already found that there is a trade-off between using too much technical language and not enough. Those in favor of using technical language point out that it makes you look more professional. Saying "wee wee" instead of "urine" just doesn't sound like a doctor!

Your language and terminology also affect the client's perception of value. What's more valuable—a shot or an injection? A "routine spay," or an "ovariohysterectomy with monitored anesthesia"? "Put on fluids," or "monitoring intravenous electrolytes and fluids"? Of course, you will *translate* those technical words to ensure client understanding.

> **Using too much technical language alienates your clients—and they won't necessarily let you know.**

Using too much technical language alienates your clients—and they won't necessarily let you know. Instead, they'll ask someone else for information about their pets' problems—on the Internet or at the pet store. Don't assume that even your clients involved in the health fields will know all of the terminology you use. You can show respect for their (potential) knowledge and still translate words they may not know, if you are tactful.

Example

"As a nurse, Ms. Grant, you probably know most of the words that I use here, but I'm just in the habit of translating, so I hope you don't take offense when I do so.

"I recommend that we perform a urinalysis on Fluffy. We'll take a urine sample and then look at it under the microscope. That will help us see whether there is infection or some other problem."

DEALING WITH DIFFICULT CLIENTS

Pleasant interactions probably don't occupy a lot of your thoughts. Those difficult interactions, though, tend to stick in your memory. How can you reduce the tension in situations where clients act uncertain, emotional, or angry?

Defining "difficult" is your first step toward resolving conflicts. What is a "difficult person" to you? Have you ever been in a situation where *you* may have been seen as a "difficult person"? Why were you behaving the way you were? What do you think the other people around you thought about your motivations?

Dealing with difficult clients is something most of us would rather avoid. Nonetheless, all veterinarians must learn to interact with people who are not showing their best side. It is to your advantage to "win over" these difficult people and to make them loyal clients. You will also reduce your chances of being the target of lawsuits, most of which are brought about because of communication breakdowns.

The first step in dealing with difficult people is realizing that *you have no idea why* they are being difficult. Don't assume that you know anything! Your assumptions are based on your own perceptions of why *you* would behave a certain way in similar circumstances. But *they are not you!* A "difficult client" might be feeling one or more of these emotions:

- Anger
- Frustration (because you aren't listening, the client is feeling ignored, or the client feels you don't trust him or her)
- Sadness
- Intense grief
- Distrust
- Conflicting desires or needs
- Confusion
- Lack of respect
- Fear
- Worry

A client could also have *any* of the above emotions in response to a situation in his or her life that has nothing to do with you.

215

If you want to be heard, you first must listen. And unless you ask, you have no idea what is going on with a difficult client. *It takes strength to listen* when all you want to do is get the client to be quiet! But if the client is out of control, then who is *in* control? You can take control by not reacting in the same way.

- First, get the client in a place where you can talk. Resolving issues in the reception area or hallway won't work. "Ms. Brakeman, I can see that you are upset, and I'd like to help resolve this problem. Can you come with me to the conference room where we can talk?"

- Ask questions to find the source of the client's anger. Don't assume that you know. A client who appears angry because her cat cannot come home today may actually be terrified that the cat is going to die. Use open-ended questions to find out all that you can. "Ms. Brakeman, please tell me more about what happened."

- Next, listen for *as long as it takes* to fully understand the client's concerns. How do you know when that point is reached? By rephrasing what the client says until she says, "Yes, that's what I am feeling."

Rephrasing a client's feelings does not have to mean that you agree with them. It means that you heard what was said. "Ms. Brakeman, what I'm hearing is that you are really angry that we didn't call you to tell you the results of the blood tests. You arranged to have your daughter drive you all the way down here only to find out that Alex has to stay in the hospital another night. That was a big inconvenience for you and for her. Now you're really worried about how Alex is going to feel being left here another day, and you're worried about how things will turn out for him. Is that right? Is there anything else?" Then be quiet—bite your tongue—and wait for the client to respond. Listen to the reply. Rephrase again if you didn't get it right the first time. If the client seems to be repeating herself, it probably means that she thinks you don't understand

or did not hear what was said. Try rephrasing again. No matter what their gripe, the bottom line is that people want to be heard and understood. Achieving that goal brings you almost all the way toward resolving problems.

- The next step is to apologize. Apologizing can, but does not have to, mean that you are accepting blame. You can say, "I'm sorry that we made you angry." If "I'm sorry" doesn't seem like the right words, try, "I apologize." At this point, do not offer excuses (even if they are truly valid reasons for your actions). Your client doesn't care *why* things happened the way they did; she only wishes things had been different. Don't make the client feel guilty for her anger by explaining the emergency that came in, causing you to be late. You may feel better for "explaining," but the client now has both anger and guilt and an even greater reason to dislike being at your hospital. "Ms. Brakeman, I'm really sorry we did not call you as promised. We should have done that, and we did not. I apologize."

- Finally, offer amends. What can you do to make things right? Making amends can be done immediately or as a follow-up. For some clients, making amends means reducing their bill, but *that's not always a necessary step.* You may want to send a card or flowers, adjust your schedule to accommodate them, or make other arrangements for them. "I share your concern for Alex, and I think it's best for him to stay another night here. I think that he will improve a lot faster if he can stay here where we can give him fluids all night. I know that it is difficult for you to arrange transportation here. I can arrange to have Linda, our technician, bring Alex home to you tomorrow, to spare you another trip down here. Would that help? Would that be all right with you?"

> People don't necessarily need you to do something specific right now—they just want you to acknowledge that something needs to be done.

MORE TIPS FOR DIFFICULT CONVERSATIONS

- **Give yourself time**—If you don't have the tools or the information to handle the situation, buy yourself some time by making a statement that lets the person know you *will* take action. People don't necessarily need you to do something specific right now—they just want you to acknowledge that something needs to be done. Giving yourself extra time helps you in two ways—you can gather more information, and you can let tempers cool. "Ms. Erikson, I can see that you are really angry, and I am really sorry we disappointed you. I am going to take steps to resolve this situation. I need to take some time to talk to Julie, our technician, about what happened. Can I call you later?"

- **Distance yourself**—It's easy to get caught up in the moment, giving a single situation more emotional weight than it deserves. Try to mentally distance yourself from the situation. Just how important is this interaction, relative to the rest of your life? Does this person's reaction reflect on whether or not you are a good, decent human being? Do you need to "win" to feel good about yourself? Do you have to prove that you are right?

- **Gather information**—Knowledge is power. Find out all you can about what happened from as many people as you can. Ask enough questions until you figure out the process that allowed the problem to occur. Find out who has the authority to take action to resolve the issue.

> Every time you hesitate to discuss the best treatment, based on your concern about the client's ability to pay, you are letting money interfere with how much you care for that pet.

- **Focus on the process, not the person**—Most people don't go out of their way to do things wrong. Focusing on blame only makes people defensive and doesn't prevent the problem from recurring. If a client was not called about lab results, was that because the technician was lazy or didn't care? (Not likely.) Or was it because there is no time set aside for her to make calls? Or because call-backs are something left for "whoever has time"?

- **Don't take the bait**—We all have "trigger points" that certain people somehow manage to "push" and set off our tempers. Know your trigger points and sensitive buttons, and don't let yourself be baited or pushed into reacting. By staying calm, you are in control. When you allow someone to push you into reacting, that person is in control. Breathe deeply, and allow the other person to vent.

- **Rehearse handy phrases**—"I can understand your concern." "I can see that you are angry, and we need to resolve this problem." "I appreciate your bringing this to my attention." "I'm sorry we upset you."

TALKING ABOUT MONEY

When we think of "difficult situations," conversations involving money top the list. Why is it so difficult for us to talk about money? Many people are brought up to think that it is not polite to discuss money. As veterinarians, we may believe that empathy and profit conflict, and to show that we care about our clients and their pets, we cannot possibly let money interfere.

Here's a new way to view money: Every time you hesitate to discuss the best treatment, based on your concern about the client's ability to pay, *you* are letting money interfere with how much you care for that pet.

How can this be? First, you have no idea how much money your clients have. Even if you did, why in the world do you assume that you can decide *for them* how they want to spend their own money? It's disrespectful to them to assume you know their priorities.

Your clients come to your clinic *because they want you to help them* and their pets. They *expect* that they will be charged for your services. What does it mean when a client says, "Wow, that's a lot of money!" You might assume that they mean, "I can't pay that," but don't jump to conclusions. "That's a lot of money" does *not* necessarily mean the customer cannot afford it, that it is more than he or she wants to spend, or that the pet isn't worth spending that amount of money on. Rather, "That's a lot of money" *might* mean, "I'm surprised," "I don't know what I'm getting for that amount," "I don't see the value for that amount of money," "Compared to what I spend for groceries, that's a lot (but I can afford it)," or "Compared to what I spend on cosmetics, that's a lot (but my pet is worth it)."

What is "a lot of money"? Think about the dollar figure that, *to you*, is "a lot." Now imagine a successful attorney in your town. What dollar figure do you think is "a lot" for that person? How about a nurse, a plumber, or a teacher?

Now, think about what, *to you*, is "a lot to spend on pet healthcare." Then imagine those same people, and what they might think is "a lot to spend on pet healthcare." The point is not that you should be able to guess—that's *their* decision—but that you realize "a lot of money" can mean many different things to many different people.

What happens when you are explaining an estimate that, to you, is "a lot of money"? Chances are, you let your emotions cloud the way you present that estimate. Do you apologetically say, "I know it's a lot of money . . ." What if the client had not thought it was a lot? Might he or she now feel uncomfortable saying, "Hey, not for me! I'm rich! That's hardly anything in my eyes!" Might they now feel stupid to spend "that much" on a pet? What is the outcome for the pet?

What's the best response to a client who says, "That's a lot of money!" How about, "What are your questions about the services we've listed here?" Then you can show the client the value of your recommendations, and you can find out what the client meant with that statement. *Don't assume that the client can't or won't pay!*

Don't Misinterpret Silence

Are you uncomfortable with silence? If so, your discomfort may be costing your clinic money, and you may be jeopardizing the health of the pets you serve. When you offer your client your best recommendation, then state the cost, the client may not respond immediately. How often do you then offer another option, assuming that the client's hesitation is because of the dollar figure?

Give people time to think and process what you've said, and don't put objections into their mouths. They can think of their own objections! Their silence may simply mean that they are considering what you've said, and that they have

some questions or concerns about the procedure. Give your recommendation, then bite your tongue and be quiet. They can't think if you are talking.

Focus on Value

Sometimes you may truly think that some of your services or products are overpriced. Before you make this assumption, spend time learning about the costs of running a practice. Refer to the AAHA publication *Financial & Productivity Pulsepoints* for more specifics concerning the financial angle of this business. Learn more about practice expenses, and about what portion of each expense is charged to clients. Learn how all the costs add up as salary for you, for the other veterinarians, and for the staff. Create your own personal budget (see Chapter 2).

Veterinarians who do this exercise find that they no longer feel guilty about charging fairly. They learn what they must earn to support a middle-class (not wealthy) lifestyle. Learn where the money goes once it is paid to the hospital so that you can decide what is a "fair" fee to charge clients for your services.

Presenting Fees to the Client in a Positive Manner

How can you present your fees in a positive manner? *Focus on the services you offer and the value of your work.* If you remember that your job is to be a veterinarian, then you can focus on the reason the client came in—to get help for his or her pet. What did you recommend to help the pet? Focus on your recommendation. Make sure that the client understands the reason for what you recommend, including the value and extent of your services. Instead of giving an "estimate," offer a "summary of treatment recommendations." That's what you *are* doing, after all.

Which of the following two procedures sounds more valuable as well as best for the pet?

"We do all our spays on Wednesday mornings. You can drop Fluffy off in the morning, then pick her up at 5 P.M."

Or

"Although the spay surgery is one we commonly do, it is abdominal surgery that requires general anesthesia. We use a very safe gas anesthesia, and we reduce risk by first taking a blood sample to check for common problems. During surgery, we monitor Fluffy's heart with an ECG, just as is done with every surgery on humans. We also have an intravenous catheter in place so that we can give fluids to prevent dehydration and maintain health. After the surgery, we administer an injection to prevent pain."

Your clients may assume that you are doing exactly the same procedure as the low-cost clinic down the road—unless you *tell* them!

GETTING CLIENTS TO AGREE WITH YOUR RECOMMENDATIONS

Do you have trouble getting clients to commit to the treatment that you recommend? Do you assume that they can't or won't pay the amount you charge for those services? Think again. Money is a handy excuse and an easy way out of a difficult situation. It is easier for a client to say, "I can't afford that," than to say, "I am terrified that Buster will die under anesthesia," or, "I don't understand the reason for doing that test." When a client says, "I'll have to think about it," what does that mean? Usually it's a way to put off a decision. Another putting-off phrase is, "I'll have to talk to my spouse."

Don't accept these statements on their own terms. Clients may have objections that they aren't comfortable bringing up. They may not perceive the need for, or the value of, your recommendations. Using money or a spouse as an excuse allows them to get out of the office without confronting their own confusion or opening the door to an awkward conversation. It's your job to open that door and ease the way to clear communication.

Example

Client: "I'll have to think about that."

You: "I sense that you may have some reservations or concerns about the procedure. Can you tell me what those are?"

The bottom line: Successful communication with your clients requires that you first listen to their concerns. Then offer them the best solution for their pet, without allowing your emotions about money to interfere. Give them your recommendations as the doctor and as the pet's advocate. Ask them about their concerns and questions. Listen to be sure they understand and agree with your recommendations. Make a plan together, as partners in the pet's care.

RESOURCES

Books

Client Satisfaction Pays: Quality Service for Practice Success by C. Smith.

Connecting With Clients: Practical Communication Techniques For 15 Common Situations by L. Lagoni and D. Durrance.

Difficult Conversations: How to Discuss What Matters Most by D. Stone, S. Heen, and R. Fisher.

Continuing Education

The Art of Veterinary Practice: Success for Life. AAHA seminar that offers practical techniques to help you improve interpersonal relationships and play a more productive role in the success of your practice. Contact AAHA at 800/883-6301 for more information or visit *www.aahanet.org.*

CHAPTER NINETEEN

Your Performance Appraisal

Karen Gendron, DVM

IN THIS CHAPTER, YOU'LL LEARN:

- **How to prepare for your review**
- **What to expect during a review**

Performance appraisals, or employee reviews, are typically annual one-on-one meetings between your employer and you, the employee, to assess your work over the past year and set goals for the next year. There are as many ways to conduct performance appraisals as there are practices. Each system has its imperfections, but all share a common goal. The purpose of an appraisal is to work together with your employer to improve your job performance.

Some practices do not provide formal appraisals at all. There is no conscious effort to evaluate your work. This employer is content maintaining the status quo even when it deserves to be changed. While this may appear to save time and avoid confrontation, it removes the opportunity for you to get a detailed critique of your work and have a discussion about your future with the practice. This employer also fails to coach you to greater success.

Other practices provide informal appraisals. Your assessments will come in small pieces, often precipitated by specific events. It may be a matter of being told that you handled a difficult case well or being given advice on handling conflict with a staff member. For example, "Dr. Smith, the receptionists have been noticing that many clients specifically request to see you. You're doing a great job building a clientele." Or, "Dr. Jones, I received a call from Mrs. MacKenzie today. At her office visit, she expressed concern about her dog's red ears. She was disappointed that you never did an otoscopic exam. I'd like that to be a part of every exam. Certainly, we shouldn't miss it when there may be a problem."

Although you do not receive comprehensive feedback, you can make some good assumptions about how your supervisor is responding to your work and areas that your supervisor sees are in need of improvement. It is still best, however, to have an open and direct conversation about your work. You may want to use the tips later in this chapter to pursue an evaluation when one is not offered.

Most practices do have a formal evaluation process. Traditionally, this is an annual meeting between you and the practice owner, manager, or medical director, referenced here as your supervisor, that lasts one-half to one hour. The meeting is often based on an evaluation form with set criteria. The criteria should evaluate everything from your medical skills to your client- and staff-relation skills.

Although your supervisor evaluates you, she may solicit input from other employees and use financial data. Some of the input will be subjective—an evaluator's perception of your work. A good evaluator will attempt to gather as much objective data as possible for your review to reduce potential bias from subjective input. For example, your supervisor may consider production data such as revenue and number of procedures performed. Client feedback forms and medical charts might also be used.

During this meeting, you will hear your supervisor's evaluation of your work and have an opportunity to discuss your perception of your work as well. Once your prior performance has been evaluated, there should also be a discussion of plans and goals for the upcoming year. These should be based on skills you could still improve on as well as plans for changes in the practice at large.

A variant of the formal evaluation process is a multirater review. This type of review is frequently called a 360-degree review, but a preferable term is "world review." Some U.S. companies use these evaluations for training and development as opposed to formal appraisals and salary advancement. These evaluations are based on feedback from everyone in your professional world. Other doctors, receptionists, technicians, and kennel and exam-room assistants all have input. Even clients and vendors you interact with may be given the opportunity to provide feedback on their experience with you. Your supervisor will collate all the feedback into your review. This process provides the most honest and thorough feedback on all aspects of your work. The review meeting will still be with your supervisor alone, who will present all the information along with her own evaluation.

TIMING OF REVIEWS

When you first start working, you may be under a trial work period. There is no hard-and-fast rule as to the length of a trial period, but it typically lasts three months. That gives all parties enough time to assess whether you, the job, and the practice are a good match.

If you are hired under a trial period, you will likely have a brief review or evaluation at the end of that time frame. If there are significant problems with your performance, the evaluation will come even sooner. That three-month meeting is an excellent opportunity for you and your supervisor to discuss expectations for your performance throughout the rest of the year.

Whether or not you have a trial period or receive an interim appraisal, you should expect an annual review. Some practices conduct reviews on your employment anniversary date. That process ensures regular and timely reviews. Many practices choose to conduct all their reviews at a certain time of year, often at year end. When all employee appraisals are done at the same time, the practice can gather all the input they need just once and concentrate on this particular effort. Reviews can also be correlated with a traditionally slow time for the business to allow the extra time needed for this endeavor. Lastly, some practices offer performance bonuses to be distributed at the end of the year. In that instance, end-of-year reviews make the most sense.

In addition to scheduled reviews, your supervisor may schedule interim meetings to discuss your progress. If the practice is unhappy with your performance, you might expect an interim progress meeting to reassess your place in the practice and redefine expectations. If the problem is serious, you may even be warned that your position is in jeopardy.

> In addition to scheduled reviews, your supervisor may schedule interim meetings to discuss your progress.

GETTING THE MOST OUT OF YOUR REVIEW

An appraisal meeting should be a two-way street. In addition to learning what your supervisor has to say, you should have an opportunity to discuss the comments, gather additional information you may need, and bring up issues important to you that relate to your work at the practice. By the end of the meeting, you should be comfortable that you understand your evaluation and support the goals that have been set for the upcoming year.

Take the following steps to maximize your experience.

Obtain a Copy of the Review Form at the Time You Are Hired

Any practice that uses a standardized review form should be able to provide you with a copy of the form on request. By reviewing the form at the beginning of your employment, you will immediately get a sense for what your employer expects of you and how your employer will evaluate your job performance.

The form is likely to include criteria ranging from technical skills and knowledge base to your ability to interact successfully with clients and staff members. The ratings in each category will also give you a sense for how your performance will be evaluated. For example, if the possible ratings are "meets expectations," "does not meet expectations," or "exceeds expectations," the standard for your evaluation is clear. You are being evaluated against your job description or what you and your employer have agreed your duties and responsibilities will be.

If you are rated on a numerical scale—a scale of 1 to 10, for example—then you are more likely being evaluated against an ideal employee. Ask your employer to clarify what numerical rating most closely correlates to someone who fulfills the requirements of the job. With a numerical scale, that number may be different for different criteria. A doctor would need to have a very high value in medical knowledge and surgical skills to meet expectations, whereas a moderate value for staff interaction or organizational skills might still meet expectations. In either case, the acceptability of your job performance should be based on whether you meet the standard outlined for your position.

Often with veterinarians, there is a presumption of responsibilities and level of care that is not specifically delineated. Unfortunately, sometimes your understanding of your duties and responsibilities does not match that of your employer. Knowing the criteria and rating system that will be used for your appraisal brings expectations into clear focus.

Determine a Date for the Review

Your supervisor should provide some notice of an upcoming review, preferably two weeks. A specific time and location for the review should be selected. Consider what time of day you might prefer for the review to take place. If you will be anxious all day while you await an end-of-the-day meeting, ask to have the evaluation done first thing in the morning. If having the review early in the day will consume your thoughts for the rest of the day and interfere with your work, or if you believe the appraisal may make you emotional, ask to have the review at the end of the day. In many practices, it is not unreasonable to conduct the review after the practice has closed for the day to eliminate distractions and interruptions.

You should also establish a comfortable meeting place for the review. You and your supervisor should agree on a private location away from interruption. If you are uncomfortable with the location your supervisor chooses for the review, suggest another location that will be more comfortable for you. Some people, for example, find their supervisor's office intimidating—enemy territory, so to speak. It might be reasonable to ask for the review to take place on neutral ground, such as an exam room or library. Even an off-site location, such as a restaurant, might be considered.

> Throughout the year, keep a record of your successes and failures.
> A short comment on your daily calendar can be a great memory booster.

Prepare for the Review

Of course, excelling at your job and responding quickly to criticism is your best preparation for a positive appraisal. In addition, there are specific steps you can take to reduce the chance of surprises and maximize what you will get out of the review.

- **Keep records**—Throughout the year, keep a record of your successes and failures. A short comment on your daily calendar can be a great memory booster. Because reviews are often given annually, it can be easy to forget events in the early part of the review cycle. Make notes of especially difficult cases that you handled well and client or staff interactions that were notable. Also keep track of interactions that could have gone better or cases that you could have handled more proficiently. By keeping notes, you build a framework for a discussion of your achievements during the appraisal period and for goal setting for the upcoming appraisal period. You can also review these notes to get a fair sense of how your appraisal will go. These notes should cue you to your strengths and weaknesses that will come out during the review. This preparation should help keep you from being blindsided by a criticism during the review.

- **Collect data**—Obtain any objective data that may be available to you that could be used in forming your evaluation. For example, many practices share production data with their associates. Although your appraisal should never be based on a comparison with another doctor, it would be fair for a practice owner to evaluate the data to determine an expected level of production for each veterinarian and then decide whether or not you meet that level. If, therefore, you are in a multidoctor practice, or if you have been advised of your production target, you can get a sense for your productivity and how that will play into your evaluation. Also consider whether you are always on time for your shifts and remain on time for your appointments, and whether your surgical time is average, slower than average, or faster than average. All of these factors may be analyzed by your supervisor to form your appraisal.

- **Do a self-evaluation**—After gathering your notes and assessing other data, complete a self-evaluation in advance of your appraisal meeting. The review is not only a time for your supervisor to evaluate you, it is a time for you to evaluate yourself. Evaluate your performance over the past year, and evaluate what you want for yourself and the practice over the next year. Start by comparing yourself to the criteria on the appraisal form your supervisor will use. Use your notes and any data you have gathered to rate yourself honestly. If you are honest about your strengths and weaknesses, it is unlikely that your ratings will differ significantly from those your supervisor gives you.

> After gathering your notes and assessing other data, complete a self-evaluation in advance of your appraisal meeting.

Consider any areas where you might expect your supervisor's perception of your work to differ from your own. For instance, you may feel that you have a good ability to relate to clients and make them feel comfortable. You know, however, that your supervisor has heard complaints from two clients about an interaction with you. You and your supervisor might then have different ratings for your client skills. You will want to be prepared for the possibility of a discussion on this issue where you can reinforce your successes and build a plan with your supervisor to minimize any future negative client interactions.

- **Set goals**—Next, consider areas for improvement. If there is any area that you consider to be a weakness or believe that your supervisor will see as a weakness, prepare a plan of attack. How will you overcome this weakness? Can you be mentored in this area? Would continuing education help? Can the practice change a policy or procedure to minimize the weakness? If your weakness, for example, is that you tend to get behind schedule when you see appointments, can the practice be a little more flexible in scheduling your appointments to give you the opportunity to catch up? Perhaps one appointment slot could be left blank every two to three hours. If your weak area is orthopedic surgery, can you assist another surgeon on staff with orthopedic procedures or spend some of your time off with a local orthopedic surgeon? Perhaps you could arrange to attend an orthopedic wet lab to improve your skills.

Use your own evaluation to set goals for your next year with the practice. Your goals should incorporate plans to overcome any weak areas you have as well as meet any professional goals you have set for yourself. Is there a new procedure you would like to learn? Is there a continuing education seminar you were hoping to attend? Do you plan to expand your responsibilities into practice management? Is there a special project at the practice you would like to take on? What you want to get out of your work over the next year is important for your contentment and success with the practice.

With your self-evaluation and goals in hand, you are now ready to sit down for the review meeting.

THE REVIEW MEETING

Let your supervisor take the lead during the review to ensure that she has the opportunity to emphasize what she sees as important for you to know. Most reviewers will follow the evaluation form, advising you of your rating for each criterion. A good reviewer will also offer some interpretation of the ratings so that you will be clear whether the ratings are considered satisfactory or not. Your reviewer should also provide examples of your performance to back up the assessment.

After evaluating your performance over the last year, your reviewer is likely to summarize the assessment and discuss any areas you should improve on over the next year. These may correlate to goals you had already considered.

Whether you should make comments throughout the review or wait until the end will depend on your supervisor. Some prefer that you wait until they have finished their major points. It is important to listen openly to what you are being told and to wait for the full context. Arguing any

points of disagreement is not likely to work to your advantage. On the other hand, if you still have questions about your supervisor's satisfaction with your performance at the end of the review, do not hesitate to make pointed inquiries. "I have listened carefully to what you have said but am still wondering what you think of my work overall." "Can you tell me, specifically, what you see as my strongest assets for the practice?" "Are there any specific areas you would like me to work on?"

Salary

In some practices, the review meeting will also include a discussion about salary. If your compensation is production based, you may find that your percentage goes up based simply on your tenure or on additional skills or value you now bring to the practice. If your compensation is salary based, you will be told your new salary and, sometimes, the basis for that decision.

You should prepare for a discussion about salary in advance of the meeting by assessing your financial value to the practice. Look at your productivity and consider national and local pay scales for a veterinarian with your level of experience. With this information in hand, as well as a sense of what you want your compensation package to be, you can negotiate with your employer for the best pay and benefits. Understand, however, that if your employer believes the practice is compensating you fairly, there may not be room for negotiation.

> You should prepare for a discussion about salary in advance of the meeting by assessing your financial value to the practice.

Some practices also tie bonuses to the appraisal. Bonuses may be a standard amount or may be based on your specific value to the practice as highlighted in your evaluation. For example, a practice might give higher bonuses to employees who receive the best evaluations. Presumably, these employees contribute more to productivity and income. Bonuses are rarely negotiable.

These negotiations and the review are usually concurrent with signing a new contract. Before you sign a new contract, be sure that the terms meet your expectations and that you are committed to

225

staying with the practice. If you are planning on leaving the practice or will not be renewing your contract, do not presume that the review has no value. Even when you are dissatisfied with your job or your employer, there will be something you can take home from this meeting to enhance your future performance with this or any practice.

Conflicts

Even after a thorough self-evaluation, you may find that you disagree with your supervisor's assessment of your performance. When that occurs, it is important to give your evaluator an opportunity to finish making her point. Make sure that you have heard comments fully and in context before responding. You want to maintain professionalism during the evaluation and not argue.

When you disagree with a comment, first consider whether the comment could be valid. Even if you believe it is not, remember that the comment is the perception of your evaluator(s). Their perception of your performance is critically important. So, instead of arguing with an invalid assessment, ask questions or make comments to precipitate a discussion of the issue. "I am surprised that the assessment of my client-relations skills is that low. Can you give me some examples of where you believe I could have done a better job?" "I hadn't realized that you thought I was taking too much time in surgery. Can you give me some time guidelines you think I should be working toward?"

Emotional Responses

It is never easy to be judged. Add to that the anticipation of the unknown, and anxiety levels can run high. Some people, because of anxiety or stress, will become emotional during a review, particularly when they hear something negative about their performance. If you are inclined to an emotional response, such as crying or anger, remind yourself to keep it in check during the review so that you can communicate professionally.

If, however, despite your best efforts, you become upset, it is best to address your feelings with your reviewer. Your comment should be limited to assuring your reviewer that you can continue and that your reviewer should not be put off by your emotion. "Excuse me, Jane. I guess I am a little more anxious about this review than I thought. I would still like to hear what else you have to say."

Requests for Changes

If there is something you believe the practice could be doing better, the review can be an appropriate forum for that discussion as well—after your professional evaluation is complete. This meeting is likely your single best opportunity to optimize your integration into the practice, and that includes letting the management know how you can work best and where services might be improved.

> If there is something you believe the practice could be doing better, the review can be an appropriate forum for that discussion as well—after your professional evaluation is complete.

Perhaps you have heard the receptionists tell several clients that your practice does not see rabbits. You are willing and able to examine and treat rabbits. Take advantage of this meeting to suggest that you start seeing rabbits, and discuss any staff training or new equipment that will be needed. If your practice does not have a blood-pressure monitor, you might suggest that a practice goal for the upcoming year is to purchase a monitor and train all veterinarians and technicians in its use.

Be prepared to discuss how often the monitor might be used, what cases it will be used for, and the cost. Although these suggestions for professional and practice growth can appropriately be made at any time during the year, the review is often the only planning meeting you can count on to have your employer's undivided attention. This part of the discussion also shows your employer that you are thinking about the big picture with the practice and are interested in expanding services. Your request may take your supervisor by surprise; therefore, it is best not to expect an immediate response to your request.

Ending the Review

Leave the meeting as professionally as you can. Summarize any lingering points as well as your goals for the upcoming year. Thank your evaluator for her time and thoughtful comments.

Often, your reviewer will ask you to sign the review form before leaving. Signing the form does not necessarily indicate that you agree with all the ratings or comments. Signing means that you have received the evaluation. You should be given an opportunity to rebut anything you believe to be inaccurate or to add any comments regarding your performance that you want to be part of your permanent record. Your comments can be written on the evaluation form that you sign or added on at a later date. You may write down your comments and submit them to your supervisor at a later date to add to your review form.

WHEN NO REVIEW IS OFFERED

If you are in a practice that does not offer a formal evaluation, you are missing a tremendous growth opportunity. It may even be difficult for you to feel comfortable that your supervisor is pleased with your work and that your skills are progressing as quickly as they should.

It can be awkward to challenge the status quo or to ask for an evaluation of your performance. If you do not ask, however, your supervisor will never know that you want one. If you are starting a new job, you can address this issue when you are hired. Ask when you will be given a performance appraisal. If you are advised that you will not receive an appraisal, simply ask if it is possible to schedule one in six to twelve months. If you sense some hesitation, you might add that you want to ensure that you are meeting the practice's expectations for performance.

If you have already been in your position for a while and are sure that your supervisor does not intend to provide a review, find a quiet time to approach her with your request. "Dr. Smith, I have been with the practice for several months

now and was hoping we could schedule a time to sit down and talk about my work and expectations for the upcoming months." That will usually be enough to get the meeting scheduled. If it is not, and you are met with a response such as, "Everything is fine," follow up with, "I'm glad to know that you think things are going well. I believe I could do a better job if we looked more closely at my work. Can you find a half hour or an hour to sit down with me?"

Because your supervisor is not accustomed to providing a performance appraisal, you may need to help steer the discussion rather than leaving it all in your boss's hands. It will be especially important to prepare for the meeting and have a list of questions and discussion points, because your supervisor may not prepare. She might just look you in the eye and say, "So, what do *you* want to talk about?" I suggest that you ask your boss to cover the following areas:

- In what specific ways have I been most successful in my job and in meeting your expectations?

- Where do you think I still need to improve the most?

- What problem areas have you seen or had someone bring to your attention?

- Is there any aspect of my work that must be improved for me to keep my job?

- What skills would you like me to work on over the next year?

- Will there be any changes in the practice that may affect me?

Let your supervisor know that you find this feedback valuable and that you would benefit from regular meetings. Add your goals and expectations for the upcoming year.

The "no-review" scenario means more work for you in the short run. In the long run, you will find that the professional feedback contributes to your best work.

RESOURCES

Books

A Practical Guide to Performance Appraisals by K. Gendron. Available through AAHA.

227

The Complete Guide to Performance Appraisals by D. Grote.

The Complete Idiot's Guide to Performance Appraisals by A. Margrave and R. Gorden.

Partners in Performance: Successful Performance Management by T. Moglia.

Websites

About.com
www.humanresources.about.com
This site offers human resources articles and links as well as a free newsletter.

www.work911.com
Hundreds of free resources on a wide range of workplace issues.

► CHAPTER TWENTY ◄

Employment Laws You Need to Know

Kerry M. Richard, Esq.

IN THIS CHAPTER, YOU'LL LEARN:

- **The basics of at-will employment**
- **What you need to know about antidiscrimination laws**
- **Your rights regarding wages, leave, and workplace safety**

A wide variety of laws govern employer-employee relationships. These laws generally come from three sources:

- Common law
- Federal legislation
- State or local legislation

It is important to have a basic understanding of the types of laws governing the employment relationship, because these laws set the parameters for day-to-day employment decisions made by you and your employer. This chapter discusses the laws that apply to most employer-employee relationships, including the general rules of at-will employment, antidiscrimination legislation, wage and hour legislation, leave laws, and workplace safety requirements. Keep in mind that laws vary from state to state; therefore, before relying on any topic discussed in this chapter, it is wise to check the statutes and cases that apply in your particular state or municipality.

EMPLOYMENT AT WILL

Since the late 1800s, most employment relationships have been presumed to be at will. Simply put, this means that the employment relationship continues as long as it suits both the employer and the employee. Either party can terminate the relationship at any time—for any reason or for no reason. This rule is the default rule of employment today. Any offer of employment that does not specify a definite term is deemed to be employment at will. Because most employees do not have contracts for a definite term, most employees are at-will employees.

The at-will rule has been defended as necessary to level the playing field for employers. Specifically, an employee, even one with a written contract for a definite term, can always quit at any time—for any reason or no reason. To require otherwise would be to condone involuntary servitude —slavery. Thus, the at-will rule has been rationalized as necessary to give an employer the same rights as an employee.

While acknowledging the meritorious purpose of the at-will rule, courts and legislatures have created substantial exceptions to the blanket at-will rule. Today, it would be more accurate to state that an employer can terminate an at-will employment relationship at any time—for any *lawful* reason, or for no reason.

Court-Created Limitations to the At-Will Rule

In an effort to avoid the seemingly harsh at-will rule, courts have looked for ways to *imply* a "definite term" in an employment relationship. For example, statements like "You will always have a job here," or "As long as you come to work, you will have a job," have been found to imply a contract for life (a definite term). In addition, courts have looked at employee manuals and other documents to find contractual promises not to discharge without cause.

Courts have also created exceptions to the at-will rule. Almost every state today recognizes that an at-will employment relationship cannot be terminated for a reason that violates public policy. The so-called Public Policy Exception has been defined in a variety of ways by courts in different states, but basically, it means that it is illegal to discharge an employee for a reason that contradicts a well-articulated public policy. Some typical examples are:

- It is illegal to terminate an employee because that employee has responded to a valid summons to perform jury duty.

- It is illegal to terminate an employee because that employee refused to falsify records that the employer is required by law to maintain.

In both of these examples, there is a well-articulated public policy in favor of the employee's behavior (i.e., encouraging juror service or encouraging compliance with laws); thus, the courts have prohibited employers from discharging employees for these reasons.

This Public Policy Exception is normally construed narrowly. If an employee cannot demonstrate

that he or she was terminated for engaging in conduct that the law requires, or that he or she was terminated for refusing to violate the law, the termination is lawful. However, this area of law continues to evolve. Some courts have recognized other specific exceptions to the at-will rule, and others have more broadly construed the definition of public policy. Where courts have not been active, legislatures have stepped in.

Legislatively Created Exceptions to the At-Will Rule

Federal and state legislatures, and in some cases, county and city authorities, have been active in creating limitations on the rule of at-will employment. For example, Congress has enacted laws forbidding the termination of an employee on the basis of race, national origin, ethnicity, religion, sex (including pregnancy), age, disability status, status as a disabled or Vietnam-era veteran, or citizenship status. Most states have enacted laws that are duplicative of the federal laws, but many of them have added additional prohibitions. For example, in Washington, D.C., in addition to forbidding termination on the basis of the protected categories set forth above, an employer cannot terminate an employee on the basis of that employee's marital status, political affiliation, sexual orientation, personal appearance, source of income, or matriculation status, among others. In addition, both federal and state laws prohibit terminating an employee who complains about an employer disregarding these laws, or who participates in an investigation of a complaint related to these laws.

> It is important to note that most of the prohibitions created by federal laws apply only to employers who have fifteen or more employees.

It is important to note that most of the prohibitions created by federal laws apply only to employers who have fifteen or more employees. State laws also have size limitations. However, some courts have found that smaller employers who are not specifically covered by federal or state statutes may still be violating public policy if they terminate an employee on the basis of a protected status created by federal or state law. For example, in Maryland, an equine veterinarian with three employees terminated a female veterinarian because he said his clients were skeptical about a woman's ability to perform as an equine practitioner. The female veterinarian sued, claiming that her termination was wrongful because it was based on sex. The employer argued that he was excluded from coverage under the federal or state laws because he was too small. The Maryland court ruled that even though the employer was not technically covered by the statutes, the statutes constituted a clear statement of Maryland's public policy against sex discrimination; thus, her discharge constituted a wrongful discharge in violation of public policy.

ANTIDISCRIMINATION LAWS

The same federal and state laws that limit an employer's right to terminate employees at will also prohibit an employer from discriminating against protected employees in any other aspect of employment. Specifically, an employer cannot discriminate against an applicant or employee in hiring, promotion, discipline, compensation, benefits, transfer, layoff, recall from layoff, access to training, or access to company-sponsored social events. As you can see, these laws affect all aspects of the employment relationship. The following sections summarize each of the major federal laws prohibiting discrimination. Where applicable, reference is also made to corresponding state laws.

Civil Rights Act of 1964 (Title VII)

Title VII prohibits employers with fifteen or more employees from discriminating in any aspect of employment against an individual on the basis of sex, race, national origin, or religion. Title VII also prohibits the harassment of an individual on the basis of that individual's protected status. This law is most commonly applied in the context of sexual harassment, where it prohibits an employer from conditioning an employment benefit on submission to sex (*quid pro quo* harassment), as well as from creating or tolerating a hostile work environment. A hostile work environment in the context of sexual harassment is one in which conduct, language, or atmosphere is so sexually charged or intimidating that it would interfere with a reasonable person's ability to work.

Again, while this law is most commonly applied to harassment based on sex, the law prohibits harassment on the basis of any protected category, including, among others, race, national origin, or religion. All states except Mississippi, Georgia, and Alabama have enacted their own laws protecting employees from employment discrimination. Many of these state laws cover employers with fewer than fifteen employees.

Age Discrimination in Employment Act of 1967 (ADEA)

The ADEA prohibits employers with twenty or more employees from discriminating against individuals who are age forty or older in any aspect of employment. Once again, many parallel state laws cover smaller employers. In addition, many state laws remove the age limit (forty), simply prohibiting employers from considering age as a factor in employment decisions. To protect older workers from layoffs and forced retirements, the ADEA imposes special restrictions on an employer's ability to lay off or terminate older workers. For example, when an older worker is being asked or offered the opportunity to retire early, the employee must be given a window in which to consider the offer, must be advised of his or her right to contact an attorney, must be given a list of other affected individuals (and their ages), must be told that he or she might have rights under the ADEA, and must be offered benefits that are no less generous than what the employee would receive if he or she retired normally.

Americans with Disabilities Act of 1990 (ADA)

The ADA prohibits employers with fifteen or more employees from discriminating against qualified individuals with disabilities. A qualified individual with a disability is one who has a physical or mental impairment that substantially limits a major life activity, but who can perform the essential functions of a job, with or without accommodation. If an individual with a disability is qualified for the job, the ADA requires employers to make reasonable accommodation, if necessary, to allow the individual to perform a job. Accommodations can include changes to the physical workspace, the purchase of assistive devices, flexible scheduling, leaves of absence, and/or a change in job descriptions, among others.

The ADA is a comparatively new law. There are many gray areas, and it is a very complex statute. It is hoped that, with time, the court will make the requirements of this statute clearer. As with Title VII and the ADEA, most states prohibit disability discrimination. Because most state disability discrimination provisions were enacted before the ADA, state laws can vary substantially from the ADA.

The Immigration Reform and Control Act of 1986 (IRCA)

The IRCA prohibits employers from discriminating against individuals on the basis of U.S. citizenship. Instead, the law focuses the relevant inquiry on whether an individual is authorized to work in the United States. Many noncitizens are lawful residents of the United States with proper permission to work. As long as an individual applicant can demonstrate that he or she is authorized to work in the United States, it is illegal to prefer another candidate simply because the other candidate is a U.S. citizen. The IRCA also requires employers to keep careful records verifying the identity and work authorization of their employees while simultaneously prohibiting employers from asking for any information or documentation that exceeds the information deemed necessary by the IRCA.

Remedial Scheme for Discrimination Claims

Almost all claims of discrimination, federal or state, must be brought first into an administrative arena. Specifically, a charge must be filed with the federal Equal Employment Opportunity Commission (EEOC) or a state counterpart.

Typically, claims are waived unless they are filed within 300 days from the date of the discrimination. These claims must then be processed at the EEOC (or other agency) for at least sixty days, before an individual can ask for a right-to-sue letter. After sixty days, if an individual prefers, he or she can obtain a right-to-sue letter and then file a claim in court. If an individual goes to court without first having filed and obtained a right-to-sue letter, the individual's claim will be barred. Discrimination statutes offer a variety of remedies, including reinstatement, back pay, attorney fees, and, in some cases, front pay, compensatory damages (pain and suffering and emotional distress), and punitive damages.

WAGE AND HOUR LAWS AND REGULATIONS

The federal Fair Labor Standards Act (FLSA) and corresponding state laws require employers to pay most employees on an hourly basis—a wage equal to at least $5.15 per hour (the federal minimum wage)—and to pay most employees at a rate of time and one-half for all time worked more than forty hours per work week.

Veterinarians are in most cases exempt from coverage under the FLSA as professionals. This means that employers can hire veterinarians on a salaried basis and can expect more than forty hours of work from a veterinarian without having to pay additional compensation. It also means, however, that employers cannot normally dock the pay of salaried veterinarians for working less than forty hours in a given work week. There are certain exceptions to this rule, such as when a veterinarian employee has used up all earned leave time and misses additional days.

The FLSA also requires employers to keep records, such as time sheets, payroll-calculation information, and attendance records for employees. Finally, the FLSA limits the employment of minors.

> **Veterinarians are in most cases exempt from coverage under the FLSA as professionals. This means that employers can hire veterinarians on a salaried basis and can expect more than forty hours of work from a veterinarian without having to pay additional compensation.**

Most states have enacted laws that supplement the FLSA. Some have set the state minimum wage at a rate higher than the federal minimum wage. In addition, some states have put limits on the number of hours per day an employee can work, some require certain meal and/or work breaks per day worked, and some states require those breaks to be paid breaks. Furthermore, almost every state legislates how often employees must be paid—not less than monthly, and frequently, biweekly or weekly. These laws also regulate what deductions may lawfully be taken from an employee's paycheck and require employees to be given notice of any deductions from gross pay. In the great majority of states, it is a misdemeanor to fail to pay wages when due, especially at the termination of employment.

> In the great majority of states, it is a misdemeanor to fail to pay wages when due, especially at the termination of employment.

LEAVE LAWS

There are a number of federal and state laws that provide employees with a right to take leave from work. These laws include the federal Family and Medical Leave Act of 1993 (FMLA) and its state counterparts, jury leave, voting leave, school leave, and military leave. In addition, there are a number of other types of leaves of absence that are not statutorily required, but that employers frequently provide, such as vacation time, sick leave, disability leave, or bereavement leave. Although an employer is not required to offer leaves of this type, if an employer does, there are certain rules concerning the provision of those leaves.

- **FMLA leave**—The FMLA requires employers with fifty or more employees in a seventy-five-mile radius to offer eligible employees up to twelve weeks of leave from work upon the birth or adoption of a child, to care for a family member with a serious health condition, or to care for his or her own serious health condition. An eligible employee is one who has worked for the employer for at least twelve months and has worked at least 1,250 hours in the past twelve

months. FMLA leave can be paid, partially paid, or unpaid, but an employer must continue to provide the employee with health-insurance coverage during the leave period. In addition, the leave may in some circumstances be taken intermittently, as long as the total leave is no more than twelve weeks in twelve months.

An employee who takes an FMLA leave is normally entitled to be reinstated to the same or a similar position, without loss of seniority or benefits, as long as the employee returns from leave in accordance with the FMLA.

Obviously, most veterinary employers will not meet the FMLA size requirements (fifty employees); thus, most veterinary employees are not entitled to take FMLA leave. There are, however, states that provide parallel leave to employees of smaller employers. The eligibility, duration, benefits, and rehire provisions of the state laws all vary but frequently provide a substantial benefit.

- **Jury leave**—Almost all states have provisions requiring employers to grant a leave of absence to an employee who is summoned to serve as a juror or to act as a witness in a court proceeding. Many, but not all, states require that the employee continue to receive pay during jury service. At a minimum, employees are not to be punished for missing work to serve as a juror.

- **Voting leave**—Many, but not all, states require an employer to allow employees sufficient time off from work (usually two hours) while voting polls are open to allow the employee to vote in county, state, or federal elections. If the employee is an hourly employee, the time generally does not need to be paid, but a salaried employee cannot be docked for voting time.

- **School leave**—School leave laws are a recent trend. Some states have enacted laws that require employers to give employees with school-age children a certain number of hours off work per year to attend school conferences and/or other functions. Although this leave time can technically be unpaid, an employer

233

cannot normally require an employee to use vacation or sick-leave time for these purposes, and, as with voting leave, salaried employees cannot be docked for taking school leave.

- **Military leave**—Federal and state laws require that employers allow employees who are called to military service or who must fulfill military-reserve requirements to take the necessary leave from work. If an individual is called to active duty, the employer must permit that individual to go, and must reemploy that individual in the same or a similar position without loss of benefits, seniority, or pay, upon his or her return—providing the individual remains qualified to perform the position, and the individual reapplies for work within the statutory window.

  These laws were last updated at the end of the Persian Gulf War, when those on military leave began returning from active duty and sought to reenter the work force. The war in Iraq has required the mobilization of a far greater number of reservists for a much longer time. To ensure the smooth reentry of those reservists into the work force, it is likely that the current military leave laws will be substantially revised. To protect your rights and ensure compliance with the law, review the military leave laws in effect at the time the issue arises.

- **Voluntary leave benefits**—Although not required by law, most employers offer certain paid or partially paid leave benefits, including vacation, sick, disability, or bereavement leave. If offered, these leaves must be applied in a nondiscriminatory fashion. For example, if an employer allows a male employee who suffers a heart attack (and therefore must miss six weeks of work) to take paid leave to recuperate, then the employer must offer the same treatment to a female who gives birth and requires a period of time to convalesce. Both conditions result in a temporary disability, and there is no legiti-

mate basis to treat the two differently. This is true even if the employer is not required to provide any FMLA leave.

WORKPLACE SAFETY LEGISLATION

The Occupational Safety and Health Act creates a general duty for employers to protect the safety and health of their employees. Relying on this authority, the Occupational Safety and Health Administration (OSHA) has issued a number of safety standards with which employers must comply. Generally, employers are required to advise employees of the existence of any known hazards in the workplace, to provide personal protective equipment, and to provide training to employees that will enable them to safely handle known hazards. In addition, employers must provide training and equipment to enable employees to respond to a fire emergency safely, as well as keep records of the existence of hazards, training provided, and safety protocols.

Employees who believe their employer is not meeting these standards can report the employer to OSHA, and an investigation will follow. If violations are found, a citation will be issued, and the employer may be fined. Employees who report in good faith are protected from any form of retaliation for reporting. Bad faith reports can be prosecuted.

In addition to the extensive safety regulations issued by OSHA, some states have issued their own safety standards and conduct their own safety inspections. States also require all employers to maintain workers' compensation insurance for employees who are injured or become sick in a work-related incident. The insurance covers an employee's medical bills and provides some salary replacement during the employee's recovery.

There are nearly 200 federal and state statutes regulating the employment relationship in a

> Generally, employers are required to advise employees of the existence of any known hazards in the workplace, to provide personal protective equipment, and to provide training to employees that will enable them to safely handle known hazards.

234

given state; this chapter has discussed some of the more common legal topics. Whenever an employment issue arises, it is safe to assume that there is some legislation or case law that defines the obligations of employers and employees in resolving the issue.

RESOURCES

Books

Every Employee's Guide to the Law: What You Need to Know About Your Rights in the Workplace—And What to Do If They Are Violated by L. Joel.

The American Bar Association Guide to Workplace Law: Everything You Need to Know About Your Rights as an Employee or Employer by B. Fick.

Websites

Americans With Disabilities Act
www.ada.gov

Occupational Safety and Health Administration
www.osha.gov

U.S. Department of Labor
www.dol.gov

U.S. Equal Opportunity Commission
www.eeoc.gov

CHAPTER TWENTY-ONE

Getting the Most Out of Association Memberships

Samuel M. Fassig, DVM, MA

IN THIS CHAPTER, YOU'LL LEARN:

- **The benefits of association membership**
- **Why it's important to be involved in a professional association**

Business today is so complicated and complex and constantly undergoing change that only the unwise attempt to go it alone. And any time people come together with similar interests and common bonds, it intensifies energy and enthusiasm. It also promotes being open to a sharing of ideas. Professional associations provide this platform for veterinarians.

WHAT'S IN IT FOR YOU?

Although you may wonder, "What's in it for me?" you might be better off asking, "What will I lose by not being a part of an organization that promotes high quality and standards in veterinary medicine?" Just remember—there are new frontiers ahead of you, your colleagues, and the profession in general.

For example, you may need protection from litigation and large settlement awards for emotional damage as companion animals no longer are looked upon as just property in the eyes of the law. If you are detached as a practitioner, you can be singled out and become easy prey for an aggressive attorney. Without the ability to show you are making an effort to maintain a standard of care, improve your professionalism, and keep abreast of knowledge that is set as the norm by your peers, you will soon be isolated and out of touch with mainstream veterinary medicine.

One of the most valuable benefits is the opportunity to interact with colleagues who understand your issues, problems, successes, and stresses. At meetings, dialogues often take on mentoring overtones, allowing you to examine what worked for others and what their approaches were to problem-solving. This exchange of information will afford you multiple contexts, professional and social, through which you can expand your perspectives, challenge your assumptions, and enjoy a sense of peer-group camaraderie. Membership provides you with opportunities to create networks and understand what is on the horizon for the industry.

If you reciprocate and interact, helping another member succeed—even in some small way—it will help you redefine and reflect on your own goals, assumptions, and ways of doing things. One of the shortcuts to success is helping others succeed.

Membership does require some form of commitment, even if it is just to pay the dues to get the journal and respond to the occasional survey. The more proactive you are, the more resources you will have available to help you in your career.

Through membership, you will also be afforded the opportunity to assume a leadership role. Depending on the type of association, its actions may influence federal or state legislation affecting practice, the animal-health industry, or the manner in which veterinarians are assimilated into society. For you, it means the chance to grow your own character.

Intangible Benefits of Membership

Some of the best reasons for belonging to and participating in associations are:

- You can tap into vast sources of winning expertise, mentorship, and camaraderie.

- You can stimulate your own personal and professional growth.

- You will receive emotional, spiritual, and holistic support from others who have been there.

- You can contribute guidance to move the profession in directions it needs to go.

- You can protect the profession in a united front from special-interest groups that have significant funding and power, yet may be somewhat misguided or uninformed in their beliefs.

- You can prevent harm from coming to the unknowing and unsuspecting.

- You can promote the features and attributes of being a veterinarian, and, in general, enrich the profession by sharing the high standards, interests, and contributions of this group of professionals with the rest of the world.

- You can contribute to unity in the profession and one-voice input on local and national issues.

As an associate, it is your privilege to seek and enjoy the benefits of membership by rite of passage, if nothing else. It is also your responsibility as long as you are a part of the veterinary medical community. Your involvement should not be just for personal-growth benefits, which will be many, but also for the collective well-being of your professional fellowship. Affiliate with groups that fuel your passions and with one or two that make you stretch or entice you to broaden your scope. Who said they all have to be veterinary-related? Anything that makes you exercise your mind will only help you in your quest to be a better person.

Associations are currently revisiting their visions, taking a good look at why their particular values and goals should be attractive to other veterinarians. This process requires hard questions, considerable membership input, and courage of the group to act, and it will test the character of the organization. Your involvement and perspective, especially as a new associate, are invaluable to the process. You are the face of change, and you may have different wants and needs than those who came before you.

If you are a member, you have the right, obligation, and responsibility to critique and be part of any leadership or change process. If you do not belong, you are most likely not part of the solution either, which, when set, may have a considerable impact on your career. When the dust settles, and you have chosen not to be a part of the proceedings, you have no real standing from which to voice a complaint. Get involved, even if it is to promote your own agenda. Such involvement adds to the mix, empowers the group, and promotes evolutionary change.

Tangible Benefits of Association Membership

The tangible benefits most people think of when they're deciding whether to join an organization include:

- Discounted malpractice/negligence insurance

- Liability insurance

- Life and premise insurance

- Disability insurance

238

- Low-interest credit cards

- Collective buying power for supplies and services

- Access to survey results, publications, newsletters, magazines, or journals

- Free or low-cost business consults

- Reduced continuing-education registration rates

- Discounts on publications

One of the best paybacks from association membership is being able to attend educational conferences. Aside from the fact that many states still require some form of approved continuing education for license renewal, where else do you have the chance to gain product and technical information on a wide spectrum of topics? Where else can you immediately question what you have heard with peers? The hallway conversations, the shuttle-ride conversations, and the coffee shop discussions frequently yield the most practical tidbits of immediately useful information.

Continuing-education experiences can take the form of lectures, pure academic short courses, wet labs, internships, and work at remote sites. Who says a discussion around a campfire during a rafting trip is less informative than a formal classroom lecture? It basically depends on your adult learning style, the skill of the presenter, and your willingness to entertain new ideas.

Seek to expand your reference base and stretch yourself. You best accomplish that by networking, belonging to professional organizations and common-interest groups, getting involved in mentoring experiences, and participating in other types of community activities. Undoubtedly along the way, you will challenge your values and beliefs and perhaps alter your perspectives.

RESOURCES

Books

Awaken the Giant Within by A. Robbins.

Enhancing Adult Motivation to Learn by R. Wlodkowski.

The AVMA Directory and Resource Manual, published annually by the American Veterinary Medical Association.

The Magic of Conflict: Turning a Life of Work into a Work of Art by T. Crum.

Magazine Articles

"Friend or Foe?" by K. Johnson in *TRENDS*, Vol. XVIII, No. 6.

"Putting 'Essence' Into Veterinary Continuing Education" (3 parts) by S. Fassig in *JAVMA*, Vol. 204, Nos. 8, 9, and 10.

▶ PART FIVE ◀

Taking Care
of Yourself

CHAPTER TWENTY-TWO

Managing Your Time

Samuel M. Fassig, DVM, MA

Shannon Pigott, CVPM

IN THIS CHAPTER, YOU'LL LEARN:

- **Basic principles for managing your time**

- **How to effectively manage time spent with patients, clients, and medical records**

Time has no independent existence apart from the order of events by which we measure it.
—Albert Einstein

The manner in which you spend your time defines who you are more than what you wear, what you say, the people whom you choose to be your friends, or what you think. What you do—not what you say—provides insight into your values. You can say you love your spouse and family and that they are the most important aspect of your life. Yet you may spend very little time playing with the kids, relating to your spouse, visiting either set of parents, or participating in family activities. Although it is an old cliché, in many respects it holds great truth—it isn't what you say, it's what you do that counts.

BASIC PRINCIPLES FOR MANAGING YOUR TIME

No two people have the same concept of what represents perfect time management. While there is no "one-size-fits-all" plan for managing time, here are some basic principles to follow:

- **Create and implement a good plan**—You need to design a plan that accurately reflects the day-to-day realities of your work and other responsibilities, allowing for the usual interruptions, crises, and delays. You should be able to handle these events with a little room to spare.

- **Schedule "free time" for leisure activities**—To achieve balance in your life, the best time-management plans are holistic. This means including dedicated blocks of time for family, friends, exercise, sports, special events, or projects. These things are often forgotten or put on the back burner for "whatever time is left" at the end of the day.

- **Underpromise and overdeliver**—Set due dates for certain types of work when scheduling time with clients. For example, set the approximate length of time it takes you to do a physical examination with vaccination and the length of surgery intervals that are not just meetable but bearable. If a receptionist or technician schedules exam time and surgeries, give this person some realistic guidelines for how long it usually takes for such an exam or procedure. If you are in a mobile or farm-call practice, try to figure out what it takes for a routine setup and exam time. If you somewhat overestimate the time it will take to complete a job or course of action, you can ensure on-time delivery even in the face of delays, and you can surprise and delight your client, boss, and family by delivering the goods sooner than anticipated.

- **Reduce big jobs into smaller, more manageable chunks**—Eat the elephant one bite at a time. By breaking a big task into manageable steps, setting a timetable for doing each step, and chipping away at the project, you can accomplish almost anything and with a lot less stress than if you try to tackle it all at once.

> Working longer and longer hours (whether for extra pay or not) upsets the balance between work and leisure that is essential to your health and well-being.

- **Measure**—If you are working on a project (like making an annual herd-improvement plan for a client's cattle), a speaking engagement, or event, it is important and easy to create some timeline guides to keep you on track. Identify the major steps or milestones on the way to completion. If you set realistic target dates, your progress should match your plan. Leave room in your schedule to make some work-in-progress notes, reminders, and a little buffer of time in case you do fall behind.

- **Delegate**—If you have all kinds of reasons for doing things yourself ("It takes too long to explain or show someone else," or "I just end up having to do it all over again"), you may be holding onto the idea that it is useless to try to delegate. Guess what? You are not as indispensable as you think. Delegate those routine, time-consuming tasks to someone else. Be aware that teaching someone else the ropes will take a bit of time. Take time to stress why these tasks need to be done and how they help with the overall animal healthcare team's mission. Not only can you become a hero for helping someone else gain more responsibility and

interest in the practice (and perhaps both of you being favorably noticed by the boss), but you will gain time, decrease your stress level, and perhaps boost staff loyalty for being interested in what they have to offer. This may be an opportunity for you to mentor a technician or coworker and stimulate this coworker's intellectual and personal growth.

- **Set limits**—Working longer and longer hours (whether for extra pay or not) upsets the balance between work and leisure that is essential to your health and well-being. Not being able to say "no" and set time limits on your work may also have a negative effect on your reputation. Almost everyone ends up working late or bringing work home once in a while. That is being a team member. However, if you find yourself doing it more and more often, it may be time to say "no."

- **Develop priority lists**—Some people make three lists at once: one for high priority (must be done), otherwise called the "A" list; a medium-priority or "B" list for less urgent or moderately important tasks; and one list for those things it would be nice to do if there is time. The key, of course, is to put the most important at the top and make the list doable. Other people make one list at the end of each day for things to do tomorrow. Set a priority. Try to at least get the top three things on the list done each day.

- **Pinpoint your hours of peak performance**—To maximize your time, group tasks according to skills required to do the work. Try to do the hardest jobs—those requiring the most focused concentration and peak efficiency from you—at the times of the day when your attention and energy levels are the highest. Even better, try to incorporate those tasks during periods of fewest interruptions. Schedule the low-level tasks for times of the day when you find it hard to concentrate and disruptions abound.

- **Develop shortcuts**—It is never too late to incorporate new and better ways of doing things into your routine. It is always tempting to do things the old way, just because it is the most familiar. Finding, adapting, and applying efficient new techniques and methodologies not only saves time, it can cut down on the overall workload and make you look good in the process.

- **Managing "face time"**—If you are expected to stick around the office until the boss goes home, say 6:15 P.M., and you have nothing to do, you could sit there and twiddle your thumbs and drink coffee, or you could ask others if they need help. You could also finish your to-do lists or start your own side project or look up something medical regarding a case you recently treated as a way of self-directed learning. Time is not an entity that can be purchased or replaced. Once spent, it's gone. Do you waste time so much during the day that you have to stay late just to catch up? If you are spending too much time at the office, ask yourself, "Am I really accomplishing something, or am I wasting valuable time I could be spending getting things done? Are there ways that I can be more efficient?"

- **Understand that it is what you do with your time that counts**—Others will not value you as an employee because of how much time you spend at the clinic. They value the results you produce, your contribution to the bottom line, and your empowerment of the group. If you dedicate yourself to focusing on the task and do not allow yourself to get distracted, you can get a lot completed in a reasonable period. You can be focused, accomplish what needs to get done, and still laugh. Just think of the operating theater portrayed in the TV series *M.A.S.H.*, where determined healthcare providers were intelligent, patient-focused, and interactively responsive as a team. This included incorporating music, humor, and laughter under very hectic and stressful circumstances. Production was incredibly high. Play was valued as a means to help the team, to cope with the adversity of persistent demands on their time, to heighten their awareness of life's value, and to reflect on the gift of being alive.

- **Value what you do**—Most of us gripe about our jobs far more than we crow about them. Did you know that children are more likely to look up to and respect their parents and want to emulate them if they think their parents like their work and what they do? Can you provide answers for these questions: How does your work contribute to the larger good? What can you do to make your days even more worthwhile? Are there ways to make your work relationships richer? As your passion grows, so does utilization of your time. Ever get that rush and notice how time seems to fly when you are actively focused and engaged in what you are doing? Those sparks help you to stay on track. Everyone faces the danger of procrastinating the things they dislike in order to get to the "fun" stuff. It takes discipline to get the "routine" bits and pieces done in order to get to the really good parts. If you are bored and not stimulated, the day drags by. When it is time to go home, all too often you may discover that you have yet to get your work done.

THE TOP TEN MYTHS ABOUT TIME SPENT AT WORK

Let's take a look at some of the assumptions and myths about time spent at work, along with suggestions for how to deal with them.

Myth #1:

Most people are overworked because of the nature of their jobs. It is not the job—it is the person doing it. Sure, unexpected events can create too much work. (Three regular and two new clients come in all at once, at closing time, each with a patient in crisis. Several technicians fall sick to the flu, and all the veterinarians are booked solid. A key staff member quits unexpectedly, leaving the clinic in the lurch.) However, if you repeatedly work too much, it is often the result of your failure to delegate and inability to say "no," as well as your failure to establish proper priorities. Or, it could be the fact that you are spending too much time on details and trivia, or perhaps you are just plain sloppy with your work habits.

If this is true for you, stand back and take a look at your job. Does the practice need additional staff? Are you delegating, saying no, and doing activities that are really your responsibility to get done? Do you need new ways to work? Do you need to train a technician how to do some of the tasks?

> If you repeatedly work too much, it is often the result of your failure to delegate and inability to say "no," as well as your failure to establish proper priorities.

Myth #2:

246

Your job is unique and does not have patterns. All jobs have patterns. To identify the work patterns of your job, you need data, and you need to think about cause-and-effect relationships. For example, people seldom know the pattern of their phone use during the day. How many calls do you field, at what times, from whom, about what? How many problems or questions are handled on the first call? How many require one or more callbacks? Are you the one who should be making the callbacks? If so, when do you make them? Do certain people call about certain things on a regular basis each month or at certain times of each week? Do you get the drug reps' calls even though you do not do the ordering for the clinic? Does the front-office staff relay calls to you that someone else should be getting?

With enough data, you can identify the patterns, anticipate events, and make schedules to accommodate them more efficiently. You can gain more control by scheduling them at a more convenient time for you and establishing what types of calls you should receive.

Myth #3:

No one ever has enough time. Time is a paradox. No one ever has enough, yet everyone has all the time in the world. The problem is not the amount of time you have, but how you spend it. There is always enough time to do what is really important.

Write out your objectives and priorities. Arrange your schedule to spend more time on the high-priority items and less time on low-priority things.

Myth #4

Delaying and taking more time to make a decision will improve the quality of your decisions.

Unnecessary delay will not enhance the quality of the decision. If you habitually delay making decisions until you have every scrap of information, you are probably just procrastinating. Sometimes, "sleeping on" a decision can be beneficial. This is especially true if others may be involved, if it has financial consequences, or if the end result will have other far-reaching effects.

Example

A veterinary distributor is offering your clinic a deal on a piece of equipment that also takes a new kind of inhalation agent your staff has never used. From what you and your boss have heard at continuing-education events and from a few colleagues, the boss is interested but not sure if this is a right move for the clinic at this time. Not one to look away from new advances in veterinary medicine, he asks you to make the determining evaluation. This is your project, and ultimately the decision will be yours. He has already informed the other associates that he will go with whatever you decide. To make your decision, you know you will need the following:

- All the available information on the delivery equipment, a list of reference contacts who already have it in place, and some competitor pricing

- Information from some key leaders in anesthesia and at a few veterinary schools to fully get the overall picture of whether this kind of system will do what you expect, including hazards and benefits

- Scientific reports of performance, gleaned from a sensible literature search

- Time to evaluate costs of purchase, daily operation, and required staff training time

- Research as to future availability of the inhalation product

- An analysis on how to pass on the higher costs to the client

- A "buy-in" from your other veterinary colleagues on staff, through informational meetings, progress reports, gathering of objections, and a presentation regarding your findings

This is a big "to-do" list. It is your first major decision for the practice and a purchase you do not want to make hastily. If you had to do it right now, you are not sure what you would recommend. It seems that reaching a decision will take a lot of your time.

First, make a written plan with timelines in your calendar to get each step done, measure your progress, and set up colleague meetings well in advance.

If you delegate parts of the information-gathering process (giving guidelines as to what types of information you need) to staff members, such as technicians, a number of side benefits may occur:

- It may actually entice staff buy-in and product acceptance before the product is actually in the clinic.

- Staff may get a "heads up" about usage pitfalls, as well as information from other clinics that are using the technology and what they experienced when training their staff and actually began using the product.

- When staff share what they are learning with other staff, the formal educational learning curve for the product may be shortened. That could save training time and money for the hospital. It will at least heighten their awareness of the product.

Guess what? The huge elephant just got nibbled down to a reasonable, plate-sized piece for you. You did not have to divert hefty amounts of your time to gather all the information. The decision-making process became a team-building event, and if it becomes costly to put into practice, everyone on the team has some awareness of why it will be more expensive to the client and why the medical team has

> Managing your time to accomplish important objectives requires making hard decisions about how to respond to particular people.

decided to implement the change. Armed with this information, the staff can more readily handle client objections for increased anesthesia fees.

Myth #5:

Managing time better is essentially a matter of reducing the time spent on every activity. Managing time better involves spending the appropriate amount of time on every activity. For some tasks, it means cutting down. For others, it means increasing your time commitment. You may want to cut down on time you spend in meetings, casual conversations, report handling, and correspondence. You will probably find it helpful to increase the time you spend planning, thinking, and developing yourself and your subordinates, your technicians, and the front-office staff. You may also want to spend more time with new clients to enhance their relationship with the clinic.

Your activities should be consistent with your objectives. Look at all your activities during your workday. How important is each in terms of what you are trying to get accomplished? Where can you reduce your time commitments? Where should you increase them? Is there some activity that you are not doing that should be added?

Myth #6:

All people are important; everyone should be treated the same. Every person is important. But all the events you're involved in are not equally important. In fact, in terms of your job, all people are not equally important.

Learn to separate people from the issues, activities, demands, pressures, and problems. Prioritizing your time does not mean you need to dismiss people or deny human dignity. You can be patient but persistent, polite but tactful, diplomatic but firm. Managing your time to accomplish important objectives requires making hard decisions about how to respond to particular people. For example, say you have two surgeries scheduled. Janet, the surgery technician, has the first one on the table, prepped and ready to go. You, however, are already eight minutes behind schedule. A regular client, Mrs. Allison, age sixty-one, comes in the waiting-room door, sees you near the front desk, marches directly up to you, and begins a dissertation regarding "Miss Molly's" itching and what happened after you saw the cat yesterday. This two-year-old, relatively healthy, spayed female cat is Mrs. Allison's pride and joy. She does not have the cat with her. You have seen the cat three times in the past two weeks. There is an owner compliance issue, because Mrs. Allison tends not to follow the flea control program you have set out for her. You can be firm, indicate your interest, yet defer her until later in one of several manners. You could say:

> "Mrs. Allison, I must interrupt for a moment. I know how much this itching distresses you and Miss Molly. I believe we are on the right track with the prednisone and flea-control products. Right now, I really need to be in surgery. Can I have Gayle schedule an appointment this afternoon to talk more about it? I will be glad to take another look at Molly then. Martha (technician) is available right now to go over again how to use the medications I gave you. Would that be all right? Thank you so much for your understanding."

Notice that there is no "but" or "however" between your acknowledgment greeting of Mrs. Allison and your **"I"** statement that you must be in surgery. It is critically important to *not* use those terms, because clients often hear "but" and "however" as negatives. They can be taken to mean you really think these clients are not important. They will tend to feel discounted and "handled." You want clients to feel very important, even though you are placing them in a lower position on your priority "to-do" list. Always try to thank them verbally in some manner for their understanding. Make your body language support a sense of urgency. Then, move on.

Managing time is managing events. Life is made of a series of events. If you take control of events that consume the time allocated to you, you take care of yourself and you manage your life. If you are taking care of yourself, you can take much better care of someone else.

Myth #7:

Most people can solve their time problems by working harder. Although sometimes working hard pays off, working smarter always beats working harder. Many people do not consider that there might be a way to shorten the task, eliminate some steps, combine some parts, and actually get more accomplished in the same amount of time.

Periodically analyze the workflow. Make the job easier and quicker. Try to find ways to reduce the number of tasks. If you create shortcuts, make sure there is sufficient time available for the really important tasks. Only the trivial activities should be eliminated.

Myth #8:

People who concentrate on efficiency are the best performers. Efficiency relates to the cost of doing something, or cost-effectiveness. It concerns itself with the ratio of costs to results, input to output. Efficiency and effectiveness are very different. Effectiveness refers to goal accomplishment. Did the job get done? You either reach your objective or you do not.

Some veterinarians believe that efficiency is performing an ovariohysterectomy on a dog with just one strand of suture. Although it might get the job done (effective) and can appear to be efficient (only costs one suture packet), is this the whole story? In some cases, even for experienced surgeons, the time it takes to fight and reposition the tiny bit of suture left on a swaged needle, to redo the suture, which breaks from being handled so much, and the extra effort it takes for a dulling, possibly bending, needle-slowing closure, may cost six to ten times as much as if a second suture pack ($3.15) had been opened and used. Both methods by definition were effective, although in this case, the use of a second pack of suture was much more efficient. In addition, if you could put a value on the frustration level of the surgeon, there were even greater costs for trying to be efficient by isolating the cost of one material item at the expense of time and attitude.

Focus on effectiveness first, then on efficiency. Evaluate the entire picture as a whole system. Determine what you should be doing to be effective, then determine how to do it most efficiently.

248

Myth #9:

Most people know how they spend their time and can easily identify their biggest time wasters. Think again. Most people really do not know how they spend their time. Don't believe this? Try remembering last week accurately. Even if you use your appointment book, you will probably be unable to accurately recount many of the things you did. This happens because so much of your behavior is habitual. When you act out of habit, you do not concentrate or pay conscious attention to your behaviors or activities. Even if your job consists of unique tasks, you probably approach them in routine ways. When you do not know your time habits, you end up wasting time. Many time-management consultants believe that most people waste up to two hours every day.

Take a week or two and record your time usage in a log. Discover your time habits and patterns. A time log should be kept in fifteen-minute segments, beginning the first thing in the morning and ending when you go to bed. Keep it in front of you or with you. Make entries as the day goes by, not at the end of the day, because you will forget what you did. Give the highlights with enough information that will allow you to rate the importance of each event. List outgoing phone calls. Record interruptions, what you were doing when you were interrupted, who was in-volved, and briefly what the interruption was about. At the end of a week or so, look for trends and patterns and peak periods of activity. Do you see any time wasters? Can you revise your schedule to accommodate routine happenings, thus freeing up time for more important tasks?

Myth #10:

All activities are equally important. Actually, most of the results you achieve are produced by a few critical activities. This is the 80-20 rule first expounded by Vilfredo Pareto, a nineteenth-century Italian economist. He indicated that 80% of the value lies in 20% of the elements, while the remaining 20% of the value lies in the remaining 80% of the elements. Simply put, 20% of what you do yields 80% of your output value; i.e., only a few activities are critical to your success.

Appreciate that some things are much more valuable than others in terms of achieving your objectives. Examine all your activities and determine which ones are really the most important. Concentrate your focus on these high-value activities.

TIME-MANAGEMENT RECOMMENDATIONS FOR DAILY TASKS

Here are some specific recommendations for associate veterinarians on how to manage time, specifically with regard to patients, records, clients, the telephone, and appointments.

Managing Time With the Patient

Evaluate all hospitalized or inpatient cases before seeing the first appointment. The most important aspect in managing the time required to observe, evaluate, and treat inpatient cases in an average workday is establishing a clear and concise plan of care for each animal. Your assessment of the patient's problems must be noted in the medical record, along with a step-by-step diagnostic and treatment plan for the day. Incorporating an individual patient treatment sheet or whiteboard (preferably a combination of both) will help prioritize treatments and ensure that each patient receives the intended care at a specified time. The advantages of an individual patient treatment sheet are that procedures and medications are recorded, along with who is responsible for the execution of the task. Once the case is finished, the treatment sheet returns to the medical record to serve as evidence of the activity.

Do not schedule elective surgeries and diagnostic-imaging procedures according to some

> The most important aspect in managing the time required to observe, evaluate, and treat inpatient cases in an average workday is establishing a clear and concise plan of care for each animal.

250

arbitrary, predetermined number per day; rather, schedule them according to the actual time each procedure requires according to historic time comparisons for each veterinarian. If an assessment of your last two months of feline neuter procedures reveals that each surgery required forty-five minutes, including preoperative lab work, induction, patient surgical preparation, and procedure, that amount of time must be scheduled in the appointment book. Of course, the forty-five minutes may be divided between technician and veterinarian columns. The point is that each procedure requires a specified amount of time for each veterinarian and paraprofessional staff person.

Before leaving the hospital for a break or for the day, check the status of each hospitalized patient by reviewing the patient treatment sheet and whiteboard. Make notations in the medical record, if necessary, and communicate instructions to nursing staff before leaving.

Managing Time Spent on Records

Every event occuring within the hospital that has a direct or indirect effect on the patient must be recorded *immediately* in the medical record; otherwise, a patient, person, or practice is vulnerable to criticism . . . or worse. Unfortunately, medical records inadequately represent the level of care delivered in most veterinary practices due to incomplete or nonexistent entries in the progress notes. Every event, from the administration of an oral medication to the parting verbal home-care instructions, should be noted in the medical record.

Most veterinarians cite lack of time as a reason for incomplete entries. The reality is that medical records save time. Patient data sheets (cover sheets that compile, in an organized manner, a patient's major health problems, past surgeries, and laboratory activity) can save valuable minutes at the beginning of an appointment by revealing past problems and treatments before you see the patient. Ask yourself how long it takes to review the complete history of a sixteen-year-old cocker spaniel. If the information was concisely presented on one form at the beginning of every medical record, an average of forty-five minutes

could be saved per day, assuming fifteen patients were seen, sparing three minutes in each review.

If you are writing up a complex case after your initial evaluation, it is not necessary to go through the formal process of ruling out a long list of possible diagnoses. Rather, commit yourself to a diagnosis if you are confident and to a tentative diagnosis if you are less sure. At a minimum, list possible rule-outs. In most cases, the final diagnosis will be apparent within a short period of time and can be clarified in the progress notes and patient data form. Too often, recent graduates are noncommittal on paper until receiving verification by means of laboratory results or ultrasound. In the meantime, another member of the practice team has had to guess what you were considering.

Also, noting the number of allowable refills for prescriptions can save considerable time for you and the staff. Additionally, various state practice acts and the AAHA *Standards of Accreditation* require that the number of refills be noted in the medical record. For instance, by noting the number of thyroid-medication refills a client can receive before reevaluating blood levels, you are reducing the number of interruptions necessary to get refill approval when the client is waiting in the reception area. This simple, but productive, habit improves client service and efficiency without consuming valuable time. Just be certain to physically verify the filled prescription before the client picks it up.

Managing Time With the Client

The reality is that veterinary medicine is practiced according to the desires and pocketbooks of clients. For the most part, your knowledge must be communicated in terms the client can understand. The following suggestions help focus the client on your recommendations.

Once you enter the examination room, spend a brief period of time talking directly to the client. The client will form an opinion of you in the first thirty seconds of the conversation. Address the client's pet by name, and convey your intentions to address the problem at hand. Make a mental note of other pets the client may own, and the names of family members.

When you have completed a thorough physical examination, take a few moments to write down your findings in the medical record. This may seem like an interruption to the visit, but it provides an opportunity for you to think through your approach in discussing needed care. This pause also allows the client to consider additional pertinent history.

Be completely clear in your communication to the client about the care of her pet at home. Provide written discharge instructions to your client for reference after the visit and so that each family member understands what the pet needs in the way of home care.

Use physical-examination report cards as a communication tool for potential health problems. Typically, animals are presented with one major problem, but other abnormalities often exist that may require further diagnostics or treatment. A patient report card provides you an opportunity to introduce other problems you may have identified and to give your client your recommendations in writing.

Managing Time on the Telephone

One of the main contributors to inefficient time management is the telephone. Most veterinarians enter the practice each morning to face a stack of messages requiring return phone calls from the day or week before. It is essential that you develop a system for placing and returning phone calls.

To reduce the number of calls you receive from clients, assign a technician working with you on each case as the patient's advocate for the term of the illness or injury. Give each client a business card listing the technician's name assigned to the case so that the client knows who to contact if there is a question. This person will be the primary contact person for the client and can field many of the client's questions after the visit. It is an expensive proposition for a veterinarian to return a client's call when the question is simply when to start the medication you prescribed. Train all patient advocates to keep you abreast of

the patient's progress and to refer cases back to you if the patient is not improving as you have described in the medical record.

Develop a simple, timely, logical system for communicating laboratory results and specialist evaluation reports to the client. Since all events center on the movement of the medical record, creating a basket or file slot for each associate is a must. When patient samples have been collected for submission to a specialist or reference lab, the record should be noted and returned to each doctor's lab-pending basket. Most reference labs send results in the morning via the FAX machine. Often, many of the previous day's lab requests are completed by the time the veterinarian arrives in the morning.

In most cases, try to finish yesterday's work before beginning another day. As a courtesy to the client and to justify the expense of advanced diagnostics, report the findings of all major lab panels, histopathology reports, and specialist evaluations to the client. The patient advocate can communicate in-hospital lab work to the client as long as she is an effective communicator and notes the conversation in the medical record. The key to making this system work is communicating to the client when you expect to receive the results and when you will be calling.

If necessary, block a twenty-minute period of time at the end of the morning to communicate results, and tell your clients that you place all your calls between 11:00 A.M. and 12:00 P.M., giving yourself a cushion if the morning becomes hectic. Once the client has been contacted, summarize your conversation either in the progress notes or on the lab report, then return the file to the reception station for filing. There is nothing more burdensome than realizing you have let down a client by not contacting him or her when you promised. Additionally, if you let diagnostic reports pile up without contacting the owner, you have done a disservice to the patient and dismissed the client's confidence in the value of your recommendation. Just consider for a moment how often people complain about not receiving notification of their

> A patient report card provides you an opportunity to introduce other problems you may have identified and to give your clients your recommendations in writing.

251

own or a family member's results from a physician.

Absolutely, the most important habit to develop in regard to the telephone is returning phone calls before leaving for the day. No one knows what tomorrow will deliver at your front door, but without doubt, it will be as busy as the day before. Never look at the appointment book and think, "Tomorrow looks slow. I'll leave early and catch up on these calls later." Get in the habit of returning phone calls, and place this activity at the same priority level as entering the exam room for an appointment. This habit alone will ensure peace of mind when you leave the practice for the evening, knowing that you contacted every client and can start with a clean slate the next day.

> Absolutely, the most important habit to develop in regard to the telephone is returning phone calls before leaving for the day.

Managing Appointment Time

In most practices, appointments are typically scheduled in twenty- to thirty-minute time intervals. Client-satisfaction research indicates that clients want to spend no more than twenty to thirty minutes at a veterinary-hospital visit. The practice's appointment book should reflect this finding with the understanding that the client's clock starts ticking the moment the client walks through the door. The most productive scheduling systems use twenty-minute time slots for routine visits and thirty-minute appointments for multiple problems, consultations, and new client visits.

Once the client enters the reception area and is greeted by friendly and eager staff member, she should be escorted to the examination room with the medical record ready for review and notation. The veterinarian should enter the examination room once the nursing staff takes the vital signs of the animal and records pertinent history. Entering the room prematurely devalues the role of the veterinary nurse and consumes time, which could be more efficiently used by finishing the record from the previous appointment or returning a client phone call. Remember—the veterinarian has just three responsibilities: diagnosis, treatment, and

prescription. The entire process should take no more than five minutes from the time the client and patient enters the hospital, completes paperwork, and receives a cursory veterinary-nurse examination.

You then have eight to ten minutes to engage in conversation with the client, perform a thorough physical examination, note your findings in the medical record, and recommend what course of action is required for the health and well-being of the patient. If your recommendations require additional procedures, the pet should be admitted to the hospital for a short period of time so that the animal receives an appropriate level of care. An unscheduled, "rushed" procedure does not serve the patient or the practice. Procedures or additional diagnostics should be worked into the day's activity, not between appointments.

The nursing staff and/or receptionist should use the last five minutes to fill prescriptions, go over client instructions, and explain anticipated future veterinary care for the pet. The veterinarian uses the last five minutes to complete the medical record *before* going to the next appointment.

It's Your Time

Because you cannot increase the quantity of time you have, it is essential to pay attention to its quality. Your time does not belong to anyone else. Only you can improve the quality.

RESOURCES

Books

The 10 Natural Laws of Successful Time and Life Management: Proven Strategies for Increased Productivity and Inner Peace by H. Smith.

Time Management from the Inside Out: The Foolproof System for Taking Control of Your Schedule and Your Life by J. Morgenstern.

Time Management: Proven Techniques for Making the Most of Your Valuable Time by M. Cook.

252

Time Tactics of Very Successful People by B. Griessman.
The Time Trap: The Classic Book on Time Management
    by R. MacKenzie and A. MacKenzie.

Websites

bguides™ by MaxPitch Media
www.bguides.com
A free resource with guides and tools on time management.

CHAPTER TWENTY-THREE

Coping With Stress and Burnout

Linda L. Black, EdD, LPC
Elizabeth I. Fassig, MA, PsyD

IN THIS CHAPTER, YOU'LL LEARN:

- Sources and symptoms of stress
- How to minimize stress in your life
- What leads to burnout

Stress is an intrinsic part of daily life. We need to keep current with email messages, have faster-paced computers, carry cell phones and pagers at all times, compulsively complete "to-do" lists, take care of the needs of others, and answer the "do-more-with-less" directive or suffer the consequences. We have become a culture that sleeps less, compulsively presses the door-close button in elevators, opts for speed dial on our telephones, and tracks investments to complete day trades on the Internet. We are always on the go and never have enough time.

Whether you call it stress, pressure, anxiety, tension, or excessive worry, there is no shortage of it in today's fast-paced, technologically advanced workplace. The young are not immune from its effects; in fact, young adults just entering the workforce or launching a career may find work extremely stressful in both positive and negative ways.

WHY DO YOU FEEL STRESSED?

You feel stressed when you are faced with demands for which you *do not* have effective coping strategies. You may have excellent coping skills in a few areas and limited resources for several others. It is important, then, for you to determine which areas are more challenging for you and make appropriate adjustments.

You "stress out" because of three basic reasons:

1. A change in your life produces an unsettling effect.

2. You feel challenged or threatened by some outside force or influence.

3. You experience a loss of personal control.

When you experience any of these factors, you can resist them, avoid and evade them, or adapt to them.

A "Stressful" Example

Whether you are in your last year of veterinary school or have been in the field for a while, you experience demands and challenges for which you may not be well prepared. Transitions, like chaos, offer both crisis and opportunity; the successful professional is one who is aware of and prepared for either. Consider the following:

Dr. Julie Hartman graduated from veterinary school two years ago filled with anticipation, excitement, and uncertainty. She is a quiet, reserved person but is amiable and warms up to people. She did not date much in school; in fact, her social activities were always in a group. Upon graduation, she joined a mixed-animal, four-veterinarian practice. During her employment interview, she indicated that her focus was on companion animals and that she had little large-animal experience. (Julie had recognized early on in veterinary school that except for the occasional "nice" horse, she did not really like large-animal work.)

As a new graduate, Julie was partial to the idea of a predictable income and work schedule with no after-hours or emergency work. The hospital was a cooperative member of an emergency service three miles away, which handled companion-animal after-hours cases. She got an apartment, and with her first couple of paychecks, she put down money to purchase a new car and some clinic work clothes.

Within the first eight months of taking this position, Julie noticed she was having headaches and backaches, her stomach was upset and tense, and she felt a vague sense of uneasiness. She passed it off as the flu or the jitters related to the new job. Occasionally, she noticed that things at the clinic were not as she had hoped or expected. She knew that she was not getting enough sleep and frequently found herself obsessing about her performance. By February, she had met Jack Gunderson, a bit of a loner but a decent guy, in the next town. He worked as a route manager for a PVC pipe distribution company. In June, they were married.

Often finding herself the only veterinarian in the building during late mornings and early afternoons, Julie feared she could not handle the more difficult internal-medicine cases she knew would come in the door, and she worried that she would totally fail in her newly assigned clinic duties (e.g., occasional coverage of a large-animal case). She was not sure she wanted to or would be able to care for large animals. Cows made her nervous, every chicken she had ever been around had tried to attack her, and pigs were the pits to even approach, with all the squealing and associated odors. Julie felt that caring for a large animal was really an unfair assignment. She had signed up for companion animals and believed it was only due to the clinic being short staffed that she was given these tasks.

Julie told herself that if she worked harder, she could overcome her anxiety and doubt. She reminded herself that even though she was not too keen on it, she had been successful during her large-animal rotation in veterinary school. This self-talk worked for a while. Her confidence, skill, and competence grew with the small-animal cases as she distinguished herself with some successes, and some clients were actually asking for her to look at their pets. Sometimes she would work beyond her regular hours to further demonstrate to her boss how dedicated she was to the companion-animal side of the business, thus entrenching her on the small-animal side of the practice.

One day, she froze in her tracks when she was told that she was being assigned a large-animal reproductive case from a new client who would arrive later in the afternoon. After hearing this distressing news, Julie had lunch at a local tavern. Lunch included burying herself in the Merck Veterinary Manual and drinking a couple of rum and Cokes just so she could calm her nerves before she saw the client. Her mind racing, she returned to the clinic only to find that the case had become an emergency and was being assigned to a senior veterinarian. Julie felt confused; she had dodged a bullet but felt guilty and incompetent for behaving as she did.

Time passed. After a year and a half, Dr. Hartman had begun to feel like she was in a pressure cooker. She dreaded going to work. Home was not much of a refuge, either, as she felt annoyed by her partner's expectations that they start a family and buy a house. He was always complaining about her working late in the clinic. That local tavern had become her refuge, a place to stop after work and have a few drinks and munchies in the back booth before enduring Jack's whining. One of his chief complaints was that she was spending less time with him. She knew that they were barely making enough money together to cover their current debts, which included her sizable student loans, the car and truck payments, and now Jack's new bass boat.

Julie felt scared and anxious when she thought about the cost (both personally and financially) of a baby and a mortgage. She did not know where to turn. And she worried that her business was nobody else's. In this part of the country, everybody seemed to know everything. Secrets did not seem to stay secrets very long.

In the last five months or so, Dr. Hartman seemed to have been in a haze, acting somewhat distant and irrational, sometimes ignoring the technicians or snapping at them for no apparent reason. Occasionally, she came to work tired, clothes rumpled, and hung over. She knew she was just going through "the motions" at the clinic and at home. Still frightened, she successfully avoided most of the large-animal cases and felt temporarily relieved, yet panicked if she was the only veterinarian in the clinic and the phone rang. She experienced feelings of guilt, incompetence, and sadness for not caring as she once did about her clients or her marriage.

Julie's experiences and feelings are common among professionals as they negotiate the transition from graduate training into their chosen field. Often these experiences, doubts, and fears are not addressed by the person they are impacting or by their support system. Transitions and

> If you find that you cannot deal with distress on your own by following certain strategies, or things are getting out of control, it is very important for you to seek professional counseling.

major life events are an expected part of human development. Often, these events require the person to pass from one identity into another. It is important to learn how to identify, address, and cope with the non-productive stressors that you may encounter during your transition and development as a veterinarian. If you find that you cannot deal with distress on your own by following certain strategies, or things are getting out of control, it is very important for you to seek professional counseling.

DEFINING STRESS

The concept of stress is such an overused and ubiquitous term in our lexicon that it has lost much of its power and meaning. Historically, scientists and theorists believed that the response to stress or trauma was unconditioned or innate—a remnant of the fight-or-flight response. Current authors support the notion that stress appears to be a systemic response that integrates a combination of conditioned (learned) and unconditioned (innate) factors.

When a person's well-being or system gets out of balance, the feelings of stress signal or warn the person of potential danger. Julie was clearly experiencing stress in several areas of her life. She felt pressured, sad, and, at times, incompetent. The combined stress of multiple demands taxed her ability to cope and left her feeling overwhelmed.

Stress manifests in an acute, chronic, or combined fashion. For example, you may experience the acute distress of not finding employment after graduation and the chronic anxiety of repaying your student loans. When these events occur simultaneously, you experience a combined type of stress. A threatening situation signals or warns you that some event is about to happen. The threatening event puts you at risk for an unwanted and perhaps unwelcome change.

In the example, Julie was told she would be seeing large-animal cases. She felt this was unfair because she explained at her interview that she did not want to see large animals. She felt she was taking up the slack for her supervisor because he did not recruit enough veterinarians with large-animal experience. This event caused stress for Julie because she did not want to see this type of patient and did not feel competent to treat them. She chose to behave in an inappropriate and unethical manner (drinking while working), which could have placed her, her colleagues, and her patients at risk.

The signals sent by stressors can be viewed positively, negatively, or in some combination. A positive reaction (productive stress) to the stressor usually signals a curiosity response in which there is less perceived threat. A negative reaction (nonproductive stress) to the stressor typically provokes an anxiety response and a heightened sense of threat. For example, you may experience a positive form of stress when you feel anxious or nervous about completing a task. The signal motivates you to complete the task and experience satisfaction. You experience negative stress when you feel fearful, threatened, or tense about a task. The ambiguous or negative feelings lead you to avoid or deny your experience. You then remain in a state of apprehension, confusion, or agitation.

Finally, when you experience a combined form of stress, like Julie did, where both positive and negative feelings are present (e.g., the excitement of securing her current position [positive] and the dread and tension she feels related to large animals [negative]), you receive signals that may lead to feelings of confusion, apprehension, and excitement. Julie's response to her stressors progressed to the point where her previous coping skills (working harder and talking to others) no longer worked, and she turned to alcohol on a regular basis to numb herself.

Because every individual identifies and responds uniquely to stressors or signals, the perceived threat or benefit of similar signals can hold a multitude of meanings. The meaning, intensity, frequency, duration, and importance of the stressor all determine its effect on you as an individual. Some of you might find Julie's story compelling and concerning, while others may view it as inconsequential. The experience, process, and management of stress are complex and idiosyncratic.

Indicators of Stress

What is important is that you recognize *your own* signals and warning signs (see Table 23-1). In general, the hallmarks of stress are:

- Disruption of personal, social, emotional, or vocational functioning to a greater degree than typically experienced
- Unsuccessful attempts to avoid, deny, or ignore the signs of stress
- Persistent and unwanted negative experiences or feelings
- Harmful emotional and physical consequences
- Traditional coping strategies not reducing discomfort

Stress signals are sent to us via physical, psychological, emotional, relational, and vocational means. Julie ignored numerous warnings or signals and the intensity of her distress. Internally, she doubted whether she wanted to have children at this point in her career and feared that she was not competent to see large animals. Although angry and disgusted with herself for her drinking behavior, she felt it was the only thing that gave her comfort. She had headaches, backaches, and muscular tension, and her stomach was upset and tense (physical). She hoped these were just symptoms of adjusting to a new job or that she was getting the flu, but she secretly feared and suspected it might mean more.

Her sleep disturbance and increased drinking (psychological symptoms) seemed to cause more difficulty between her and her partner. She was besieged by feelings of sadness, hopelessness, fear, pressure, and misunderstandings (emotional symptoms) in most areas of her life. She felt annoyed by and isolated from her husband and misunderstood by her family and friends (relational symptoms). She used to obsess about her performance at the clinic and now is occasionally embarrassed and ashamed of her casual attitude toward the animals and their companions (vocational symptoms).

Identifying and understanding the personal meaning of your stressors are difficult and critical components to effectively coping with the inevitable stress of a professional transition.

258

SOURCES OF STRESS

Whether managing the competitive nature of veterinary school or balancing your new career and personal life, it is safe to say that you have personally experienced nonproductive stress. Chances are that you, like Julie, have struggled to effectively manage the tension, anxiety, and discomfort that accompany transitions and stress. As you reflect on these and other experiences, consider how well or poorly you handled stressful, tense, or traumatic situations in the past. The obvious question is: If we all experience stress, why do so many of us struggle to manage or cope with it?

Sources of stress abound. Much of the time you may feel as if your life is in balance or homeostasis. Yet, a partial response to the above question is that most people fail to:

- Adequately identify the true source of stress in their lives

- Understand the meaning of their stress

- Develop appropriate coping resources, even if they have correctly identified the sources of stress in their lives

Currently, you are in the midst of a life and career transition. It is potentially an unsettling experience. Take a moment to consider how many of the following categories may be a source of productive or nonproductive stress in your life:

- Your individual personality style or temperament (e.g., easygoing or easily upset)

- Your new professional role

- Your immediate and nuclear family

- Your health

- The employment setting

- The demands of success or promotion

- Finances

- The continual updating of your training and specialization

- Adapting to changes in the field (promotion of specialization, corporate veterinary medicine, increased use of technology)

- Your responsibility for patient and human care and the potential death of a patient

> Identifying and understanding the personal meaning of your stressors are difficult and critical components to effectively coping with the inevitable stress of a professional transition.

This partial list is provided to heighten your awareness and understanding that stress can originate from anywhere.

PRETENDING NOTHING IS WRONG

After you have identified the meaning and scope of your stress and you attempt to understand or cope with your experiences, you may inadvertently create roadblocks via your own thoughts and behaviors. In an effort to reduce feelings of uneasiness, some people may seek to avoid identifying and dealing with stress by cognitively distorting an experience. Julie tried this by telling herself to "work harder" and "avoid large-animal cases."

Initially, you may not be cognizant that you are distorting your thinking. Cognitive distortion is not always an intentional process. It is an ineffective coping strategy in which you attempt to meet the demands (stress) in your life with inadequate or yet unknown resources. Examples of cognitive distortion strategies are:

- Denying there is a problem; denying that the problem affects you and that it is not your responsibility to act on it

- Repressing how you feel about the experience; persistently ignoring or avoiding feelings of tension, sadness, or worry

- Rationalizing your experience by providing a plausible but inaccurate explanation for your experience

- Displacing your feelings and experiences on a "more acceptable" activity (such as using drugs, drinking alcohol, having sex, or overspending) to numb the tension or worry of stress

259

Table 23-1
SYMPTOMS OF STRESS

Physical*	Emotional and Mental	Social and Behavioral
Headaches	Depression	Isolation
Muscle tension	Anxiety	Teeth grinding
Backaches	Forgetfulness	Increased smoking
Neck pain	Poor concentration	Procrastination
Stomach problems	Confusion	Nagging
Frequent colds or flu	Mood swings	Increased number of mistakes
Fatigue	Anger	Fewer contacts with friends
Insomnia	Irritability	Nail biting
Constipation	Crying spells	Poor grooming
Ringing in the ears	Worrying	Increased use of alcohol and/or drugs
Weight gain or loss	Feeling overwhelmed	Change in eating habits
Diarrhea	Negative attitude	Being late or missing appointments
Dizziness	Tension	Decreased sex drive
Cold hands and/or feet	Panic attacks	Being uncommunicative
Heart palpitations	Indecisiveness	Loneliness
Excessive sleeping	Lethargy	Nervous laughter
Increased allergies	Aggressiveness	Overreaction to little things
High blood pressure	Low productivity	Finger or foot tapping

* Consult your physician if any of these symptoms are intense or persistent.

Julie engaged the strategies of distorted thinking. For example, she used denial (e.g., working harder so that things would be okay), repression (e.g., ignoring her headaches and upset stomach), and displacement (using alcohol) in an effort to manage her experience. Sadly, these strategies did not work. Her stress increased, and she began to increase her drinking.

As her stress increased, she tried to reduce her feelings of inadequacy and anxiety by working harder, often staying well past her scheduled workday. Remember—she wanted this job, in part, because of its regular hours. It seemed to Julie that the more she worked, the more it seemed to create turmoil at work and home. Her coworkers wondered why she remained after her shift, and her husband questioned why she was not at home with him.

She felt unappreciated, misunderstood, and torn between home and work. She thought that working harder would please her supervisor, her peers, and Jack, yet all she seemed to do was anger and annoy all of them. She tried to manage an unrealistic workload and expected perfection from herself and from those around her. As a result, she suffered chronic headaches, upset stomach, and muscular tension.

Julie's behavior (e.g., working longer and harder) backfired on her. She ignored the signals of stress (headaches, backaches, irritability, and increased drinking), which compounded her distress and pain. By failing to recognize her stress, her behavior became more self-destructive (alcohol misuse), which led to increased emotional disturbances (feelings of depression and/or anxiety) and increased health risks (alcohol dependence and sleep disturbance). As the stress increased, Julie became overwhelmed by her situation and chose ineffective methods to manage the multiple and complex demands of her life and career. She felt out of balance, constantly under pressure, and misunderstood by those around her. These feelings led her to feel isolated and alone.

Julie's ineffective responses to her stress (acute, chronic, or combined) had a dramatic impact on her physical health. For example, research indicates a relationship between unmediated stress and the following conditions: chronic muscular tension or pain, coronary heart disease, cancer, hypertension, substance use and abuse, and emotional disturbances, including suicide. Julie had at least three of these well-recognized conditions (muscular tension, substance abuse, and emotional disturbance), and if she continued to ignore the stress in her life, chances were that these conditions would only worsen.

Julie's downward spiral could have been averted. She needed to recognize the signals of stress so she could begin to seek out more useful coping strategies. Coping with stress means changing how to think, feel, and interact during stressful situations. For example, Julie may have coped successfully with her stress if she had been more assertive in communicating with her employer, with Jack, and with herself. Clear, consistent, and persistent communication would have allowed her to ask for help.

Julie could have initiated a conversation with her supervisor regarding the specifics of her work performance. This way, she could have verified what she was doing well and identified areas for improvement. In this discussion, she could begin to openly acknowledge her concerns regarding treating large animals. Second, she could have spoken openly with Jack about their relationship; specifically, her worries about work and about their finances. Finally, she could have gotten professional consultation and treatment for her substance use. A counselor or social worker could help her learn how to express herself more directly and reduce her reliance on alcohol.

MINIMIZING STRESS IN YOUR LIFE

Prior to outlining strategies and resources for coping with stress, it is important to acknowledge the importance of minimizing the negative effects of stress in your life. It seems inappropriate to speak of "preventing stress," because stress is as funda-

mental to the human condition as is love. Each has the capacity to entice, excite, and incite, as well as to frustrate, confuse, and hurt. To minimize the negative effects of stress, you must live with intent and purpose. This means it is essential to examine and to be accountable for the manner in which you care for yourself and for those who are significant to you.

Julie let events and assumptions control and influence her. If she had accurately identified and acted on her concerns at work and home, she would have experienced more control over and less fear about the events in her life.

These guidelines will help you minimize stress in your life.

- Eat a balanced diet, get regular exercise in consultation with your physician, and have a stable, meaningful, intimate love relationship. These all contribute positively to physical and emotional health.

- Get adequate sleep in accordance with your own individual needs.

- Don't take yourself too seriously. A well-timed and appropriate sense of humor can temper difficult and stressful events.

- Become self-literate. Reflect on and understand how you experience your surroundings. This includes emotional, relational, volitional, and intellectual curiosity and understanding. This can help you understand the meaning and purpose of your stress.

- Practice effective calming and relaxation strategies on a regular basis. Find a quiet place to focus so that you can understand how and why you feel the way you do at that moment.

- Acknowledge that change is an expected life event, and realize that any event can produce stress if you appraise its meaning (attribution) as a threat. You have choices in how or if you choose to deal with potentially stress-producing events.

- Develop a network of trusted colleagues for professional consultation and connection to others in the field. Making contact with other professionals reduces isolation, provides the opportunity to compare experiences, and is a major factor in reducing professional burnout.

- Find a mentor. This could be a practicing veterinary professional, a former faculty member, or a retired veterinarian. Be open to his or her guidance and support. Mentoring has numerous personal and professional benefits (e.g., increased earning power, sponsorship, give and take between the protégé and mentor) (see Chapter 15).

- Seek continuing education and training after graduation. This serves several functions: it maintains your licensure, keeps you in regular contact with other professionals, and may lead to specialization and association-based leadership opportunities.

- Take time to balance your personal life and career. This is a symbiotic, mutually reinforcing relationship. When you grow and thrive, so should your career.

- Build and enhance your network of social support.

- Seek and accept feedback about your personal behaviors from persons whom you trust. They may see your stress before you do.

- When appropriate, seek counseling or other personal-support relationships. Professionals can treat stress (e.g., biofeedback, massage therapy, talk therapy, substance-abuse counseling, financial consulting, relaxation training, meditation training, and prescription medication) and its related manifestations.

- Monitor your use of alcohol and drugs. The warning signs of misuse or abuse include, but are not limited to, frequent and persistent attempts to secure the substance(s), relationship conflict related to substance use, financial problems when funds are used to purchase the substance(s), health problems related to substance use, disruption of job-related activities due to substance use (missing work or lack of productivity due to the effects or aftereffects of the substance), and legal problems related to substance misuse.

- Get in touch with your value system, your beliefs, and your goals.

- Try different approaches to problem-solving.

- Spend time with animals and people you value.

- Do career and financial planning.

- Don't smoke (at least restrict smoking).

- Incorporate something you enjoy into each day.

- Develop a hobby.

- Keep a journal.

- Talk out your problems—don't try to "protect" others by keeping things to yourself.

- Use relaxation techniques such as hypnosis, biofeedback, and visualization.

> Making contact with other professionals reduces isolation, provides the opportunity to compare experiences, and is a major factor in reducing professional burnout.

COPING SKILLS

No matter how well you minimize negative stress in your life, you will continue to face it frequently. Coping with stressful events, like anything meaningful in life, takes time. Effective coping depends on many factors: personal temperament, the nature of the threat, the proximity of the threat, the intensity and duration of the threat, and personal resources (e.g., emotional, physical, and financial). Coping is a process that involves an integration of cognitive and emotional skills with awareness. Although this section lists seven stages to this process, it is important to note that these steps are not necessarily linear or discreet. Coping is a dynamic, multilayered, integrated, and complex course of action. But, there's the rub. It requires you to act.

The seven stages described here are awareness followed by appraisal, association, attention, acknowledgment and acceptance, alternatives and action, and assessment. Each stage described is followed by a series of questions.

Keep a notebook of your thoughts and your answers as you progress through each stage. This should help you reflect, remember, and hopefully act on your personal understanding of negative stress.

Awareness

Stress signals may be clear and defined or ambiguous and elusive. A cell phone is successfully activated or "signaled" only if the equipment is in working order, turned on, and in range. At times, the call is clear and sharp, and at other times, you get a garbled, unintelligible contact. The same is true for your stress signal. You must be partially available, conscious, and alert to your emotional and physical states. Remember that Julie's stress manifested in many ways (physical, psychological, emotional, financial, relational, and vocational). She was receiving simultaneous signals on many channels. She was aware that she was overwhelmed, but she did not identify this as stress. Awareness requires availability (a quiet time with no distractions) and alertness (the ability and desire to focus).

Answer the awareness questions, and as you think about them, be alert to what may be out of balance for you and what message you might be receiving. Now you have to investigate what the message is and who is sending it.

AWARENESS QUESTIONS

- What do I feel? Am I stressed (whatever this means to you)? If the answer is yes, or maybe, or I don't know, continue to answer the questions in this list.

- How worried, fearful, scared, tense, or threatened do I feel right now? List all the things that may cause you to worry. Do not edit or leave anything out, however inconsequential it may seem. Have I included all areas of my life (e.g., work, work relationships, work performance, family, friends, partners, finances, health, housing, transportation, emotions, pets)?

- How concerned or bothered am I about each thing that causes me worry (on a scale of 1 to 10, with 1 being *not at all* and 10 being *completely*)? Write down your rankings.

- Within each area *specifically*, what or who is bothering me?

- Am I denying, minimizing, or avoiding the importance of this concern? Am I blaming others?

- What reasons do I have for not paying attention to what I think and/or feel?

- Who (besides me) is most impacted by my worry?

Appraisal

The primary behaviors in the appraisal phase are cognitive and emotional curiosity and an unrelenting spirit. The appraisal phase of coping is like being a detective. Your goal is to ask accurate and focused questions, free from cognitive distortions.

The answers to the questions , we hope, will lead you to an understanding of the nature, meaning, and purpose of your stress. Julie never seemed to stop and ask the who, what, when, where, and how questions that guide this phase. She seemed to resign herself to be a casualty of poor coping and increasing negative stress. The questions she was likely asking herself were: Why is this happening to me? Why don't people understand me? Why am I in this situation? She was attempting to make sense out of her experience, but her questioning strategy focused on finding out who was responsible (blame and rationalization) for her situation.

Asking a "why" question is an ineffective strategy. This type of question almost always gets you a "because" answer as you feel the need to justify or defend your actions or beliefs. More effective questions seek understanding as their outcome, rather than blame.

APPRAISAL QUESTIONS

- How long have I felt sad, tense, scared, worried, and/or angry?

- What will change if I pay attention to how I feel?

- What will I get; what am I willing to give up?

- What are my priorities (e.g., feel better, improve relationships, avoid confrontation)?

- Who is involved in my concern?

263

- Who may be the source of my concern, and how do I react to him or her?

- Who will support me in feeling better?

- What specifically happened? Do I have accurate information?

- To what degree are my feelings impacting all areas of my life?

- Am I engaging in other behaviors (alcohol, drugs, sex, overspending) as a substitute for dealing with how I feel?

- Have I received feedback from people whom I trust that I seem different (tense, tired, irritable, distant)?

- Am I distorting how I feel or think about this issue to avoid dealing with it?

- What proof do I have that I have taken direct action to address my concerns?

- What would successful coping with this problem look like?

- What do I want to have happen, and do I have the desire and power to make that change happen?

- Where does my stress occur? Where in my body do I experience stress?

- When do I feel the most stress? The least?

- Who or what do I fear most?

This list of questions is not meant to be complete. Its purpose is to get you focused. Concentrate on your situation and see if the answers to these questions fully describe the who, what, when, where, and how of your particular situation. Questions specific to your situation may emerge from your reflection.

Association

Correctly identifying the source, purpose, and meaning of your stressor is essential. The attribution or meaning you give a stressor is unique and determined (at some level) by you. Examples of attributed meaning include the importance, the value, the intensity, the significance, and the anticipated consequences you believe will result from your situation.

Association is intimately connected with awareness and appraisal. For example, Julie needed to sense (awareness) that she felt sad, dejected, and hopeless (assessment). For her, it meant that she was not doing her job and that her dream of being an excellent small-animal veterinarian was dying. She failed to recognize and question the genuine source of her distress (that she was not measuring up and not speaking up).

Answering the following questions will aid you in determining what stress may mean to you.

ASSOCIATION QUESTIONS

- Is there any connection between how I am feeling physically and emotionally?

- In what situations do I anticipate that I will feel tense, sad, or stressed?

- Do I know what it is that I am feeling?

- Are my feelings of anger really anger, or are they something else (e.g., sadness, shame, or regret)?

- What is the stress preventing me from doing or feeling?

- Prior to this, where or when have I felt similar feelings?

- To whom can I go for help?

- What, if anything, am I doing to contribute to my own stress?

- What happens if I cope with the stressor?

- What happens if I deny or delay coping with the stressor?

- Who or what is in control of me, and do I want it to continue?

- What prevents me from acting on what I know?

- When I am attending to my stress, what else am I avoiding, feeling, or thinking?

- Does recognizing and/or coping with my stress mean that I am a failure or weak?

- Do I believe others have stress? What does theirs look like?

- Am I the only one who feels this way?

- What have I learned from others (family and significant others) about coping with stress?

These questions require that you take an honest appraisal of your situation, of the beliefs and feelings you have about it, and of the impact it has on your life and career. This phase may require you to seek someone else's perspective so that your cognitive distortions do not keep you from facing your reality (you're worried about something and are avoiding dealing with it).

Attention

Attention requires you to recognize the events in your life as *stress* and commit yourself to working through them. This phase of coping seems simple, yet is one of the more difficult ones in which to engage.

Up to this point, you have increased your awareness of your distress; assessed its origins, scope, and degree; and understand (to some degree) how it impacts you. You may feel some relief and hope that the stressor has passed. As Julie's anxiety began to rise, she felt that working harder and avoiding large-animal cases would help. She failed to maintain her attention on how she felt by ignoring the underlying feelings that she was unhappy at work and, to some degree, at home. She thought she was handling things by focusing on what she felt on the surface. She did not seem to give herself the time or the space to really attend to and examine her experience. Her use of alcohol further distanced her from her experience. The following are questions she could have asked herself:

ATTENTION QUESTIONS

- What is the worse thing that could happen to me if I told the important people in my life how I really feel?

- How will I choose to focus on what I need?

- What am I choosing to do instead of attending to how I feel?

- Have I begun drinking or using drugs to manage how I feel?

- How often am I angry or moody?

- How do I focus on a problem? Do I know how?

- Have others told me I look or am acting differently?

- How do I relax?

- Who listens to me? Do I talk with him or her?

- What will it take for me to pay attention to myself?

- When I avoid how I feel about stress, what do I do?

If Julie had asked and honestly answered any of these questions, she may have been able to interrupt the downward spiral she was experiencing. By not seeking a quiet and focused place, she kept up the cycle of worry and stress. Coping would have required Julie (or you) to do something different (interrupt the process of worrying) and to behave in a more productive manner (deep breathing or going for a walk) for some period of time. Change in behavior and beliefs takes time. The reality is that it took Julie years to get that stressed; it is now going to take some time and work for her to learn to cope with the stress that her career and life will inevitably bring.

Acknowledgment and Acceptance

Julie's situation was difficult but not impossible. She did not acknowledge or accept that what she *was* experiencing was stress and disappointment. Up to this point, she blamed herself and others for how she felt and was not coping well (e.g., she had not spoken directly to her supervisor or to her husband). In fact, she was creating more problems for herself by choosing to drink nightly.

Successful coping is learned and takes time. Too often, like Julie, you may try to deny or ignore the pain or concern you feel. Delay and denial only make most situations worse. Here are some questions for you to consider at this stage.

ACKNOWLEDGMENT AND ACCEPTANCE QUESTIONS

- Stress is a part of my life; what role do I want it to play?

- How can I take stressful situations and manage them so I feel some control?

- As I review the process of coping, what have I learned about myself and how stress works in my life?

- What does this current stress tell me about where I am out of balance? What is the signal saying to me?

- What are my strengths in dealing with stressful situations? How have I changed my thinking or behavior related to stress-filled events?

- How aware am I of how I am feeling?

- Do I stay connected to my emotional experiences?

- I am going to have stressful times; what strategies do I have in place to cope with stress so I am not caught off-guard?

- What makes me feel in control during times of stress?

- After becoming more aware of negative stress, what am I doing to minimize it in my life?

If Julie had acknowledged and accepted her feelings as stress rather than her employer's unfairness or her own perceived incompetence, she may have been able to assertively advocate for herself. She could have spoken directly with her partner about the pressures she was experiencing regarding work, building a family, and their financial situation. This may have been uncomfortable for her at the time. Right now, she feels resigned to her fate. Julie's failure to acknowledge and accept her needs and feelings inadvertently set up herself (and others) to feel trapped. It was as if she was saying, "I feel too badly to tell you how I feel and I am upset with you for not knowing I am unhappy!" Acknowledgment and acceptance help you to integrate your awareness and understanding so that you can determine your alternatives and plan a course of action.

Alternatives and Action

Assuming Julie had learned effective coping strategies, she would be feeling some relief. She could begin to think about what alternatives she may have regarding work. For example, she could consider talking directly with her supervisor about her fears, describing her feelings of confusion over her apparent reassignment, examining what caused her to feel less competent with large animals, or asking to be assigned only to small-animal cases.

With respect to her home life, she could consider openly discussing the finances and family-planning concerns she has with her partner and asking for his help and support as she begins her new career.

Another consideration is for Julie to enter counseling if she is not feeling heard by significant persons in her life and her alcohol misuse is moving toward abuse or dependence. She could benefit from counseling because she could test out her beliefs and feelings. This reality testing and support could provide her with the clarity she needs to then prioritize what she would like to do next.

ALTERNATIVES AND ACTION QUESTIONS

- Now that I have identified, understand, and recognize my stress, what do I want to have happen?

- What is my first step, and the second and the third?

- What resources or support do I need to act?

- What if I get a result I do not like? What adjustment will I make?

- Whose support do I need as I change my behavior? How can he or she be helpful?

- Do I need to seek professional support, counseling, or coaching?

- What will prevent me from acting?

- What would successful coping look like? What would failure to cope look like?

Julie's identification and selection of an alternative action plan must be focused on her beliefs about and experience of her stressor. She will have to continue to challenge herself not to cognitively distort her experience or believe that it will just go away. The alternatives and action phase is an active and energetic one. She needs to be prepared that as she changes her behavior (speaking up for herself or identifying how her needs conflict with others), some people may want her to remain as she was before. The problem is that before, Julie was miserable.

Personal change, while eventually beneficial to Julie, will cause her and those around her some discomfort. Furthermore, she will need to prepare herself that change in herself and others takes time. She may not be as accepting of previous unacceptable working and relationship conditions. People in Julie's life will respond to her changes and may also need to change. This is the essence of coping.

Assessment

As Julie begins to act, she will enter the final phase of coping, which is assessment. Here she asks if what she is doing (*her action plan*) is working. Because stress is a constant in life, the process of coping is constant and circular. Hopefully, each time Julie goes through this cycle, she will gain new awareness about herself and learn more effective coping strategies. Assessment questions include the following:

Assessment Questions

- Who is responsible for my success?

- How will I know my action plan is working?

- What steps will I take to keep my plan in place?

- What behaviors are working for me?

- What behaviors or thoughts do I need to refine?

- What changes in my health, emotional state, work setting, or relationship demonstrate that I am successfully coping?

- How will I recognize stressors the next time they happen?

- What have I learned about myself and how I handle stress?

- Do I like how I am coping? What would I wish to change?

Julie's ability to learn successful coping strategies will depend on her willingness and desire to reduce the negative feelings and outcomes in her life and to challenge herself to engage in assertive and self-care behaviors that may be unfamiliar to her. Rather than avoiding or denying how and why she feels the way she does, she can deal with her distress in the moment and hopefully reduce the myriad negative consequences that unrelenting and unrecognized stress can bring.

267

STRESS AND NEGATIVE THINKING

Understanding where your stress originates is an important step toward gaining control over it. You could do wonderful relaxation exercises every day, go on regular vacations, and never work more than forty hours per week and still be incredibly stressed if you don't address your negative thinking. Included in this thinking are assumptions, generalizations, negative expectations, and self-criticisms that guarantee higher levels of stress. You must find a way to reprogram your critical, self-defeating thinking in order to begin shifting your individual experiences of stress.

In order to change the habit of negative thinking, you first need to practice recognizing when you are having negative thoughts or when you are being self-critical. You want to identify the negative thought, the situation that prompted the negative thought, and the feelings you are experiencing in relationship to the thought.

Example

John had the negative thought that he had become incredibly boring. This thought occurred in connection with turning down an invitation to go camping with his close friend, Brian. The feeling John experienced in relationship to his negative thought was one of depression.

You must also look at the ways that your thoughts might be twisted or distorted, and reframe those thoughts into ones that are positive and empowering.

Example

John could take the next step of examining and challenging the negative thought that he has become incredibly boring. Taking just a moment, he could recognize that this thought of his is a very global generalization. When he really thought about it, he knew he was a great storyteller, could carry a tune better than most, and was one of the best two-steppers in town—certainly not the description of a boring person. By gaining this more accurate perspective, John recognized how his negative, self-critical thought was distorted, and not an accurate description of him at all. He then could reframe his perception into a thought that was positive in nature. John might say to himself, "I can see that I am distorting my thinking by greatly overgeneralizing. I'm really not a boring person. What I'm disturbed about is that I did not let Brian know what a valued friend he is to me, and how much I appreciate him. I can begin to turn that around by calling him back right now."

> Choosing to be positive doesn't miraculously eliminate difficulties from your life. It does, however, give you a sort of shock absorber, making the bumps in the road a lot easier to maneuver.

When you use these techniques of reprogramming your negative thoughts into positive, empowering thoughts, and use the question series in the previous section, you will begin to reduce your feelings of stress. Practicing the technique of reframing—shifting a negative thought into a positive statement—requires you to focus on the things that are good in your life—the things you feel a sense of appreciation and gratitude about. The result is that you are far less likely to experience stress and anxiety.

Choosing to be positive doesn't miraculously eliminate difficulties from your life. It does, however, give you a sort of shock absorber, making the bumps in the road a lot easier to maneuver. It puts you in the driver's seat when it comes to reducing and regulating your perceptions and, thus, your experiences of stress.

BURNOUT

Remember the old saying, "All work and no play makes John a dull boy?" Well, all work and no play is a sure way to invite burnout into your life. Burnout doesn't need years to develop. A minor case of burnout can occur after just a few weeks of pushing yourself hard and not balancing your efforts with necessary relief. You find yourself feeling tired, irritable, and short-tempered. A more serious case of burnout can occur after a few years of all work and no play. This can result in serious outcomes, such as significant depression and even suicide.

Researchers have found that symptoms of burnout include a "lack of" the following: energy, enthusiasm, concentration, motivation, joy, satisfaction, zest, interest, ideas, play or permission to play, humor, and self-confidence.

Based on work by Ann McGee Cooper in *You Don't Have to Go Home From Work Exhausted*, there are at least three symptoms of burnout that can be called dysfunctional:

- **Sexuality**—You may temporarily lose interest in sex or have a strong sex drive but find yourself unfulfilled, no matter how much you experience.

- **Appetite**—You may lose interest in eating or may want to eat everything in sight – primarily junk food. Again, you seem to be eating without feeling fulfilled.

- **Sleep**—You may not be able to sleep or you may oversleep, using sleep as an escape from life, which has lost its interest. Again, this kind of sleep is unfulfilling, and even though you sleep for long periods, you awaken tired and listless.

Burnout can happen to anyone, and it can happen more than once. Experiencing burnout does not make you immune to ever experiencing it again; it can occur over and over. Take a moment to complete the questionnaire in Figure 23-1 about burnout and job stress, reproduced here with permission from Sheila Hayward's book *Relax Now*.

268

Work-Related Issues That Can Lead to Burnout

There are many possible sources of stress related to your work. One of these is the physical environment in which you work. As you look around your office area, notice the setup for your desk, computer, telephone, etc.

- Does your chair provide adequate support for your back? Is it adjusted for your height, allowing your legs to make a ninety-degree bend at the knees?

- Is your keyboard positioned at a height that allows your arms to make a ninety-degree bend at the elbows?

- Do you have a wrist rest with your keyboard to help your wrists to remain level, not bent, while you are working at the computer?

- Is your computer monitor placed so that you are looking straight at it, as opposed to having to turn your head to the side or tilting the screen up or down?

- Do you have the habit of freeing up your hands while on the telephone by scrunching the receiver between your head and shoulder instead of using a headset?

These are just a few things to look at when ergonomically evaluating your workplace. Without attending to these and other details, you will undoubtedly experience a higher level of physical stress on the job, and physical stress can increase your level of psychological stress.

Feeling bored or overworked, or not having enough work to do can all lead to burnout. The beliefs you carry with you to work each day are the greatest source of job stress and possible burnout. Perfectionism is one such stress-builder. Perfectionists never feel they have done enough, no matter how many hours have been expended at work or on a special project. They are quick to criticize themselves when something doesn't go quite perfectly, and sometimes even at the anticipation of an error. They are masters at pressuring themselves to achieve bigger and better results. Perfectionists will almost always give up fun, relaxation, or other pleasures in order to work harder and achieve more to be the best.

Another stress-building work attitude involves thinking you must keep everyone happy—that you must please everyone else. These workers derive their self-esteem from other people's opinions, not from themselves. They put themselves last on the list, always caring for other people's needs and requests first above their own. A great source of their fear and stress is the concern they will somehow disappoint their boss or coworkers.

Additional stress-building beliefs include feeling the need to be in complete control at all times, or feeling you will never do as good a job as your coworkers. What is important to remember is that all of these beliefs, which serve to increase your stress levels at work, originate in your thoughts. You can achieve great results in combating these negative thoughts when you begin consciously recognizing the specific thoughts and actively replacing them with positive, empowering ones. For example, if you tend to carry the thoughts of a perfectionist into your work, try reframing any mistakes by looking at what went wrong, what you learned as a result of the mistake, and what needs to happen in order to do it differently in the future. In this way, you are reinforcing the possibilities instead of emphasizing any sense of failure. The experience becomes empowering rather than depleting.

Burnout Checklist

Healthcare workers suffer a high rate of burnout because of the intensity of their work and emotional investment in patients. There are some personality traits that put a person at risk. People are most at risk of burnout if they:

- Do not know how to say "no" to demands on their time and energy

- Assume added responsibility when they are already working at capacity

- Consistently sacrifice their personal lives for work

- Lack control in their positions in the workplace

- Regularly suppress their emotions

Figure 23-1
COPING QUESTIONNAIRE

HOW WELL ARE YOU COPING AT WORK?

We all need a challenge at work, but too much becomes stressful. Find out how well you are coping at work, answering "yes" or "no" to the following questions.

	Yes	No
I feel enthusiasm for my job.	☐	☐
I feel my efforts at work are appreciated.	☐	☐
I feel tired at work even after a night's sleep.	☐	☐
I am forgetful.	☐	☐
Recent changes at work have been for the better.	☐	☐
I can communicate easily with colleagues and supervisors.	☐	☐
I feel a sense of dissatisfaction most of the time.	☐	☐
I feel emotionally, physically, or spiritually depleted.	☐	☐
My health is not as good as it was six months ago.	☐	☐
I am not as efficient as I would like to be.	☐	☐

SCORING

If you have answered "no" to questions 1, 2, 5, or 6, score 1 point each.
If you have answered "yes" to questions 3, 4, 7, 8, 9, or 10, score 1 point each.
Now add your total.

1 to 3 Points
You seem to be coping adequately with your job.

4 to 7 Points
You are probably suffering from some job-related stress and need to take preventive action.

8 to 10 Points
You are burning out and need to make a comprehensive plan.

- Do not and will not discuss problems or feelings
- Routinely criticize themselves
- Have not learned how to manage or reduce stress effectively in their lives

A good question to ask yourself is, "Do you work to live or live to work?" If there is no sense of fun or excitement in your work, and you do not have a balance between work and play, then your levels of energy and passion are likely waning and you are on the road to burnout. You could make a conscious choice to get off that road and instead begin getting back in touch with your sense of purpose, with your dreams, and with your excitements in life.

You could stimulate yourself and renew your energy by:

- Taking a class at a local community college or university

- Spending more private time in activities such as meditation and other forms of relaxation

- Exploring new hobbies

- Putting more thought, time, and energy into relationships with family and friends

- Taking time to experiment with different ways you can unleash your creativity

Most important, you need to understand that stress at work or at home is not something that others can give you. Your level of stress begins with your thoughts and your perceptions. You can learn to control your thoughts, replacing negative, self-defeating thoughts with positive, empowering ones.

LAUGHTER, BALANCE, AND WISDOM

It seems for most of us that our default setting for dealing with stress is to buckle down and try harder. We might tell ourselves that if we can just do all ninety-eight things on our "to-do" list by Friday, then we can kick back and relax over the weekend. When we begin to organize all of these things, somehow more get added to the list until we find ourselves with 119 things to do by Friday and only four get completed.

We then continue to work through the weekend, never relaxing, and the negative thoughts begin to multiply in our mind. "I'll never be able to get everything done" is one such thought. Richard Carlson and Joseph Bailey touch on this in their book, *Slowing Down to the Speed of Life*: "In order to feel less stress in your life, you must at some level realize that getting what you want isn't

> **Stress is a major cause of unrest in our lives, but we don't have to surrender our lives to it. If we understand where stress originates (in our minds), and its relationship to our thinking, we can begin to eliminate it, regardless of ourcircumstances.**
>
> **—Richard Carlson**

usually the ultimate answer. Instead, the only answer is to experience thinking that allows you to feel peaceful whether or not you get what you want."

Most people say that they simply don't have time in their lives to relax. What most of them come to realize is that they don't have many ways to relax that take just a few minutes of time. After all, you don't have to find an entire day or even half a day to achieve relaxation. There are many things that take just a matter of moments and that are refreshing and rejuvenating for you. This list might include the following:

- Closing your eyes, taking a few deep breaths, and imagining all your tension and stress floating away each time you exhale

- Listening to a favorite song

- Leaving a loving message on your spouse's voice mail

- Taking a short walk

- Planning something fun for the weekend or one evening during the week

- Laughing—it has a physiological and psychological benefit

- Talking and venting to a trusted friend

- Getting in your car, turning on the radio or CD player, and singing at the top of your lungs

Once you get started, your list of possible mini-breaks will get longer and longer. It is important to balance these mini-breaks with longer pauses, and most of you will have no trouble at all thinking of things you would like to do when you have a larger block of time available. If for some reason you feel at a loss as to possibilities, ask a friend for help. This is a great way to come up with ideas you may not have thought of yourself.

271

A Few Additional Ideas to Lessen Your Stress

- Change your thought patterns. We often think the worst is going to happen, yet it usually doesn't. Initiate your thinking in a more positive manner. Each time a negative thought goes racing through your mind, consciously change it to a positive one.

- Learn to say "no" when you really don't want to do something. Conversely, say "yes" when you do want to do something.

- Guilt serves little purpose. So stop it! Being honest with yourself about your feelings is a good place to start. Expressing them to others is even better.

- Write down the things that bother you. Writing often helps to put problems into perspective.

- Help someone less fortunate than you or a friend in need.

- Put yourself first. Healthcare workers who continually put the patient's needs above their own will experience compassion burnout. Taking care of yourself first is not selfish and means you will have more energy for others.

- Start a brag file. Keep those cards, letters of appreciation, and thank-you notes from clients. When you get down, take them out and reread the impact you have made.

You can gain knowledge of all these techniques, which can help you reduce your experience of stress and feel as if you are flowing with life. However, if you do not interpret these techniques in ways that are most appropriate for you, and if you do not actually use them or apply them, you are not exercising the wisdom that is available to you. There is no "quick-fix" for long-term stress or burnout. The only way many people can combat long-term stress or burnout is by changing their lifestyles or improving their working situations.

One way you can effectively and gently move into this place of wisdom is to begin practicing compassion for yourself. Developing the skill of compassion is an integral part of enhancing your self-esteem and reducing your perceived experience of stress.

In their book *Self-Esteem*, Matthew McKay, Ph.D., and Patrick Fanning write: "Most people think of compassion as an admirable character trait like honesty, loyalty, or spontaneity. If you have compassion, you show it by being kind, sympathetic, and helpful to others." *Compassion is actually a skill*, not an unchanging character trait. It is a skill that you can acquire if you lack it or expand on if you already have it. Compassion should inspire you to be kind, sympathetic, and helpful to yourself as well as something you feel for others.

The skill of compassion has three essential elements: understanding, accepting, and forgiving. Consciously being compassionate with yourself provides a tremendous boost in eliminating negative and self-defeating thoughts. When you truly apply the qualities of understanding, accepting, and forgiving that together make up compassion, it is nearly impossible for critical, negative, stress-inducing thoughts to sneak into your mind. In this regard, compassion is like a secret weapon against stress.

As Richard Carlson states in *You Can Be Happy No Matter What*, "When we feel stressed, we lose our psychological bearings, wisdom, and common sense; we tend to take things too seriously; we lose site of the big picture and often get lost in the details of our problems." Living a life of balance, and achieving just that right level of stress for you, does not have to remain a distant dream. By applying the techniques outlined in this chapter, you are making a decision to take charge of your life, to shift self-defeating, stress-inducing thoughts into positive, opportunity-creating thoughts. You are moving away from the pattern of feeling tired and unfulfilled to feeling optimistic and grateful. The choice is yours.

> Compassion is actually a skill, not an unchanging character trait.

RESOURCES

Books

Awaken the Giant Within by A. Robbins.

Beyond Anger: A Guide for Men: How to Free Yourself from the Grip of Anger and Get More Out of Life by T. Harbin.

Brain Workout by A. Winter and R. Winter.

Coping with Stress by C. Snyder.

Don't Sweat the Small Stuff at Work: Simple Ways to Minimize Stress and Conflict While Bringing Out the Best in Yourself and Others by R. Carlson.

Emotional Intelligence by D. Goleman.

Getting Things Done: The Art of Stress-Free Productivity by D. Allen.

Relax Now by S. Hayward.

Slowing Down to the Speed of Life by R. Carlson and J. Bailey.

Stress and Emotion: A New Synthesis by R. Lazarus.

The Stress Management Handbook by L. Leyden-Rubenstein.

Stress Management: Psychological Foundations by S. Auerbach and S. Grambling.

The 10 Step Method of Stress Relief: Decoding the Meaning and Significance of Stress by A. Crum.

Time Management from the Inside Out: The Foolproof System for Taking Control of Your Schedule and Your Life by J. Morgenstern.

You Can Be Happy No Matter What by R. Carlson.

You Don't Have To Go Home From Work Exhausted by A. McGee-Cooper.

Magazine Articles

"Earnings, Feminization, and Consequences for the Future of Veterinary Medicine" by G.Y. Miller in *JAVMA*, 1998, no. 3.

"Graduate Student Academic and Psychological Functioning" by C. Hodgson and J. Simoni in *Journal of College Student Development*, 1992, Vol. 36, No. 3.

"Is the Veterinary Profession Losing Its Way?" by N. Nielsen in *Canadian Veterinary Journal*, Volume 41.

"Major Life Events and Minor Stressors: Identifying Mediational Links in the Stress Process" by D. Pillow, A. Zautra, and I. Sandler in *Journal of Personality and Social Psychology*, 1996, Vol. 70, No. 2.

Websites

Conscious Living Foundation
www.cliving.com
Offers a number of products to test and measure stress as well as educational resources on the topic of stress.

McKinley Health Center at the University of Illinois-Urbana
www.mckinley.uiuc.edu/health-info/stress/vul-stre.html
A questionnaire designed to help you discover your stress vulnerability quotient and to pinpoint trouble spots.

Alcoholics Anonymous
www.aa.org
Information about their programs and links to local chapters.

Cocaine Anonymous
www.ca.org
Information about their programs and links to local chapters. Includes a self-test for cocaine addiction.

Narcotics Anonymous
www.na.org
Information about their programs and meetings. Includes articles on narcotics recovery.

SoberRecovery
www.soberrecovery.com
Information on various addictions. Includes a comprehensive directory of drug rehab centers, alcohol treatment programs, and detox centers.

273

▶ CHAPTER TWENTY-FOUR ◀

Dealing With Death and Grief on the Job

Laurel Lagoni, MS

IN THIS CHAPTER, YOU'LL LEARN HOW TO:

- Prepare families for euthanasia
- Effectively deal with your own grief over the loss of a patient

---

Today's pets are often considered to be family members. In fact, according to a survey conducted by the American Animal Hospital Association, 70% of respondents said they thought of their pets "as children," and 29% said they relied on their pets more than anything else for companionship and affection.

As a veterinarian, you would probably agree that the foundation of your profession is the family-pet bond. After all, if families didn't feel deep levels of attachment for and commitment to their pets, they probably wouldn't seek medical care for them. Thus, providing high-quality medical care for family pets is one of the primary ways you can help pet owners preserve and strengthen the very important relationships they share with their pets.

However, in today's marketplace, providing high-quality medical care is often not enough to meet your clients' needs, particularly when the family-pet bond is broken by the pet's death. Under these circumstances, many clients also want and expect you to provide them with the kind of skilled emotional support that will guide them through their feelings of grief.

In spite of a growing knowledge base confirming companion-animal loss as a significant life event, it's unlikely that you've been trained how to provide skilled emotional support. This lack of training extends to the procedures surrounding euthanasia. For example, you most likely did not receive adequate instruction in the emotional-support protocols known to provide effective, sensitive care for people during family-present euthanasias. Furthermore, you probably were not taught how to attend to the emotional ramifications that patient death and euthanasia can have for you and for the members of your staff.

PATIENT DEATH AND CLIENT GRIEF

Companion-animal death is an inevitable part of veterinary medicine. Due to the short life spans of animals and the option of euthanasia, it is estimated that veterinarians experience the deaths of their patients five times more often than their counterparts in human medicine. One study reports that 3% of the companion animals treated by veterinarians die over a period of one year, and 66% of these deaths are due to euthanasia. Grief, then, is an issue of central importance to the field of veterinary medicine.

Grief is one of our most common human experiences; yet, it is also the one most of us know the least about. This gap between experience and knowledge exists because conversations about personal loss and feelings of grief are usually considered to be morbid, morose, painful, taboo, and even unhelpful. In truth, when conversations about loss and grief are conducted with sensitivity and skill, they are the opposite. They can be uplifting, comforting, and very helpful.

Normal Grief

Feelings of grief occur naturally and spontaneously as a response to loss. Grief is the normal way people adjust to death, as well as to all kinds of endings and change. The grief process is necessary for healing when emotional wounds are caused by loss. Normal grief may last for days, weeks, months, or even years, depending on the significance of the loss.

The intensity of the grief response is based on several factors. These include the nature of the loss, the circumstances surrounding the loss, the griever's "preloss" emotional status, and the availability of emotional support before, during, and after the loss. If grief is progressing in a healthy manner, the feelings, thoughts, and behaviors related to it lessen in intensity over time.

Each of us grieves in unique ways. There is no right or wrong way to grieve. The nature of grief varies according to societies, cultures, age, gender, and other factors. For instance, research shows that women shed more tears and cry more often during grief than men. This is probably due to the fact that men are socialized to maintain their composure during emotional times, while women are socially conditioned to express their feelings more openly.

Research has also proven that children grieve just as deeply as adults. Their grief is more sporadic, though, due to their shorter attention spans. Until children reach the ages of eight or nine, they do not possess the cognitive development and language capabilities necessary to verbally express grief. Thus, most children express their grief through behaviors instead of through words. They act out their grief through artwork, play behaviors, or expressions of anger and irritability.

Clinical experience shows that, when the expression of grief is restricted, the healing time for recovery is prolonged. Likewise, when grief is expressed freely, the healing time for recovery from loss is, in general, greatly reduced. As a veterinarian, you can best help your clients by encouraging them to openly express their grief-related thoughts and feelings about their pets' deaths. You can do this by giving your clients "permission" to grieve. Encourage them to cry, to ask questions, to view their companion animals' bodies, and to reminisce about their pets' lives. This sort of "permission" from you, an authority figure, normalizes grief and reassures your clients that their feelings are not immature, overly sentimental, or crazy.

FAMILY-PRESENT EUTHANASIA

Veterinary medicine has always accepted the responsibility of patient euthanasia, believing it is a privilege to help severely injured or terminally ill animals die in a humane, painless way. The option of active euthanasia for patients is unique to veterinary medicine, and it puts you and your staff members in a special position. Like your human-medicine colleagues, you are morally and ethically obligated to save lives. Yet, when quality of life ceases to exist for an animal, you are also morally and ethically obligated to put an end to suffering and pain. Euthanasia allows you to legally and humanely end the very lives you once saved.

> When you are prepared to skillfully and sensitively conduct both the medical and emotional-support procedures associated with euthanasia, the experience becomes more positive for everyone involved.

The presence of a client's family at their pet's euthanasia puts you in an even more unique position because, during the procedure, you witness what very few human medical professionals ever see—the planned death of a family member—and the family members' immediate displays of grief. When you are prepared to skillfully and sensitively conduct both the medical and emotional-support procedures associated with euthanasia, the experience becomes more positive for everyone involved. The key is being prepared.

Over the past decade, protocols have been developed to guide veterinary teams through both the medical and emotional aspects of euthanasia. These protocols are designed so that you are prepared to facilitate family-present euthanasias with minimal medical side effects and maximum emotional support. Providing effective emotional support related to euthanasia consists of preparing families to face their pets' euthanasias, facilitating a sensitive family-present euthanasia, and providing effective follow-up care after euthanasia.

Preparing Families to Face Euthanasia

When it comes to preparing families to cope with the painful feelings surrounding a pet's death, a preeuthanasia consultation is essential. Clinical experience shows that, when people have time to plan and prepare for a death, they are less likely to have regrets about the way death unfolds. The key concept to keep in mind during a preeuthanasia consultation is choice. When people make conscious choices, they feel they have an element of control and are making decisions that are right for them.

Research shows that choices and longer preparation times diminish the intensity of grief after a loved one dies. This anticipatory grief—grief that begins before death has actually occurred—aids the healing process. For this reason, it's important for your clients to have a thorough understanding of their pet's prognosis and to have as much time as possible to plan and prepare for the death. This means it is usually up to you to introduce the subject of euthanasia and to explain it in such a way that clients don't feel pressured to make an immediate decision, but feel prepared to decide once the timing is right for them.

Preeuthanasia consultations should take place in a quiet, private room where clients will not feel

> Preeuthanasia consultations should take place in a quiet, private room where clients will not feel hurried or pressured to make decisions.

hurried or pressured to make decisions. Many practices use specially designed comfort rooms for this purpose. During the conversation, you should expect that a variety of emotions might arise (including your own). You can support and normalize emotions by making tissues, water, and other "comfort" items readily available.

During the preeuthanasia consultation, you or a well-trained member of your staff should discuss several topics with the family and help the family make as many decisions as possible prior to the pet's death.

FAMILY PRESENCE

The first decision to discuss with pet owners is whether or not they wish to be with their pet during the euthanasia procedure. It's important for owners to make this decision for themselves. There are several reasons why owners may want to be present when their companion animals die. These include the following:

- Families feel their pets have always "been there" for them. In turn, they don't want to "abandon" their pets at death.

- Families want to know for themselves that their pets died peacefully and that their deaths actually occurred.

- Families want to hold their pets and say goodbye at the moment death occurs. They want the last thing their animals hear and feel to be the owners' soothing words and loving touches.

If you are like many of your colleagues, having your clients present during euthanasia may cause you some anxiety. Some of your anxiety probably stems from the following concerns:

- If owners become emotionally upset while present at euthanasia, they may increase the anxiety levels of their animals, and, subsequently, make the pet more difficult to handle and the euthanasia procedure more difficult to complete.

- If animals become more difficult to handle, something is more likely to "go wrong" during the euthanasia procedure (e.g., you might miss a vein or there might be unpleasant side effects of the drug).

- Actually witnessing their companion animals deaths may be more than most clients can handle, causing them to faint, get sick, or even become hysterical if they are present during euthanasia.

- Client-present euthanasias may take too much time and be too emotionally draining for all involved (including you).

278

- Seeing your clients' grief may trigger your own, and you might cry in front of your clients. You may feel that crying in front of clients is unprofessional and inappropriate. You may also be concerned that, if you are upset, you may not be able to support your clients.

> No other part of veterinary medical care engenders more loyalty to your practice than well-planned and sensitively conducted, client-present euthanasias.

Although these are legitimate concerns, the experiences of veterinarians who regularly conduct family-present euthanasias suggest that, when euthanasias are well planned and facilitated, the opposite of these predictions is what actually happens. When both patients and clients are adequately prepared for euthanasia, these difficulties *rarely* occur. And, if they do occur, you have prepared your clients (and your staff) to face them.

There are several things you can do to ensure that these concerns will not be realized. For example, a drug combination or a mild sedative (e.g., thiopental) followed by the euthanasia solution (e.g., pentobarbital sodium) has been proven to minimize side effects like patient anxiety, agonal gasps, and body twitching. Placing an intravenous catheter in one of the animal's hind legs also minimizes the possibility that you will miss a vein or that the animal will pull away from the injection, making it seem to the family like their pet is struggling against the procedure. If you decide to use a catheter, you should also use a saline flush to test the catheter before you make the other two injections.

Many people, including veterinarians, do cry during euthanasias. But it is important to remember that emotions are normal responses to loss and are to be expected in response to death. Most clients report that it meant a lot to them that their veterinarian cried, too, when their pet died.

Client-present euthanasias do take more time. There is no getting around that fact. However, no other part of veterinary medical care engenders more loyalty to your practice than well-planned and sensitively conducted, client-present euthanasias. When clients feel they have been given choices about how and when their pets die and are able to witness their pets' peaceful death, surrounded by people who love and care about them, they are forever grateful.

In order to decide whether or not to be present, clients usually need information about what the actual euthanasia procedure entails. Your role during this time is to provide detailed information about the process of euthanasia and to support your clients' decisions to the best of your ability. The following is a sample script for informing clients about both the medical and emotional processes surrounding euthanasia.

"Marcy, Paul, Jake, and Jimmy . . . I know Pepper is very important to each of you. Therefore, I am committed to making this experience as meaningful and as positive for you as possible. In order to decide whether or not you want to be with Pepper when he dies, I want you to completely understand what we're going to do. Would you like me to explain the procedure to you now?" With the family's permission, you continue.

"The first thing I will do in preparation for Pepper's euthanasia is to take him back to our treatment area, shave a small area of fur off his hind leg, and place an intravenous catheter in a vein. The use of a catheter simply means that I can administer the euthanasia solution more smoothly, without causing Pepper any further discomfort. It also means that I can accomplish what I need to do medically without interfering with your way of saying goodbye to Pepper, like holding his head in one of your laps, talking to him, maybe even holding his front paws like you would hold someone's hand.

"After I've placed the catheter, Pepper will be brought back to you and you will be given time to spend with him, if you want to. Then, when all of us agree that it is time to proceed, we will begin the euthanasia process. The method I prefer to use involves three injections. The first is a saline-solution flush. This ensures that the catheter is working. The second is a barbiturate, usually thiopental, which places Pepper into a soothing state of relaxation. The third injection is the euthanasia solution, usually pentobarbital sodium. This injection will actually stop Pepper's heart, brain activity, and other bodily functions, and ultimately cause his death. Many people are surprised by how quickly death takes place, as it occurs within a matter of seconds.

"You should also know that, although humane death by euthanasia is painless and peaceful, Pepper may pee, poop, twitch, or even sigh a bit. He will not be aware of any of this, though, and he will not feel any kind of pain. In addition, Pepper's eyes may not close. It takes muscles to make eyes close, and Pepper will not have use of his muscles at that time.

"Do you have any questions about any of this?" If the family expresses understanding, you can conclude with, "After Pepper has died, you can stay with him for as long as you want to."

It's important to remember that this conversation will most likely elicit a range of strong emotions, and you will need to be prepared to deal with and support them.

Although client presence has value, encouraging client presence must be done with care. You should never aggressively talk a client into being present at a euthanasia. Some clients very clearly decide to leave their animals in their veterinarian's hands to be euthanized. This option is as acceptable as any other if it is what your clients choose. Your clients should not be deterred from this decision when the choice is an informed one.

Timing

Pet owners use many methods to decide when the time is right to euthanize their pets. Some let the medical signs point the way, while others ignore the medical evidence and allow themselves to be guided solely by emotions. Although it can be emotionally difficult, it is best for all involved to schedule an appointment time for euthanasia. An appointment is the only way your clients can ensure that you will be available to help their pet die in the way that they have chosen.

Location

The site for a family-present euthanasia might be outdoors, at the family's home, or in a specially equipped comfort room inside your veterinary hospital. When you have prior knowledge about where the procedure will take place, you and your staff can prepare the site ahead of time. For example, if the family prefers to say their last goodbyes outdoors, tissues and some type of ground covering can be brought to the space prior to their arrival. If your exam rooms are large enough, you can place a large mat on the floor so that the euthanasia doesn't have to take place on a sterile-looking exam table or countertop. Floor mats allow families and staff alike to gather around a pet in a comfortable, intimate way to say good-bye.

Body Care

Before death occurs, owners should be offered all of the body-care options you can make available to them, and each should be explained with honesty and sensitivity. The cost of each option should also be disclosed. It is helpful to use visual aids during this explanation. For example, if your practice makes caskets or urns available for owners to purchase, samples can be shown to them. If cremation is an option, sample cremains can be available to view if clients choose to see them.

Memorializing

Before their pets die, families should be encouraged to think about and to plan how they will want to pay tribute to their pet. If pet owners aren't encouraged to think about memorializing *before* their pets die, they often miss out on opportunities to spend special times with their pets, to take pictures or videos of their pets, or to schedule "funerals" or tributes for their pets. Planning ahead helps minimize regrets—the things families wish they would have said or done, but find that now it is too late.

279

Facilitating Family-Present Euthanasia

Scheduled euthanasias should be given first priority over all other appointments, except medical emergencies. Upon arrival, the family should be immediately escorted to wherever the euthanasia will take place. Prior to euthanasia, the euthanasia consent form should be signed, arrangements for payment should be made, and, if you prefer to use a catheter, the pet should be taken to a treatment room for catheter placement. Once they are settled, the family should be asked if they would like some private time with their pet before the procedure begins. It's important for you to ask about your clients' wishes rather than to assume all of your clients will want more time alone. Some clients have said their good-byes at home and feel ready to proceed immediately when they arrive at your clinic. Forcing them to wait when it isn't what they want or expect can cause them great anxiety.

When the family is ready to proceed with euthanasia, each drug should be injected with little or no lapse of time between them. As the drugs are injected, each should be named so that owners understand how the procedure is progressing. For example, you might say, "First, I'm using a saline flush to make sure the catheter I have inserted is working properly. Now I am using a barbiturate that will make Pepper sleepy and relaxed. Now I am injecting the final drug." Aside from these statements, it's best to remain silent. Most owners want to focus on saying goodbye to their animals and find comments, questions, and chatter distracting to this profound, private conversation.

Once the procedure is completed, it is very important for you to use a stethoscope, listen for a final heartbeat, and pronounce the animal dead. A clear, simple statement, such as, "Pepper has died," will often trigger sobbing and even feelings of relief. Owners may make remarks about how quickly death came and about how peaceful the experience was. Some may express feelings of guilt, and others will tell stories, reviewing the pet's life. This is a good time for you to reassure families about their decision to euthanize and to express your own feelings of affection and grief for your patient.

Some veterinarians offer families the chance to clip some of their pet's fur or to make a clay imprint of their pet's paw. Keepsakes like these are meaningful links to pets in the days and weeks of adjusting to life without their long-time companions.

Post-Euthanasia Follow-Up Care

If the family is not taking their pet's body with them, a staff member should stay with the animal's body at the euthanasia site. Almost all owners take one last look back at their pet before they actually leave the euthanasia site. When they see their pet accompanied by a friendly, familiar face, they feel reassured that their companion animal will not be forgotten or treated with disrespect once they leave. Condolences (sympathy cards, flowers, memorial donations) should be made as soon as possible following the pet's death.

There are many other aspects of euthanasia and patient death that are important for you to feel you can facilitate with confidence. For a more complete and detailed discussion of these topics, take time to read one or more books about pet loss and grief written specifically for veterinarians. See the resources section at the end of this chapter.

YOUR STRESS RELATED TO PATIENT LOSS AND GRIEF

Stress can be specifically related to helping others deal with loss and grief. Many stressors are uniquely associated with caring for terminally ill patients and their families. Researchers Vachon, Lazare, Cook, and Oltjenbruns identified some of the common stressors that arise when working with dying patients. With some adaptation to veterinary practice, those stressors are:

- Difficulty accepting the fact that the patients' physical problems cannot be controlled or cured

- Feeling frustration and failure when a patient in whom you have invested large amounts of energy dies

- Difficulty deciding where the limits of your involvement with patients and their owners, particularly during off-duty hours, begin and end

280

- Feeling overwhelmed when several patients die within a short time span

- Continuing to feel guilty and responsible for a misdiagnosis or mistake that was made concerning patient care

- Holding on to the belief that veterinarians are supposed to be strong and not give in to or show their emotions

Like most veterinarians, you probably experience at least some discomfort when you deal with these issues. It is normal to be touched by the pets and pet owners you care for and to struggle with the feelings that arise in practice. Yet, feelings related to patient loss and grief can sometimes be so intense or persistent that they affect your overall work performance and peace of mind. The following strategies represent some ways you and your staff can cope with patient loss and the subsequent feelings of grief on a day-to-day or at least regular basis.

Stress Management Strategies

Information about stress management theories and practices abound (see Chapter 23 for additional information on stress). There are thousands of ways to cope with life's hassles. Yet, some strategies are more relevant to dealing with patient loss and grief than others. A sampling of these strategies follows.

SEEK THERAPY

An important part of managing your grief-related stress involves learning from your loss experiences. Malenik et al., in an article in the *American Journal of Psychiatry*, interviewed fourteen adults whose parents had died during the two years preceding the study. About 50% of the participants reported that, even though the deaths of their parents had been very painful, they had experienced a beneficial outcome from the experience. For example, participants reported benefits like greater caring for friends and loved ones, increased emotional strength and self-reliance, and deepened levels of appreciation for life. Participants also said they now placed more value on the present rather than investing so heavily in the future.

You may find that particular cases involving patient death and client grief touch you and cause you to react more strongly than others. Mental-health professionals call this being "triggered" or "hooked" by cases. This is normal. It happens to everyone who works with people who are experiencing emotional pain. These are the cases, though, that you may want to look at more closely with the help of a therapist, asking questions like, "Is this animal similar to one I lost? Does this client remind me of someone I loved and lost, or someone for whom I have negative feelings? Does the decision at hand remind me of a loss I have faced in my personal life?"

Objective opinions from mental-health professionals or even discussions with other trusted veterinarians may normalize your grief or heightened emotions and help you resolve conflicts about troubling cases. It may also help you set realistic limits in the future. When selecting someone to consult or debrief with, do so with care. A nonjudgmental listener will provide support and validate feelings and will do so without advice-giving or asking questions about your competency.

DEVELOP COMMUNICATION SKILLS

Knowing how to communicate authentically and effectively is an important aspect of providing grief support. There are three types of communication-skills training that may help you feel more comfortable providing emotional support to grieving clients.

- General training allows you to practice (through role playing) many of the basic communication skills necessary for grief work and pet-loss support. This training is often provided at national conferences or through continuing-education seminars associated with universities or professional organizations.

- Training in paraprofessional crisis intervention is available through community crisis centers.

- Paraprofessional grief counseling is usually offered by community hospice programs.

Your staff members should also be included in training experiences, because they spend a relatively large amount of time with pets and pet owners. Many times, pet owners will tell receptionists and technicians things they are unwilling to tell you. This can put additional pressure on the technical staff; therefore, it is important to adequately train them how to effectively intervene in pet loss.

ALLOW FOR TRANSITION TIME

Transition time is the time needed to pass from one thing to another—to "finish" what just occurred and "focus" on what is about to take place. Transition time is used to recover your emotional composure and clarity of thinking. Transition time is generally brief. As it relates to veterinary medicine, it may be the time between appointments, between surgeries or treatments, or between meetings with your staff.

Transition time is particularly significant when the activity you are moving from or to involves an emotional experience. The key to regular use of transition time lies in building in time to "finish" one activity and ready yourself to "focus" on the next. Two techniques are especially helpful for this—deep breathing and spending time in natural settings.

> Transition time is the time needed to pass from one thing to another—to "finish" what just occurred and "focus" on what is about to take place.

Deep Breathing. Deep breathing has both calming and revitalizing effects. Noticing your breathing pattern and changing it from tension-producing to relaxation-producing is one of the most crucial—and simplest—relaxation techniques. As little as five minutes of deep breathing can refresh you on even the most difficult days.

Breathing deeply means you inhale from deep within, pushing your abdomen out and moving your diaphragm up. This is different from the more shallow breathing that takes place in your chest cavity. As you exhale, you forcefully release your breath through your mouth rather than through your nose. This is often referred to as a cleansing breath. Be careful not to do too many cleansing breaths at one time, because you may hyperventilate.

When a case involves patient death, taking time between appointments to spend a few moments alone calming your breathing, reflecting on what has just transpired, and moving your focus to the next activity can make a huge difference in how you are able to communicate and support your clients. Regulating your breathing can help you feel calmer and more able to handle your own emotions. When you don't feel "rattled," you are more able to handle the anxiety and emotional states of others.

Spending Time in Natural Settings. In a 1991 study, Ulrich et al. monitored the physiological stress responses of university students as they watched an unpleasant film about work accidents. Immediately after the students viewed the film, they were shown a color/sound videotape of an environment—a nature scene or an attractive urban environment lacking nature. Findings revealed that students recovered much faster and more completely from the stress of observing the accident film if they were then exposed to nature settings rather than to urban environments. Monitoring devices showed that the restorative benefit of nature took place within three to four minutes. Ulrich also indicated that what people responded to as a natural setting was not necessarily limited to wilderness. Agricultural fields, wooded parks in cities, and even golf courses were defined as "nature" by the survey participants.

If a case, or just the hectic pace of your day, has caused you to feel depleted and emotionally drained, try to spend a few minutes outdoors between your cases. If the weather or your environment makes this impossible, design a corner of your staff room or office space to resemble a natural setting. Place plants, an aquarium, and even posters of natural scenes in the area, and designate it as "off-limits" to the rest of the staff when it is occupied by someone in need of restoration.

ALLOW FOR CLEAN TIME

Clean time is exactly what it sounds like—it is time that is free of demands and responsibilities. It is time that is not cluttered with the worries of work or home. Everyone needs clean time, yet most say it is hard to find.

You should try to find clean time on a daily basis, but it is especially important when your day has involved a lot of loss or emotional strain. Read books or watch television programs that stimulate discussion about other subjects. Avoid "shop talk" during breaks or when socializing with colleagues. Avoid taking paperwork home, because this habit contaminates clean time. Also, take time away from the clinic to pursue personal interests. Go fishing, take a dance class, volunteer, or travel.

Ensure that your staff gets clean time, too. Allow them to take a "mental-health day" once or twice a year. With mental-health days, staff members call in "well" rather than "sick" and spend the day doing something nice for themselves. Mental-health days can be scheduled a bit ahead of time out of courtesy for others. This kind of support for one another strengthens relationships in the clinic.

DRAW CLOSURE

Of all the stress-management ideas discussed in this chapter, none are more important for dealing with grief on the job than this one. Drawing closure means that you take steps to intentionally bring your cases to an end. In other words, you work hard to resolve your nagging questions and to stop the "what ifs" and "if onlys" from invading your thoughts. When your cases are emotionally resolved, you can realize that your best efforts were put forth, you understand what you would change or do differently next time in a similar situation, and you are able to turn your energies to new patients and clients.

Sometimes, all it takes to draw closure to a case is to send condolence cards to clients or to follow up with clients by phone. Other times, it requires more "digging." For instance, you may need to track down necessary medical information to better understand your patients' illnesses or deaths.

There are two main ways to draw closure to cases—creating purposeful endings and debriefing.

Creating Purposeful Endings. Purposeful endings are ceremonies or rituals, intentionally created by you, that signal that a case, a life, a day, or a year has been brought to a close. Purposeful endings are vehicles for cele-

brating successes, honoring efforts, grieving losses, and saying thank you. They can be thoughts, actions, or events. The only guideline for creating a purposeful ending is that it be meaningful to you, respectful of the other coparticipants in the process, and realistic in terms of time and resources.

There are many ways to create purposeful endings. You probably already participate in some without realizing it. For example, when you verbally or even mentally say goodbye to the animals you euthanize, or when you make a donation to an animal-oriented organization in memory of a patient, you are participating in a purposeful ending.

Here are some examples of purposeful endings in terms of patient euthanasia.

- Say your own goodbye.

- Write about the events of the day in a journal.

- Meet weekly with your staff to discuss what you all did well and what you could improve in terms of the cases you had that week.

- Plan an annual memorial ceremony for all the animals that died throughout the year; invite your clients.

- Sponsor a yearly "Blessing of the Animals" day with the support of religious leaders in your community.

Purposeful endings can take place individually and in groups. Be sure to encourage your staff to draw closure in a way that is meaningful to them.

Debriefing. Debriefing takes place when you talk openly with your staff about the emotional aspects of your cases. It involves talking about new or challenging events in your practice, sharing thoughts and feelings, and getting feedback and support for your actions.

Evaluating cases through debriefing allows you to acknowledge what was done well and what was not. It encourages your veterinary staff to talk about frustrations in not being able to cure or save particular animals. In a good debriefing session, whether it is one

> Evaluating cases through debriefing allows you to acknowledge what was done well and what was not.

on one or in a group, basic communication skills are used to listen to and to acknowledge the feelings of the speaker(s) without judgment. Open-ended questions are asked to help each staff member thoroughly understand the problem. Open-ended questions are phrased so that they cannot be answered with a simple "yes" or "no." Here are examples of open-ended questions:

- "What is it about this particular case that is bothering you?"

- "What do you wish you could do about it?"

- "How do the rest of us handle situations like that?"

Listed below are other keys to debriefing:

- Don't wait until problems are overwhelming. Debrief on a regular basis. Regular debriefing helps prevent stress build-up and helps people build knowledge and skills.

- Practice until all of your staff can be nonjudgmental listeners.

- Meet in a private, quiet place where you won't be interrupted. This way, your conversation will be conducive to an open discussion and a display of emotions.

- Come prepared. Try to clarify your needs before the debriefing begins. For example, "I need to hear from each of you about what you think I did well on this case and what you think I could do differently next time."

- Set time limits for the discussion before starting.

- If you are going to deal with the stress associated with grief on the job, you need debriefing time to process information, share memories, and express personal feelings about your patients' illnesses and deaths. This is essential for avoiding burnout.

IT TAKES PRACTICE AND COMMITMENT

Dealing effectively with grief on the job takes practice. It takes commitment to confront sensitive issues rather than walk away from them. It also takes dedication to ongoing skill building and training.

When you possess the ability to provide effective emotional support (for yourself as well as for others), you maintain confidence that you and your staff can move through the numerous interpersonal crises that commonly arise in practice. When your emotional-support and stress-management protocols work, you are freer to do more of what you love—practice high-quality veterinary medicine.

REFERENCES

Crying: The Mystery of Tears by W. Frey and M. Lanseth.

Dying and Grieving: Lifespan and Family Perspectives by A. Cook and K. Oltjenbruns.

Grief, Dying, and Death: Clinical Interventions for Caregivers by T. Rando.

Guidelines for Bond-Centered Practice by L. Lagoni, D. Morehead, C. Butler, and J. Brannan.

Helping the Bereaved: Therapeutic Interventions for Children, Adolescents, and Adults by A. Cook and D. Dworkin.

The Human-Animal Bond and Grief by L. Lagoni, C. Butler, and S. Hetts.

New Perspectives on Our Lives with Companion Animals by J. Harris.

The Practical Guide to Client Grief: Support Techniques for 15 Common Situations by L. Lagoni. Available through AAHA.

Ulrich, R. S., Simons, R. F., Losito, B .D., Fiorito, E., Miles, M. A., and M. Zelson. "Stress Recovery During Exposure to Natural and Urban Environments." *Journal of Environmental Psychology* 11: 201-230, 1991.

Ulrich, R.S. "Human Responses to Vegetation and Landscapes." *Landscape and Urban Planning* 13: 29-44, 1986.

RESOURCES

Books

The Practical Guide to Client Grief: Support Techniques for 15 Common Situations by L. Lagoni. Available through AAHA.

Magazine Articles

"Couples' Perceptions of the Stressfulness of the Death of the Family Pet" by G. Gage and G. and R. Holcomb in *Family Relations*, Volume 40, No. 1, 1991.

284

"Grief and Stress from So Many Animal Deaths" by L. Hart and B. Hart in *Companion Animal Practice*, Volume 1, No. 1, 1987.

Products

ClayPaws™, the original pawprint kit, is a low-cost, no-mess way for veterinarians and pet owners to make clay impressions of companion-animals' paws. This tool shows clients that the bond they share with their pets is recognized and valued. In turn, they bond clients to the veterinary practice. It is very meaningful

for honoring pets at their deaths as well as when they first join a family. Call World by the Tail, Inc. at 888/271-8444 for information or to order.

ComfortMats provide a way for veterinarians to gather patients and their families together in a relaxed, comfortable setting. The standard ComfortMat kit includes one large floor mat, one small examination-table mat, two large cloth covers, two small cloth covers, and a tip sheet. Each component may be purchased separately. For more information, or to order ComfortMats or cloth covers, contact World by the Tail, Inc. at 888/271-8444.

CHAPTER TWENTY-FIVE

Substance Abuse and Violence in the Workplace

Dee Strbiak, MS, LPC, CACIII, MAC

IN THIS CHAPTER, YOU'LL LEARN:

- How to identify and deal with staff who abuse substances
- About workplace hazards associated with substance abuse
- How to deal with acts of violence in a veterinary practice

PROFILES OF ALCOHOLISM AND SUBSTANCE ABUSE

Published data reported by Paul Hersey and Kenneth Blanchard in the early 1990s indicated that in the U.S. workforce, at any given time, chemicals impair three out of every ten people. One of these is a full-blown alcoholic. Combinations of prescription medications, alcohol, or other mood-altering chemicals will impair the other two to some degree.

Alcoholism affects more than 10 million Americans; at least three million are women. The National Institute on Alcohol Abuse and Alcoholism reported in 1990 that 10% of the workforce has problems related to alcohol abuse, and these staff function at a *minimum* of 25% reduced efficiency. Although there is debate on the issue, some sources state that nearly 17% of the workforce has alcohol-abuse problems. That is a 7% increase in less than ten years.

The average alcoholic is a man or woman with a good job, a home, and a family. Invariably, this is a person who has a meaningful lifestyle, has

people who care about him or her, and has valuable possessions that may have taken a lifetime of hard work to accumulate. Forty-five percent of employed alcoholics are in professional management, 30% are manual workers, and 25% are white-collar workers. Alcoholics may perform poorly on the job for as long as ten to twelve years before their alcoholism becomes publicly obvious. They are often the most valued in the organization, averaging fifteen to thirty years of service. The cost to replace their skills, expertise, and experience is incalculable.

The causes of alcoholism are still in dispute. Some experts attribute alcoholism to environmental factors, while other authorities lean toward genetic influences. Psychiatrist Dr. Donald Goodwin, in his book *Is Alcoholism Hereditary?*, provides evidence that a predisposition toward alcoholism is passed from parent to child through genetic transfer and is related to an individual's physiology, hormones, enzymes, and brain chemistry.

There is also the question of gender and tolerance to alcohol. Dr. Eleanor Z. Hanna, director of the alcohol clinic at Massachusetts General Hospital in Boston, showed that women can begin to suffer cirrhosis of the liver with only one third as much alcohol as might cause the disease in men. This is partly because of differences in size, but also because men maintain a fairly constant tolerance to alcohol. Women's tolerance varies with the menstrual cycle and use of oral contraceptives.

Female alcoholics, according to Mona Mansell of the Freedom Institute in New York, are usually closet drinkers; they rarely get dead drunk, but they are never truly sober either. They manage to drink during the day at a steady pace, using soft drinks to disguise the alcohol. Sometimes they refuse drinks at parties, thinking this will convince people they do not drink.

Other groups adept at hiding their addiction are the affluent, the young, and the highly intelligent. Father Peter Sweisgood, a Benedictine monk who works with problem drinkers in New York, states that these groups have the greatest potential for rationalizing their behavior. The young believe they can "handle" their liquor, and the very intelligent simply are more clever at concealing their dependency. Those with money have servants, secretaries, and other hangers-on who will protect them from the real world. The threat of losing a job, which is still the single most potent factor in getting an alcoholic to treatment, is just not as compelling to someone who is financially secure.

Alcoholism is a disease that can be arrested and treated. It is, however, a staggering, overwhelming problem in our society and one of the largest contributors to on-the-job injuries.

Alcohol, though legal, available, and socially acceptable, is a highly addictive drug. As an associate in practice, not only may this issue present itself in your workplace via a coworker or a spouse of a coworker, but also by many of your clients. They, too, are represented in those workforce statistics. Clients' ability to understand what you tell them may be compromised by an addiction.

288

HOW SUBSTANCE ABUSE AFFECTS A VETERINARY PRACTICE

Some concerns that you may face as a new associate regarding drug and alcohol use and violence at the veterinary practice include the lack of authority to take action and knowledge of the correct method of handling an issue. It might be your job to develop or review what policies and procedures the practice has in place. If the practice does *not* have a policy in place, the development of substance-abuse and violence-prevention policies can be the first step. This can help your practice maintain a healthy workforce, increase the practice's growth, and provide a basis for action when needed. Two sample policy statements (Figures 25-1 and 25-2) are included in this chapter as groundwork.

Alcohol is the most used and abused drug in the world, and its use raises several concerns for a practice. The bottom line is that substance abuse will affect the productivity and profitability of a practice. With regard to illicit drug use in the workforce, it is estimated that more than 10 million people, or 71% of employed individuals, currently use illicit drugs. According to the Department of Labor, it costs companies more than $100 billion annually to deal with substance-abuse issues in the workplace. Substance abuse contributes to an increase in workdays missed, work-related injuries and accidents, workers' compensation claims, sick leave, and overtime pay. In addition, drugs cause workers' work quality to be inconsistent. Drugs and alcohol are one of the top four causes for violence in the workplace and add a hidden cost to the practice in diverted manager-supervisor time and personnel turnover.

> With regard to illicit drug use in the workforce, it is estimated that more than 10 million people, or 71% of employed individuals, currently use illicit drugs.

Dealing With Staff Who Abuse Substances

As a new associate, it might be your job to deal with staff, or even the practice owner, when alcohol or drugs affect their performance. This can be an

Figure 25-1
DRUG-FREE WORKPLACE POLICY

SAMPLE DRUG-FREE WORKPLACE POLICY

In accordance with the federal Drug-Free Workplace Act of 1988, (practice name) has adopted the following policy to maintain a drug-free workplace. The unlawful manufacture, distribution, dispensation, possession, or use of a controlled substance in the workplace is prohibited. As a term of employment, the employee shall:

1. Abide by the terms of this policy statement and
2. Notify the appropriate personnel office of any criminal drug statute conviction for a violation occurring in the workplace no later than five days after such conviction.

DISCIPLINARY ACTIONS

Staff who violate the foregoing standards of conduct shall be subject to disciplinary actions which may include, without limitation, completion of an appropriate rehabilitation program, reprimand, probation, temporary adjustment of pay, reassignment with or without a salary adjustment, suspension with or without pay, demotion, and termination. In addition to the foregoing disciplinary actions, violations may be reported to law-enforcement authorities for criminal prosecution.

DEFINITIONS

Illicit drugs shall mean controlled substances listed in Schedules I-V of the Controlled Substances Act, 21 U.S.C. § 812, and the related federal regulations, 21 C.F.R. §§ 1308.11–1308.15, as they may be amended from time to time.

Alcohol shall mean any beverage containing not less than .05% ethyl alcohol by weight.

Property shall mean any property owned, leased, chartered, or occupied by the practice, including motor vehicles, boats, and aircraft.

IMPLEMENTATION

The practice shall implement drug- and alcohol-abuse prevention programs and shall review the programs biennially to determine their effectiveness, implement changes if needed, and ensure that the actions authorized by this policy are consistently enforced.

This information is not a substitute for legal analysis or interpretation. It is given to provide a general understanding of the importance of legal issues and workplace violence. The services of a competent attorney should be used to interpret the current laws and regulations that apply to your practice as well as for the legal implications of your draft policy.

Figure 25-2
WORKPLACE VIOLENCE POLICY

SAMPLE WORKPLACE VIOLENCE POLICY

It is (practice's name) policy to promote a safe and nonthreatening workplace environment for its staff. While this kind of conduct is not pervasive at our practice, no practice is immune. This practice is committed to working with its staff to maintain a work environment free from any form of violence, whether actual or perceived. This includes, but is not limited to, the following:

- Threats (intimidating or hostile), fighting, or disruptive behavior

- Threats via email, mail, or voice mail

- Possession of a weapon (not job-duty required)

- Gestures or expressions that communicate a direct or indirect threat of physical harm or verbal abuse

- Stalking

- Sabotage or misuse of practice equipment or property

- Any behavior that is perceived as threatening

An employee who observes or experiences such behavior by anyone on practice premises, whether he or she is a(n) employee, customer, family member, or someone else, must report it immediately to a supervisor or manager at XXX/XXX-XXXX.

Managers and supervisors are responsible for taking action against any form of violence. The supervisor is responsible, once knowledge of an incident occurs, to contact a member of the violence-response team or specified practice contact regarding investigating the incident and initiating appropriate actions. **(PLEASE NOTE: Threats of violence that require immediate attention by security should be reported to XXX/XXX-XXXX or to the police at 911.)**

This practice will not retaliate against any employee who complains about violence. The employee will not be adversely harmed by means of job position, title, discrimination, or termination because of the complaint. This policy will be monitored to assess whether it is being implemented effectively.

This information is not a substitute for legal analysis or interpretation. It is given to provide a general understanding of the importance of legal issues and workplace violence. The services of a competent attorney should be used to interpret the current laws and regulations that apply to your practice as well as for the legal implications of your draft policy.

unpleasant task, but being able to identify the early signs of a problem caused by alcohol and drugs can facilitate an early intervention. Figure 25-1 lists various substances and possible workplace consequences.

When someone's use of alcohol and drugs begins to interfere with the quality and professionalism displayed in the veterinary workplace, significant steps must be taken so that the business does not suffer irreparable damage. The practice manager/owner can find help through:

- An employee assistance program

- A veterinary practice owner's policy statement or handbook

- An AVMA model program to assist chemically impaired veterinarians, veterinary students, animal technicians, and their families

- AVMA state committees organized to assist impaired veterinarians (see the AVMA *Directory and Resource Manual* for contact listings)

- Informal and formal meetings

Table 25-2 provides a quick-reference guide for dealing with disruptive and intrusive issues.

SCENARIOS YOU MAY FACE

The following three scenarios present an overview of potential substance-use issues that might arise. The options include many possible responses to the problem but are not all-inclusive. These options range from no action to the most restrictive measures that can be taken.

Scenario A

You are the new associate in the practice, but it does not take you long to figure out that Suzie, a veterinary assistant, arrives late to work on a consistent basis and returns from lunch smelling like alcohol. Suzie, a part-time employee, is a full-time college student who is studying to be a vet. Suzie is quite hostile and shuts down when anyone tries to talk to her about her drinking and states that she is twenty-one and can drink if she wants to. The rest of the staff is tired of dealing with Suzie and does not want to cause more tension at the practice. The staff has dropped it in your lap to deal with. What are you going to do?

Options

- Do nothing and hope that Suzie will address her drinking problem by herself.

- Have an informal meeting to discuss the practice's needs and how the staff sees Suzie's role at the practice. No written statement will be added to her personnel file.

- Schedule a formal meeting to discuss Suzie's attendance issue and place a written statement in her personnel file about the meeting, current actions that need to be taken, and future action that will be taken if this happens again. Current actions can include:
  - If your practice is large, refer her to the practice's Employee Assistance Program.
  - Suzie will be asked to leave if she is intoxicated at work and given a three-day leave without pay.
  - Create a contract that states Suzie must not come to work or be at work intoxicated.
  - Sign a contract that she will seek outside help for her drinking and that the practice will be involved as part of the treatment plan.
  - Sign a contract that states Suzie will resign or be terminated after one more incident of being intoxicated at work.

- Terminate Suzie due to her repeated lateness.

Scenario B

You have been working with a client, Allen Walker, and his dog, Chester, for a few visits now. The dog is in good health and you administered his yearly immunizations after a physical exam. When you were talking with the dog's owner, you noticed that he smelled like alcohol, was somewhat distracted, and was slurring his words. You state that you need to run one more test. You leave the exam room and ask your assistant if he or she noticed the smell of alcohol also. The assistant states that he or she smelled the alcohol and asks you what you are going to do. What are you going to do?

Options

- Do nothing.

- Ask the client to leave the practice.

Table 25-1
WORKPLACE HAZARDS ASSOCIATED WITH SUBSTANCE ABUSE

Substance	Common Name	Workplace Hazards
Alcohol	Beer, wine, liquor	Lack of coordination Impaired judgment and concentration Excessive absenteeism, lateness Undue stress on coworkers Inability to solve work problems effectively
Marijuana	Pot, THC, grass, weed	Lack of depth perception Loss of time and space Slowed reflexes Impaired memory and concentration
Tobacco	Cigarettes, chew, cigars, snuff	Risk of fire Complaints from coworkers or customers Secondhand smoke
Cocaine and crack	Coke, rock, white lady	Mood swings, emotional problems Absenteeism Impaired decision-making Decreased work performance Increased risk of workplace violence and crime
Stimulants	Speed, crank, amphetamines, methamphetamines, crystal meth	Anxiety and impaired vision, coordination, and concentration Increased hyperactivity Insomnia that can decrease work performance Increased irritability among coworkers
Depressants	Barbs, downers, valium, ludes	Impaired coordination, reflexes, judgment, and concentration
Narcotics	Heroin, smack, morphine, demerol, T-3, codeine	Lack of interest in work performance and quality Increased medical claims Increased risk of workplace violence and crime
Inhalants	Paint, aerosol sprays, butyl nitrite	Impaired judgment and perception Impaired decision-making and concentration
Hallucinogens	LSD, PCP, mushrooms, angel dust (Ketamine HCl)	Distorted perceptions of time, space, and judgment Increased likelihood of violence toward coworkers
Designer Drugs	China white, synthetic heroin, ecstasy	Mimic narcotics, stimulants, and hallucinogens in their hazards
Steroids	Roids, juice	Aggressive behavior Occasional psychotic behavior Depression

- Express your concerns and see if there is anything that you can do.

- Ask the client to stay until he is not intoxicated and offer him a quiet room in which to wait.

- Ask the client to call someone to pick him up, since you will call the police if he tries to drive away from the practice intoxicated.

Scenario C

One of the staff confides in you that he has a problem with Valium. He has not taken any from the med room but feels that he might in the future. He states that he really needs this job and that he would like to get some help for his pill addiction. He pleads with you not to talk to the practice owner, because he will surely be fired. What are you going to do?

Options

- State that you can and will not keep anything of this nature from the practice's owner, but you will talk with the owner confidentially about it.

- Encourage him to seek professional help and be supportive.

- Refer him to the practice's Employee Assistance Program.

- Create a contract that he will not be at work under the influence, and if he is, he will have ten days of suspension or be terminated.

- Create a mutual agreement that he will take random drug tests and give you a copy of the results.

- Make sure that he does not have access to the med room, and if he does, that he is not allowed to be there unsupervised.

- If he has been taking Valium from the med room and he is a licensed professional, he must be referred to the state's professional diversion program.

Are You the One With the Problem?

If you want to see if alcohol or other drugs are affecting your life, the following checklists may help.

The Michigan Alcoholism Screening Test (MAST) (Figure 25-3) gives a rapid, effective screening for lifetime alcohol-related problems and alcoholism. The MAST is a self-administered, twenty-five-item questionnaire that takes fifteen minutes to complete and score. Another checklist that you can use is the twelve-part self-assessment listed below.

SELF-ASSESSMENT CHECKLIST

In addition to the MAST, this quick checklist can help you determine if you may be a substance abuser.

Intoxication

- Are you frequently high or intoxicated?

- Do recreational activities center around the use of alcohol or drugs?

Social Settings

- Do you drink alone?

- Do you avoid social gatherings where alcohol is not served?

- Do your friends encourage drinking and using drugs?

Intentional Heavy Use

- Has your tolerance for alcohol or other drugs increased (you can use more without appearing intoxicated)?

- Do you take social drugs in addition to prescribed medication?

- Do you take more than is prescribed with over-the-counter or prescribed medication?

Symptom Drinking

- Do you have a predictable pattern to your drinking or using?

- Do you rely on alcohol or drugs as a method of coping with stress?

- Have you made a lifestyle change, yet your drinking and drug use have stayed the same or increased?

Dependence

- Do you rely on alcohol or drugs as a means of coping with negative emotions?

- Do you consume alcohol or drugs more than you intend to?

- Do you use alcohol or drugs to relieve pain?

Health Issues

- Do you have a medical problem that is aggravated by alcohol or drug use?

- Have you ever had an injury while under the influence of alcohol or drugs?

Job Issues

- Have you missed work or been late due to the use of alcohol or drugs?

- Do you blame your alcohol or drug consumption on work problems?

Family Issues

- Have family members or friends expressed concern about your drinking or drug use?

- Have you lost any relationships due to your drinking or drug use?

Legal Issues

- Have you had any legal issues related to alcohol or drug use?

- Have you ever had an instance when you could have been arrested for alcohol or drug use and weren't?

Financial Issues

- Do you pay your bills on time?

- Can you account for your money easily?

Anger

- Do you get angry or defensive when confronted about your drinking or drug use?

- Do you get easily angered and do not know why?

Isolation

- Are you giving up social functions or getting together with friends in order to drink or use drugs?

- Do you tend to use more heavily when alone?

If you responded "yes" to more than five of the questions, you may need to assess the degree of substance use in your life. The evaluation of a professional addictions counselor can provide further assistance.

USE OF AN EMPLOYEE-ASSISTANCE PROGRAM (EAP)

Staff members are vital to the practice, and, being human, they come with problems that can affect their work performance. Issues that affect work performance include substance use, family concerns, financial matters, emotional upsets, and health issues.

Implementing an employee-assistance program can address these issues and help increase staff work performance and contribution to the practice. The use of an EAP is confidential and short-term focused. Programs are between one to five visits, and the focus is on getting the employee back to being productive at work. The employee usually remains working and uses personal or work time for the sessions.

There are many different ways for a practice to take advantage of EAP services. A practice can establish its own EAP program, it can buy EAP services from an outside source, or it can join together with other small businesses to offer EAP services.

SUBSTANCE-ABUSE POLICY

A written substance-abuse policy should be individualized for the specific practice. It needs to clearly state the practice's stance, give a definition of substances, state what is expected from the staff, and explain what help is available. The practice can create a substance-abuse policy by following the guidelines of the federal Drug-Free Workplace Act of 1988, which requires a practice to maintain a drug-free workplace. The practice must then adhere to the following two conditions:

Table 25-2
DEALING WITH DISRUPTIVE AND INTRUSIVE ISSUES RELATED TO SUBSTANCE ABUSE: A QUICK REFERENCE GUIDE

General Incident	Possible Response
A staff member comes to work intoxicated or high or becomes intoxicated or uses drugs at work.	**Step 1.** Hold an informal meeting with the employee and tell him or her to go home, with pay, and that you will discuss this with him or her tomorrow. Make arrangements to drive the employee home. **Step 2.** The next day, express your concerns, provide any appropriate referrals, and create a plan of action that includes actions to be taken if this occurs again. **Step 3.** The employee has continued to come to work intoxicated or high. Have a formal meeting with the employee and the supervisor that spells out consequences of this action. Document all conversations and actions taken. (Possible consequences are random drug screen, inpatient or outpatient therapy, five days leave without pay, and termination.)
The employer comes to work intoxicated or high or becomes intoxicated or uses drugs at work.	**Step 1.** Have someone who knows the employer well talk informally to the employer about his or her concerns. **Step 2.** Contact any member of the practice who has voting rights (i.e., owners) and express the staff's concerns. **Step 3.** If necessary, contact the employer's spouse or family members and express the staff's concerns. **Step 4.** Contact an outside consultant who will make contact with the employer and express the staff's concerns and offer options to the employer.
A client comes into the practice intoxicated or high.	**Step 1.** Ask the client to leave. Call the police and give them a description of the individual.

Figure 25-3
MAST

This document is also available on the companion CD.

MICHIGAN ALCOHOLISM SCREENING TEST (MAST)

The MAST is a simple, self-scoring test that helps you assess if you have a drinking problem. Please circle the answers to the following YES or NO questions:

1. Do you feel you are a normal drinker? ("normal"—drink as much or less than most other people)

   YES   NO

2. Have you ever awakened the morning after some drinking the night before and found that you could not remember a part of the evening?

   YES   NO

3. Does any near relative or close friend ever worry or complain about your drinking?

   YES   NO

4. Can you stop drinking without difficulty after one or two drinks?

   YES   NO

5. Do you ever feel guilty about your drinking?

   YES   NO

6. Have you ever attended a meeting of Alcoholics Anonymous (AA)?

   YES   NO

7. Have you ever gotten into physical fights when drinking?

   YES   NO

8. Has drinking ever created problems between you and a near relative or close friend?

   YES   NO

9. Has any family member or close friend gone to anyone for help about your drinking?

   YES   NO

10. Have you ever lost friends because of your drinking?

    YES   NO

11. Have you ever gotten into trouble at work because of drinking?

    YES   NO

12. Have you ever lost a job because of drinking?

    YES   NO

13. Have you ever neglected your obligations, your family, or your work for two or more days in a row because you were drinking?

    YES   NO

14. Do you drink before noon fairly often?

    YES   NO

15. Have you ever been told you have liver trouble such as cirrhosis?

    YES   NO

Figure 25-3 (continued)
MAST

MICHIGAN ALCOHOLISM SCREENING TEST (MAST) (continued)

16. After heavy drinking have you ever had delirium tremens (D.T.s), severe shaking, or visual or auditory (hearing) hallucinations?

    YES   NO

17. Have you ever gone to anyone for help about your drinking?

    YES   NO

18. Have you ever been hospitalized because of drinking?

    YES   NO

19. Has your drinking ever resulted in your being hospitalized in a psychiatric ward?

    YES   NO

20. Have you ever gone to any doctor, social worker, clergyman, or mental health clinic for help with any emotional problem in which drinking was part of the problem?

    YES   NO

21. Have you been arrested more than once for driving under the influence of alcohol?

    YES   NO

22. Have you ever been arrested, even for a few hours, because of other behavior while drinking?

    YES   NO

Scoring for the MAST Test
Please score one point if you answered the following:
1. No
2. Yes
3. Yes
4. No
5. Yes
6. Yes
7 through 22: Yes

Add up the scores and compare to the following score card:

0–2	No apparent problem
3–5	Early or middle problem drinker
6 or more	Problem drinker

- It must publish a statement notifying staff that it is unlawful to manufacture, distribute, dispense, possess, or use a controlled substance in the workplace and that action will be taken if this is done.

- It must establish an ongoing drug-free awareness program, which utilizes educational workshops, makes counseling programs available, provides education on the practice's policies, and describes the consequences of violation of the policy.

DRUG-TESTING PROGRAM

For practices with more than 500 people, federal regulations dictate a drug-testing procedure; however, smaller practices are beginning to start drug-testing programs for multiple reasons. It reduces medical claims, on-the-job injuries, and absenteeism. Ultimately, it is the best business decision.

A drug-testing program must meet several requirements, including:

- Statutory or regulatory requirements

- Disability discrimination provisions

- Collective bargaining agreements

Other considerations include:

- Who will be tested (new hires, safety or sensitive-job only, or all staff)

- When and how often staff will be tested (once a month, biweekly, quarterly, only after an accident, when performance decreases)

- Which drugs are tested (marijuana, cocaine, alcohol, multi-drugs, single drug)

- Actions and procedures for positive tests (termination, referral, job-duty evaluation)

- How confidentiality is maintained

- How the "chain of custody" with the sample is maintained

VIOLENCE IN THE WORKPLACE

Prevalence of Workplace Violence

During 1994, approximately one million people were victims of workplace violence, representing 15% of all victims of violent acts in the United States (Bachman, 1994). Women constituted some 60% of the victims. In addition to these victims of violence, another 2.2 million experienced theft at work. According to 1994 Department of Justice reports, 879,000 assaults, 13,000 rapes, and 80,000 robberies were reported. All together, on average, these acts of violence resulted in five days of missed work per person (BLS, 1996).

Categories of violent workplace actions included in the Bureau of Labor Statistics (BLS, 1996) are hitting/kicking/beating, biting, threat/verbal assault, squeezing/pinching/scratching/twisting, shooting, stabbing, and others.

These figures do not include the numerous incidents that go unreported, nor do they include threats made at work. Unfortunately, when an injury incident does not result in lost work, it may not be reported to any supervisor or authority. It may never be tracked and remains, all too often, unaddressed. Quite frequently, the same pattern exists for domestic violence that extends to the workplace. Researchers suggest that the measuring of violent acts is vastly understated in that the figures do not reflect verbal, indirect, and passive-aggressive behaviors, which are more pervasive.

Workplace violence occurs in a wide variety of settings and locations. Sixty percent of the violent acts occur in private companies. Thirty percent occur in government jobs, which is only (18%) of the workforce. Nonfatal acts against women are 8.6 times higher in state government and 5.5 times higher in local government than in the private sector.

Companies that appear to have a higher probability of workplace violence include those with authoritarian management policies. With this style of management, staff do not feel free to participate in decision-making and view supervision as strict, unreceptive, and uncaring.

Definition of Workplace Violence

According to Webster's *New World Dictionary*, violence is defined as "a physical force used so as to injure, damage, or destroy, violating another's rights, sensibility, etc." Workplace violence has a specific meaning. The California Occupational Safety and Health Administration (Cal/OSHA,

298

Table 25-3
DEALING WITH DISRUPTIVE AND INTRUSIVE ISSUES RELATED TO VIOLENCE: A QUICK REFERENCE GUIDE

Incident	Possible Response
An employee becomes violent toward a coworker, employer, or customer.	**Step 1.** If any physical violence is involved, call the police and get any bystanders out of the immediate area. Do not be a hero.
	Step 2. Talk to the individual in a normal, calm tone of voice and ask him or her what is going on. Do not judge or argue with the individual.
	Step 3. If no physical violence is involved, try to get the violent individual to come with you and another individual to your office or a quiet place.
	Step 4. Explain the consequences of becoming violent in a clear, reality-bound manner that is not condemning.
A customer verbally or physically threatens or abuses an employee or employer.	**Step 1.** Call the police immediately. Do not be a hero.
	Step 2. Ask the customer to leave.
	Step 3. Take action to protect yourself and any other staff, customers, or bystanders.
The employer becomes violent toward an employee.	**Step 1.** If there is any physical or perceived violence, call the police. Do not be a hero.
	Step 2. Contact your supervisor, manager, or coworker and explain what happened. Document all conversations.
	Step 3. If necessary, bring in an outside consultant to act as the mediator.

1995) has developed a classification system to help define workplace violence.

- **Type I**—This is violence by people unrelated to the workplace. The violent person is not a member of the practice, but a staff member is hurt. Most fatal workplace violence falls into this category. This would include people employed as retail workers, taxicab drivers, armored-car services, police officers, and security guards.

- **Type II**—This is comprised of acts committed by people who are related in some way to an employee. This can be a person who is a spouse, family member, or friend of the staff member. This category accounts for the greatest percentage of people who are seriously and nonfatally injured in the workplace. This would include domestic and partner abuse, workplace harassment, stalking, and office obsessions.

- **Type III**—This is violence between staff members and is the rarest form of workplace violence, but it's also one that instills the most fear in people. An example is the revenge killer who comes to the office and shoots coworkers, the supervisor, then commits suicide. The more common form of this type is comprised of the nonfatal threats to coworkers and supervisors where the perception of violence is unpredictable and close by.

Potential for Violence

Some practices make a mistake in thinking that staff violence will not happen to them and do not make an assessment of their workplace environment for the potential for violence. Veterinary-hospital owners and managers are no exception. They believe violence will not happen within their business or on their premises. Like closing the barn door after the horse runs off, the majority of practices, especially small practices, seem only to do an analysis of their vulnerability to potential workplace violence *after* an incident has occurred.

In order to be effective, an assessment must be conducted before any violent acts take place. This can be a simple or long process. For the small practices, having a policy that all staff members

understand is a good start. You can purchase a ready-made violence training program, or you can contract with a violence consultant to create a specific program for your needs.

Staff Reporting Mechanism

When staff are encouraged to report all incidents of violence—minor incidents, as well as major incidents—the system works. The process works best when reports are also handled in an effective and efficient manner. It is important to decide who will handle the reports. In a larger business, breaking down the reports into broad categories may help to direct the reports to the appropriate person, because several managers or supervisors may be involved.

The Practice's Legal Responsibilities

DUTY OF CARE

The "duty of care" is based on current federal laws and regulations under the Occupational Safety and Health Act of 1971. It requires that a practice provide a safe and nonthreatening workplace environment. The practice is responsible for the safety of its staff. The practice can also be held responsible for an injury or illness as a result of violence in the form of physical threats, harassment, or creation of a hostile work environment. In addition, an employer must make every reasonable attempt to provide a safe work environment and take all measures to provide benefits once an incident of violence has occurred.

NEGLIGENT ACTS

According to civil law, a practice can be found liable if it is negligent in hiring, retention, and job-recommendation practices.

- **Negligent hiring**—Employers are liable if they do not make an effort to maintain and hire individuals who would *not* present a danger to others on the job.

- **Negligent retention**—Employers are liable for failing to take action when an employee has threatened others, has a pattern of violence, or poses a risk of violence to a coworker.

- **Negligent recommendation**—Employers are liable for a manager's recommendation of an employee who was terminated due to violence or violation of the company's violence policy. An example involves company A, which terminated an employee due to the employee bringing a gun to work. The manager of company A gave a good recommendation to the terminated employee. This employee was hired at company B, where his violence pattern began again. Company B terminated him for this behavior. He returned to company B and killed several coworkers. The family members of the deceased workers are suing company A based on the recommendation of company A's managers.

SCENARIOS YOU MAY FACE

The following three scenarios present an overview of potential violence-in-the-workplace issues. The options include many possible responses to the problem but are not all-inclusive. These options range from no action to the most restrictive measures that can be taken.

Scenario One

Don and Becky are both veterinary assistants. Becky works the morning shift, while Don works the evening shift. It is Becky's job to leave Don a written progress note on any animal that has come into the practice that day and will be staying overnight. Becky is always busy and does not leave Don a detailed note most of the time because she is rushing out to catch her bus. Don does not address this with Becky; rather, he talks about Becky behind her back to the other staff. He also occasionally takes his frustrations with Becky out on the animals that she has admitted by not caring for them and stating that Becky left no instructions. What do you do?

Options

- Do nothing.
- Talk with Becky and have her schedule thirty minutes every day to complete her written progress notes. If she finds that she has run out of time, she is to contact someone personally to leave a verbal note.

- Talk to Don and set up a contract stating that if he neglects an animal again, he will be terminated. If he needs information that was not provided by Becky, he is to call you or another staff veterinarian for the information.

Scenario Two

You have been seeing a nine-year-old cat and her owners for a few visits now. The cat presented with a broken tail last month, and today she has a broken hind leg. The owners are a sweet older lady, who shows great affection toward the cat, and her new husband, who is quiet and standoffish. They state that the cat jumped from the balcony and hurt herself. You consult with the practice's owner, and she states that since the couple's marriage a few months ago, the cat has come in with several injuries. The recommendation is that you address your concerns with the owners and inform them of the decision to contact the humane society. When you advise the couple of your concerns, the husband becomes very loud and threatens to physically harm you and everyone at the practice. What do you do?

Options

- Do nothing and say nothing to the rest of the practice because you don't want to frighten them.
- Allow the couple to leave, and call the police and notify them of the threat.
- Have a meeting with the staff and discuss what happened and the steps the practice will take to ensure safety.
  - If the husband returns, the police are to be called immediately.
  - No one is to walk out to their cars at night alone.
  - Doors are to be locked after business hours.
  - Staff members will continue to work with the police if necessary.
  - Time off will be allowed if staff members feel unsafe and do not want to work for the next few days.
- Take precautions over the next few weeks with all staff members.

301

Scenario Three

Joe, the owner of the practice and the head veterinarian, is intense and a perfectionist. When he is with an animal and the animal's owner, he is the picture of professionalism and caring, but he tends to be very short fused with the veterinary assistants and the front-office staff if something is misplaced or not ready. He slams his office door and you can hear him throwing books and yelling. The staff is afraid of him but accepts his behavior because he is the owner. They have asked you for help. What do you do?

302

Options

- Do nothing and put up with it.

- Talk to Joe about his behavior and risk being yelled at or even fired.

- Contact his wife, family, or friends and talk to them about his violent behavior at work. Ask for their help in confronting him.

Crisis Response

How should you respond once violence or a tragedy has occurred? With all the preventive measures a practice can take and planning it can go through, there are no guarantees that violence or a tragedy will not occur. When a practice experiences a violent or tragic incident, it can affect the practice, the staff, and their families. A post-crisis incident intervention can assist in the restoration of the practice by making staff feel that their practice cares and is looking out for them. For the employer, such an intervention might well help to decrease time off, insurance claims, and litigation, and maintain an overall sense of practice loyalty by the staff. There are many companies and individuals who offer crisis intervention as a service. Described below is a "typical" scenario that could happen in any business.

SCENARIO YOU MAY FACE

When you arrive at work, you are informed that an assistant's wife was killed in an auto accident. You learn she was run off the road and beaten by a man after she accidentally cut in front of him on the highway. He apparently rammed his car into her, dragged her out of her car, and began beating her head into the hood of the car. When police arrived, she was dead and the man had fled. The police have a description and are following up on the homicide. The staff at the practice are stunned and are taking this death very personally. What do you do?

Options

- Gather the entire staff and fill them in on all the information you have so that rumors are controlled.

- Give assignments to the staff for ordering flowers, making meals, being supportive, etc.

- Give personal time to people who really need it and request it.

- Coordinate with the practice management to close the practice for the funeral.

- Allow people to deal with this tragedy in their own way. People will be angry, sad, depressed, in shock, and confused.

- Allow for the staff to talk and process this event.

No practice can completely prevent or eliminate workplace violence, but the cost of just one incident of workplace violence far exceeds the relatively minor cost of proper planning and training. Therefore, it is essential to invest in building awareness of these issues.

RESOURCES

Websites

The Internet offers a wide resource for additional information on substance abuse and workplace violence. The sites listed below offer a starting point for additional information and links to more sites.

Substance Abuse Issues

U.S. Department of Health and Human Services
www.os.dhhs.gov or *www.nida.nih.gov*
The U.S. Department of Health and Human Services is the principal agency for protecting the health of all Americans and providing essential human services, especially for those who are least able to help themselves.

National Clearinghouse for Alcohol and Drug Information
www.health.org
The National Clearinghouse for Alcohol and Drug Information is a national resource for professionals seeking alcohol and drug information.

Drug Testing News
www.drugtestingnews.com
This site provides the most comprehensive source for up-to-date news and information on the drug- and alcohol-testing industry.

Institute for a Drug-Free Workplace
www.drugfreeworkplace.org
The Institute for a Drug-Free Workplace is an independent, self-sustaining coalition of businesses, business organizations, and individuals dedicated to preserving the rights of employers and employees in drug-abuse prevention programs and to positively influencing the national debate of these issues.

Working Partners
www.dol.gov/workingpartners/
The Department of Labor's Working Partners has gathered facts and figures about alcohol and drug abuse and developed information on how to establish an alcohol- and drug-free workplace. In addition, Working Partners offers a kit of industry-specific materials designed to help small businesses understand how substance abuse impacts workplace safety and productivity.

Alateen
www.al-anon.org
Alateen is a recovery program for young people. Alateen groups are sponsored by Al-Anon members. The program of recovery is adapted from Alcoholics Anonymous and is based upon the Twelve Steps, Twelve Traditions, and Twelve Concepts of Service.

Alcoholism Research Group
www.arg.org
The Alcohol Research Group (ARG) website provides information concerning the ARG research publications, the library, and the training program. The ARG Library is one of the oldest and largest alcohol and drug libraries in the United States.

Alcoholism Center for Women
www.home.earthlink.net/~acwla/
The Alcoholism Center for Women is an acknowledged leader in recovery services to women. ACW provides one of the most comprehensive recovery programs for women in the country. Special emphasis is dedicated to outreach and treatment services to underserved women, including women of color, homeless women, and women of diverse sexual orientations. Prevention and treatment services are designed to include both social- and medical-model concepts, providing a holistic, individualized approach to recovery.

Hazelden Library Collection
www.hazelden.org/library
Here is a good starting place for those seeking information and/or researching in the addiction field. Included is the Hazelden Library collection of books, videos, audios, and government documents; links to two journal databases, ETOH and DRUG; links to NCADI alcohol and drug fact sheets; links to the premiere addictions information organizations SALIS and RADAR Network; and access to the International Master list of Addictions/Substance Abuse Databases.

National Council on Alcoholism and Drug Dependence
www.ncadd.org
The National Council on Alcoholism and Drug Dependence fights the stigma and the disease of alcoholism and other drug addictions. NCADD's website provides objective information, statistics, facts, referral, and advocacy, as well as highlighting awareness and prevention programs and campaigns.

Workplace Violence Issues

National Institute for Occupational Safety and Health
www.cdc.gov/niosh/homepage.html
NIOSH is the federal agency responsible for conducting research and making recommendations for the prevention of work-related injury and illness.

Partnerships Against Violence Network
www.pavnet.org
The Partnerships Against Violence Network is an interagency, electronic resource created to provide information about effective violence prevention.

Safe and Drug-Free Schools Program
www.ed.gov/offices/OESE/SDFS/
The Safe and Drug-Free Schools Program is the federal government's primary vehicle for reducing drug, alcohol, and tobacco use, and violence, through education and prevention activities in our nation's schools.

National Crime Prevention Council
www.ncpc.org
NCPC is a national nonprofit organization whose mission is to help America prevent crime and build safer, stronger communities. Their website contains useful information about crime prevention, community building, comprehensive planning, and even fun stuff for kids!

Prevention First, Inc.
www.prevention.org
Prevention First, Inc. believes that health and well-being are basic human rights. Through the highest quality training, consultation, information services, and advocacy, they promote health and wellness among individuals, organizations, and communities.

CHAPTER TWENTY-SIX

Sexual Harassment on the Job

Samuel M. Fassig, DVM, MA

IN THIS CHAPTER, YOU'LL LEARN:

- The two forms of sexual harassment
- What actions constitute sexual harassment
- How to handle inappropriate behavior at work

Sexual harassment is a form of sex discrimination that violates Title VII of the Civil Rights Act of 1964. Although sexual harassment on the job has been illegal since 1965, few cases were filed until the hearings on the confirmation of Supreme Court Justice Clarence Thomas. Sexual-harassment allegations made during those hearings made the public aware of this aspect of the law. In the three years prior to those hearings, 18,300 sexual-harassment complaints were filed with the U.S. Equal Employment Opportunity Commission (EEOC). In the three years following the hearings, nearly 40,800 cases were filed.

In January 1997, the EEOC defined sexual harassment in the following manner: *Unwelcome sexual advances, requests for sexual favors, and other verbal or physical conduct of a sexual nature constitutes sexual harassment when submission to or rejection of this conduct explicitly or implicitly affects an individual's employment, unreasonably interferes with an individual's work performance, or creates an intimidating, hostile, or offensive work environment.*

Does sexual harassment occur only when the victim has experienced unwanted physical contact or sexual advances? No. Sexual harassment may take one of two forms:

- **Quid pro quo**—Harassment occurs when a supervisor conditions the granting of an economic benefit upon receipt of sexual favors from a subordinate or punishes the subordinate for refusing to submit to his or her request(s). Generally, an employer is strictly liable for acts of "quid pro quo" harassment committed by a supervisor who has the power to make or recommend significant employment decisions affecting the subordinate-victim, such as hiring, promotion, discipline, or discharge. This liability would exist even if the supervisor violates a clearly articulated company policy prohibiting sexual harassment.

- **Hostile work environment**—This exists where supervisors and/or co-employees create an atmosphere so infused with unwelcome sexually oriented conduct that an individual's reasonable comfort or ability to perform is affected.

The EEOC also states that sexual harassment can occur in a variety of circumstances, including but not limited to the following:

- The victim as well as the harasser may be a woman or a man. The victim does not have to be of the opposite sex.

- The harasser can be the victim's supervisor, an agent of the employer, a supervisor in another area, a coworker, or a nonemployee.

- The victim does not have to be the person harassed but could be anyone affected by the offensive conduct.

- Unlawful sexual harassment may occur without economic injury to or discharge of the victim.

- The harasser's conduct must be unwelcome.

It is helpful for the victim to directly inform the harasser that the conduct is unwelcome and must stop. The victim should use any employer complaint mechanism or grievance system available. However, if the employer has no complaint procedure, the lack of reporting the complaint will have little impact on the employee's case.

An isolated comment will not constitute harassment. Courts have stated that: "mere utterance of an . . . epithet that engenders offensive feelings in an 'employee' is not unlawful." When the EEOC investigates allegations of sexual harassment, it looks at the whole record—the circumstances, such as the nature of the sexual advances, and the context in which the alleged incidents occurred. All determinations are made on a case-by-case basis.

State laws apply to all employers within the state including veterinary practices. Federal law applies only to employers who have fifteen or more full- or part-time employees. However, it is not uncommon to have a suit filed in both state and federal court.

Is all conduct of a sexual nature in the workplace unlawful? No. The touchstone of whether harassment has occurred is whether the challenged conduct is unwelcome and a reasonable person might find it hostile. Such unwelcome conduct might include any of the following:

- Repeated offensive sexual flirtations, advances, or propositions

- Continued or repeated verbal abuse or innuendo of a sexual nature

- Uninvited physical conduct such as touching, hugging, patting, or pinching

- Comments of a sexual nature about a person's body

- Display of sexually suggestive objects or pictures

- Jokes or remarks of a sexual nature in front of people who find them offensive

- Prolonged staring or leering at a person

- Making obscene gestures or suggestive insulting sounds

Most workplaces will not be free from conduct that is not objectionable to someone. Most courts recognize that the world is not a pristine place. A single incident or isolated event will not support a hostile-work-environment claim. A hostile work environment usually requires multiple offensive acts or a pattern of offensive conduct.

> A hostile work environment usually requires multiple offensive acts or a pattern of offensive conduct.

Clinical veterinary practice is vulnerable to claims of sexual harassment. The care-giving aspect of practice brings people together emotionally as well as physically. In many veterinary practices, small teams of animal-health-care professionals frequently work long hours, under arduous conditions, in isolated treatment and surgical rooms in close proximity to each other. In rural, housecall, and emergency practices, emergency calls require time-consuming treatments and nursing procedures. Team members maintain close quarters well into the night and early morning. In these types of close-contact conditions, employees tend to form more tight-knit groups than employees of larger, less personal businesses.

Unresolved legal issues remain. These concern the amount and kind of proof required to establish certain elements of sexually harassing conduct by someone other than a managing or supervisory employee. Issues also arise in applying the law to the factual circumstances of a specific case, testing the credibility of the parties' claims and proof, conceptualizing relief, and valuing damages.

When the conduct in question does not directly involve the abuse of authority, the employer may be liable for the acts of its employees (supervisory and nonsupervisory) and perhaps others visiting the business premises on a regular basis (including nonemployees like distributor sales representatives). Liability is incurred when the employer knows or should have known of the conduct and failed to take prompt and effective remedial action.

One of the most effective ways for a veterinary employer to avoid a claim regarding a hostile environment and sexual harassment is to confront the issue openly. It is important to communicate clearly to employees that sexual harassment will not be tolerated and to adopt a sexual-harassment policy for the practice. This policy should include the establishment of an effective complaint or grievance process, taking immediate and appropriate action when an employee complains. Such a policy might be stated in an employee handbook or other such mechanism, and employees should be asked to review it annually. The repeated use of offensive language on the job does create legal grounds for a complaint. Be aware that a coworker can file a complaint against you as well as against the employer.

As an associate, you are an employer representative. If you are faced with a situation in which an employee in your work group is using inappropriate language, one approach is to diplomatically point out that this behavior offends both men and women and is not appropriate for use in a business environment. You can also inform the person that if he or she continues to use street language, he or she will be subject to the same type of disciplinary action as what is stated for violating other practice work rules (which, depending on your practice's policies, may include or contribute to the employee being fired). Be sure to document the counseling session in the employee's file, inform your superior, and make a record of the incident for your own files—just in case.

In general, unless you know someone well, other than the traditional handshake, *don't hug, don't pat, don't squeeze, and definitely do not kiss.* The best rule is: "Do unto others as *they* would have you do unto them." Even then, be careful and respectful. Remember what was said about our senses and how we communicate through verbal and nonverbal means: "If it looks, feels, sounds, or seems offensive, it probably is offensive."

As a veterinarian, your reputation in the community is extremely important. If you were involved in an incident, or an event occurred on your premises, and the staff is hostile or discusses the situation in public, clients may take sides and become alienated, and customers may be lost. In addition, you may find yourself the target of some unsolicited overtures and advances from clients, or other staff members may make your life more challenging than it already is. Just the allegation of sexual harassment can have far-reaching and potentially long-lasting consequences and impact on your career.

RESOURCES

Books

Complete Employee Handbook by M. Holzschu.
Human Relations: Productive Approaches for the Workplace by M. Garrison and M. Bly.
Unwritten Rules for Your Career by G. Graen.

Magazine Articles

"Avoiding Sexual Harassment Liability in Veterinary Practices" by C. Lacroix and J. Wilson in *JAVMA*, May 15, 1996.
"Issues in Workplace Sexual Harassment Law and Related Social Science Research" by S. Burns in *Journal of Social Issues*, Vol. 51, No. 1, 1995.

► **PART SIX** ◄

Looking Ahead

► CHAPTER TWENTY-SEVEN ◄

Searching for a New Job

Samuel M. Fassig, DVM, MA

IN THIS CHAPTER, YOU'LL LEARN:

- How avoid making the same mistakes in your job hunt
- Tips on giving notice
- How to find job number two

According to the results of the National Survey of Graduates conducted by the Canadian Veterinary Medical Association, 45.8%—or almost half—of newly graduated veterinarians working as associates will work in more than one hospital within their first two years of practice. They reported that: "For the average graduate, there is a 60% chance that they will remain in their first hospital in their first year of practice. After one year, the chances of remaining in that same hospital drop to 54% and after two years the chances of being in the same hospital since graduation drop to 43%"

Statistical comparison data for U.S. graduates is not available at this time. However, there is likely a similar trend.

REASONS FOR SEEKING A SECOND JOB

In any event, there is a good probability that you will move on to a new job within two years after graduation. Some of the reasons may be:

- The money promised by the employer was not there. The employer is slow to make paychecks out and/or there is always some disagreement as to productivity payments or bonus expectations.

- The time/work schedule was more demanding than first stated or anticipated.

- There were disagreements with the employer over what was actually expected on the job.

- The employer made promises that she did not keep.

- You started working for the employer before the contract from the lawyer arrived. When it did arrive, it was not what you had agreed to verbally. The employer expressed a take-it-or-leave-it sentiment.

- There was a personality conflict with the employer or with a long-standing staff member—perhaps a technician, a receptionist who has been there a long time, or an owner's spouse who is involved with the business.

- You underestimated the cost of living in the area. You cannot make ends meet and you believe there is no way to negotiate for more compensation.

- The time and expense related to commuting to work was higher or more physically demanding than expected.

- A personal situation changed (divorce, loss of a relationship, or entry into a new relationship requiring a change in physical location).

- You became homesick for the part of the country from which you came.

- You had health concerns or a change in physical status.

- You experienced a lack of confidence in your own abilities and felt that the employer was always "on your case" and less supportive than you expected, and you did not feel included in the culture of the practice, no matter what you did.

- You got a better offer from a competing practice or a hospital in another area.

- You had an unidentified sense or urge to move on. You felt restless and not attached or committed to this practice.

- You felt that the working conditions were terrible.

- You felt abused. As a new associate, you were allowed to do only technician-type work. As an associate, you had envisioned more.

The list can go on and on. For whatever reason, you want a change and now you are looking for job number two. The trend for many young professionals is to continue to repeat the same entry-level experience—same job, same duties, just about the same everything, including the same frustrations. This does not mean improvement. It means that you will approach employment just like before, often with the same results.

HOW TO AVOID REPEATING THE SAME WORK EXPERIENCE

To avoid repeating the same work experience, disillusionments, and dissatisfactions, give some thought to these suggestions.

- **Think about your vision**—what is your preferred future, and what are the initial steps you might want to consider taking to get there (see Chapter 4 for a discussion on creating a preferred future)?

- **Remind yourself of all the good things you have done**—the successes on difficult cases, the clients you helped, and those who were appreciative. What did that feel like? Concentrate on the positives; avoid the negatives (although they will be dealt with later). A positive attitude is a common thread among all winners. It empowers you to separate yourself from those who simply settle for less, or who just give up. Nothing is more tantamount to success than keeping your will to succeed.

- **Reexamine your expectations**—what you expect to happen plays a dramatic role in how things turn out. For example, if you are an athlete and expect that you will win the contest, you have a much better chance of doing just that. If you go into a work situation thinking and feeling that this job is for a loser, it will be.

- **Do something to make yourself feel better physically**—start to exercise more regularly. Consider taking vitamin/mineral supplements. If you feel better, it will translate into actions that will ultimately lead to success.

- **Visualize yourself achieving high goals, bringing in new business, and being welcomed in to the community**—whatever you visualize as positives, work on them every day. They are a source of newfound power and confidence.

- **Project internal positives to the outside world**—display good posture, put a spring into your step, deliver a firm handshake when meeting people, and exude self-confidence in a humble yet positive manner. The more you practice it, the more you will believe it, and the more you will embrace it as true.

- **Motivate yourself**—people who achieve the unusual and unexpected success also constantly motivate themselves by setting goals and focusing on those things they can control.

PERFORMING A SELF-ASSESSMENT

Career counselors refer to self-assessment as the "backbone of career management." It is a systematic process of exploring values, interests, skills, and personal style. Self-assessment tools help you

312

to understand the environments that let you excel, the interests that excite you, and the roles you like to play (big fish–little pond, helper behind the scenes, know-it-all, good guy, Good Samaritan, pet detective, etc.). It provides insights into how these roles help or hurt you in the workplace and to understand the skills you enjoy using that permit you to express yourself in ways that are personally rewarding. To reduce stress and enjoy what you do for a living, work needs to fit your personality. Getting to know yourself is the first step in career management.

Some people enjoy making high-level management decisions; others want to make a contribution to society. For some people, money and status are top priorities, while for others, expressing themselves creatively is what brings joy to their everyday life. Some people would rather sit at their computer analyzing data than deal with clients or patients.

The right job fit is personally gratifying because it nourishes the most important aspects of your individual personality. Most people, when thinking about a career, focus on a subject matter, industry, or job title that interests them, yet they pay little attention to what really makes them happy. Many will not have given any time to creating a preferred future.

It is helpful to revisit self-assessment questions to visualize the work environment and tasks that will help make the second work experience much more pleasurable than the first. To do so may also involve evaluating your past performance. Some questions addressing these areas include:

- Did you like working with people, or did you prefer to deal with computers and paper? Did you want to work with animals but not people? (Since veterinary clinical practice is all about people, how do you see a job that only deals with animals? Is it pathology? Isolated ranchwork?)

- Did you want to do something different every day? Or, did you prefer more repetitive tasks?

> To reduce stress and enjoy what you do for a living, work needs to fit your personality. Getting to know yourself is the first step in career management.

- Did you like being part of a controlled organization, or did "shooting from the hip" better meet your style?

- Which did you prefer—freedom and flexibility, or structure and security?

- What work environments allowed you to do your best work? Indoors or outdoors? Hectic and chaotic? Recurring and routine?

- Did you enjoy high visibility? Or, did you like to work quietly behind the scenes?

- Did you like working with large groups? Did you prefer to work with children rather than with parents? Or, did you favor working with only one or two other people?

- Did you have trouble working for a female boss? A male boss?

- Did you prefer situations where you were the sole authority?

- Did you need a lot of interaction with other people?

- Did you enjoy a collaborative decision-making process, or did you prefer working alone?

- How much of a team player were you?

- What were your pet peeves about the workplace? Make a list. Do you need to work on these areas?

- Are you full of knowledge but still inexperienced in a clinical setting? How do you assess your client skills? Did you use a lot of big words without explaining them? Did you talk to the pet and not to the client? Did you present treatment options in an apologetic or disparaging manner? Was it hard to ask your client for money and charge appropriately? Were your client transaction charges much lower than the other doctors?

- Did you consider seeking a mentor? Did you find one? What did that relationship turn out like?

Knowing your personal values is as important as knowing your skills and environmental work setting. Values are emotional power pills and exist at the core of every career choice.

What Are the Values That Drive You?

- Is it recognition, pride, status, or the thrill of meeting new challenges?

- Do you crave intellectual stimulation?

- Do you enjoy coming up with new ideas, being driven by responsibility, or being your own boss?

- Do you prefer being part of a team?

- Do you prefer supervising or being supervised?

- How loyal to your employers are you really? Or, is everything you do all about yourself?

- Why are you attracted to purchase some products and not others? Does vanity drive your consumer purchases? If so, to what extent?

- How ethical are you? Will you cut corners for a friend? Will you fill out a health certificate without examining the animal thoroughly? Will you use outdated drugs and vaccines? Do you turn a client away with an animal in pain because it is time to go home? At what point will you cross the line? Would you quit your job if the owner/employer was unethical and refused to improve?

If you were to ask several of your friends about your values, what would they truthfully say? If you have some close friends who love you, try it out. Consider asking them: "If you were to describe the things I value in my life to someone we do not know, what would you say?" "If you were to describe the things I value in my life to someone really close to us, what would you really want to say about me if I wasn't there to hear it and there would be no repercussions?"

Another essential part of the information-gathering process is to access available self-help and professional resources. Self-assessment tests are available through counseling services. They give you a good handle on your personal profile and assess your personality tendencies, ability to adjust to a job, communication styles, management

styles, and coping skills. A number of these tests are listed at the end of this chapter.

There are also excellent books and helpful aids available at the local library, bookstores, through professional career counselors, and, depending on the source, on the Internet. Many university psychology departments offer free assessments and evaluations for students and local residents.

These are all personal tools so that you can get to know yourself better. The ultimate goal is to gain a better understanding of what you prefer, how you react while under the influence of stressors, how you choose to engage others, and what your defaults are in approaching social integration.

Self-assessment vehicles are an opportunity for you to become aware of how you create what happens to you and the roles you play in creating your life situations. These are not judgments. Rather, they are a way to help you understand yourself.

A PERSONAL CHALLENGE

Let's say you have done some reflection and self-assessment. Here is another challenge for you to consider before you begin to go after job number two. Think back and reflect about every work experience you have had, whether as an employee or volunteer, and ask yourself these questions:

- Would you hire yourself?

- Are you really a willing worker?

- Do you ever unconditionally stay overtime to finish up a particular task or help a coworker?

- Are you punctual and dependable? Do you show up every day on time, prepared to work?

- Do you get along with people?

- Do you offer to help others when you have some extra time?

- Do you admit it when you make a mistake? Do you take the initiative to correct it and avoid making the same mistake again?

- Do you follow the rules and observe the policies and procedures of your place of employment? Are you a "safe" employee who follows safety guidelines?

- Do you bring your personal problems to work, or can you leave them at home?

- Do you keep yourself groomed and neat? How are your personal attire and appearance?

- Do you insist on a "coffee break" even if your work is really behind schedule and clients are waiting?

- Do you take pride in your work? How can you tell? How can others tell?

- Do you tell your coworkers "thank you" for helping you or for a job well done?

- Do you take credit for someone else's work, or do you put praise where it belongs?

- Do you work well under pressure? Can you handle angry and upset clients? Can you adjust to the pressure?

- Do you manage your time well? Are you on time for appointments, or do you chronically make the clients wait?

- How well do you work without close supervision?

- Do you treat your employer's equipment and supplies like they were your own? Do you give a lot of things away (medications, bandages, extra samples, your time) or consistently not really charge for small services like fecals, nail trims, anal-sac expression, ear cleaning, and the extra exam?

- How responsible are you? Do you see things that need to be done, or do you wait until someone tells you what to do?

- Do you respond to messages and return telephone calls in a timely, courteous manner?

- Can you demonstrate compassion for owners when they experience the loss of a loved one? Can you do so and retain your professionalism?

- Would you do business with you? Why? Why not?

Understanding your internal barriers—those psychological barricades that keep you from moving

> Seek out that particular mental attitude which makes you feel most deeply and vitally alive, along with which comes the inner voice which says, "This is the real me," and when you have found that attitude, follow it.
>
> —James Truslow Adams

forward—is the critical but often disregarded aspect of career management.

Unfortunately, there are times when you may have difficulty implementing a plan of action because of internal resistance, fear of change, overcommitment to routine, problems with authority, or other interpersonal issues. Outside stressors such as family demands and needs also put pressure on you to stay stuck in the familiar or in someone else's concept of what you should be doing.

Getting to know yourself is the long-term solution to creating opportunity to fulfill that which you really need and what you think you want out of life in order to enjoy it more fully. Self-awareness is the key to preventing burnout, self-created stress, and dissatisfaction. It guides how you earn a living, carry on your personal life, and feel social experiences. It is an important continuous growth-development process. Self-understanding imparts and permits the development of wisdom, better judgments when making choices, and what is traditionally called "maturity" in both your professional and personal lives.

When you take responsibility for your role in a problem at work, you are in a strategically better place to do something about it to prevent a recurrence. The self-assessment process, although sometimes painful and blunt, is ultimately liberating. It expands a personal definition of your self. It allows you to take risks and make changes that you would otherwise not be able to do. When you marshal this all together, making conscious choices about managing your career so that you will find both personal fulfillment and financial success, the pathway becomes clear, open, and gratifying.

Career management today is seldom simple. It is an ongoing, complex, subtle, internal, and external process. It means getting to know yourself, gathering information, and creating and exploring opportunities in order to match those opportunities appropriately to your self-profile.

Ultimately, the search for job number two goes back to the same questions visited when you first job hunted. What do you want? What do you have to offer?

STEPS IN YOUR SEARCH FOR JOB NUMBER TWO

Understanding Yourself

- Answer the self-exploration questions in this chapter.

- Review and revisit your preferred future (see Chapter 4).

- Acknowledge your part in the last employment experience. What were the good things you helped create in the job? What did you learn? What were the bad and ugly things you helped perpetuate in the job? What did you do to sabotage your working there?

- Review your skills and attributes.

- Revisit the steps to finding a job and the resources to find opportunities.

- Make a plan of action for discovering opportunities.

- Implement the plan.

Marketing Yourself

- Visit and negotiate with potential employers

- Situate yourself in an advantageous position. What special skills and value do you bring?

- Set high targets. If you ask for more, you reinforce your high value in the mind of the potential employer. Set high aspirations in keeping with your self-assessment. Ask for what you need. Go after what you want.

- Skillfully manage information. Explore what your potential employer really needs to solve his or her problems. Plan a strategy for getting that information from the employer during the job search, the interview, and the negotiations. Probe deeply to uncover and address underlying needs of the employer, which will increase the value you are offering.

- Identify the full range and strength of your power. Many new associates enter the employment negotiation thinking the employer has all the power. This often leads to low self-confidence for the associate. Realize you have power in the negotiations by positioning your value.

- Satisfy the employer's needs over her wants. The employer may really *want* to get an associate to work for low wages and long hours. However, she may *need* something different.

- In negotiations, make concessions according to plan. Many new associates give away too much too soon to the potential new employer. This happens because of lack of experience or confidence in an associate's negotiation skills. Most are uncomfortable with the natural tension of the "sales" process (in this case, selling themselves). Employers think they *want* something for nothing. What they *need* is a valuable employee. It is important to understand that if you give in on compensation too quickly and do not negotiate, the employer may think that you are not really worth it and that you lack self-esteem or self-confidence. In addition, when you do make a concession, it is important to get something of value back from the employer. This encourages the employer to pay a fair price for a valuable product (in this case, you).

> It is important to understand that if you give in on compensation too quickly and do not negotiate, the employer may think that you are not really worth it and that you lack self-esteem or self-confidence.

- Realize that you also must deliver that value. Whatever you told the employer regarding the value you bring to the business, you must, as a minimum, provide it. In order for you to build a relationship with that employer, you *need* to provide it willingly and cheerfully.

GIVING NOTICE TO YOUR BOSS

How you leave your employer can follow you and cost you unemployment benefits. Telling your boss: "You can't fire me, I QUIT!" may give you some sense of "one-upsmanship" and emotional gratification, but it will show up as a voluntary quit on your permanent job record. Unemployment benefits and separation packages hinge on the conditions of your dismissal. Quitting before you are officially fired is never a good option for most employees.

In addition, taking out your frustrations by berating the boss in public or to her face at the time you leave is also not a good idea. Your "former" employer may well indeed be all that you say she is. However, once the termination-of-employment decision has been made, it is time to make the exit with as little disturbance as you can. Many practitioners, and employers in general, have long memories, and they have various acquaintances in many arenas—people you have not had the pleasure of meeting yet. There is the risk, and it happens more often than not, that your potential future employer has just enjoyed lunch or a social function with your current boss, who may have shared a horrendous story about what you, as a disgruntled employee, told her two days ago, two months ago, or two years ago.

If you give notice, and the employer wants you to work to the end of your two weeks (or whatever time period you stated), you should. You may not feel loyal (or as loyal) to the employer, but you can often feel a sense of loyalty to the position which kept you fed for the time you were there. Working out a smooth transition goes a long way in case a former employer is contacted as a reference (even though you did not list her as a reference). A boss or supervisor tends to remember the last thing you *did not do* or accomplish for the practice, not what you did do. This all means not "burning bridges."

It is also wise for you to leave your personal decisions for leaving the job or the circumstances surrounding your termination between you and the employer. Coworkers do gossip. They like to vent or otherwise spread the news to anyone who comes near (including drug salesmen, distributor reps, etc.). They may talk a good story about supporting you, but remember, they still work there. Keeping your circumstances as private and professional helps keep you from being the "talk of the town."

GENERAL RULES FOR BEING SUCCESSFUL IN JOB NUMBER TWO AND OTHERS TO COME

- Love what you do. Do what you love. You're going to have to work very hard at it.

- Accept surprises. A seemingly off-the-wall opportunity in another industry or with a different type of employer may be just the thing to bring out the best in you and make you blossom into a star. Training in veterinary medicine has been a stepping-stone for many into other areas —some in animal health, some not.

- Be proactive and consider being more mobile. Geographic change is becoming a norm. Exploring, traveling, and changing cities may be just what you need to put some pizzazz in your life and help you get "unstuck."

- Most important, build your skills. Skills are what matter to employers today, not just experience. Can you really provide the skills you promised as part of your value?

- Skills, plus the value you bring (meeting the employer's needs), will determine your worth to the practice. The combination will become the basis for how you are compensated for your efforts. Remember—you can have great skills and little value to the employer if you do not meet her needs. If you have mediocre skills, even if you meet most of the employer's *needs*, you may never reach the level of compensation you desire. Advancing your skill sets is paramount to growing your worth.

REFERENCES

Bazerman, M., and Neale, M. *Negotiating Rationally.* Free Press, 1992.

Cohen, H. *You Can Negotiate Anything.* Bantam Books, 1982.

317

Fisher, R., and Ury, W. *Getting to Yes: Negotiating Agreement Without Giving In.* Houghton Mifflin Company, 1981.

Freund, G. *The Negotiator's Handbook.* Prentice Hall, 1991.

Karrass, C. *Give and Take: The Complete Guide to Negotiating Strategies and Tactics.* T.Y. Crowell, 1974.

McCormack, M. *What They Still Don't Teach You At Harvard Business School.* Bantam Books, 1989.

Ury, W. *Getting Past No: Negotiating With Difficult People.* Bantam Books, 1991.

RESOURCES

Professional Help Materials

These tests require a trained psychologist or psychiatrist to interpret. When you make a request for such a test, ensure that the tester (psychologist or psychiatrist) is trained and experienced to administer and interpret the instrument. Such instruments include:

- Minnesota Multiphasic Personality Inventory (MMPI-2)

- California Psychological Inventory (CPI)

- Personality Research Form-E

- Strong Interest Inventory™

- Guilford-Zimmerman Temperament Survey

Self-Help Materials

Learning Skills Profile and Adaptive Style Inventory—proprietary tools from McBer & Company, Training Resources Group, Boston, Massachusetts (617/437-7080) on improving your job-skill performance by understanding how you learn, assessing gaps between your personal learning skills and job-skill demands, and comparing your self-assessment with feedback from others. It will also confirm your awareness that certain situations are more difficult for you to adapt to successfully or that you have an over-reliance on one particular style that may limit your interactions with others, your problem-solving ability, your communications, and your perceptions.

Self-directed Search® from Psychological Assessment Resources, Inc., Odessa, Florida (800/331-TEST). Tests include The Occupations Finder, You and Your Career, and the Assessment Booklet.

CHAPTER TWENTY-EIGHT

So You Want to Be the Boss

Larry McCormick, DVM, MBA

> ### IN THIS CHAPTER, YOU'LL LEARN:
>
> - **What to consider before buying a practice**
> - **How to use consultants**
> - **The methods of valuing a veterinary practice**

Starting your own practice is not an easy endeavor. There is a considerable price to pay beyond money—it takes a lot of time to identify a suitable location, build a facility, establish a functional business enterprise, develop a viable clientele, and deal with the myriad of anticipated and unanticipated problems. The time lapse from start-up to an established and financially sound practice is frequently several years. The risks of being marginally successful, or even failing, are real. Quality-of-life issues, such as personal freedom and time for family, are often affected. But for some people, the challenge of creating and nurturing a successful practice is a thrilling, satisfying venture and is worth the risk.

In the right circumstances, buying all or part of an existing practice provides an attractive alternative to establishing a new one. The current owners or their predecessors have previously expended the personal and financial resources associated with practice start-up. If it is a successful practice, there is usually a well-equipped facility with a seasoned workforce serving a well-established client base.

These important attributes potentially allow you, as the purchaser, to spend more time as a practicing veterinarian. You can utilize established resources to generate revenues more quickly without the inherent risks associated with a practice start-up. For this established practice, however, you must pay a price that is usually greater than the dollar cost of starting a new business. Is it worth the price differential? Frequently, the answer is yes.

However, it is inadvisable to purchase some practices. So, how do you know whether a particular practice is a feasible buying opportunity or not? You arrive at an answer by:

- Performing adequate due diligence

- Using the services of qualified consultants

- Becoming knowledgeable about the factors that drive and ultimately determine the worth of a practice

- Understanding the methods used to value veterinary practices

PERFORMING ADEQUATE DUE DILIGENCE

The following is a partial list of factors that you should consider before contemplating the purchase of a practice.

- Quality of equipment
- Years in existence
- Location and parking
- Consistency of growth in earnings
- Expected future earnings
- Quality and stability of existing client base
- Level and quality of fees and fee structure
- Number of new clients per year
- Workforce in place
- Employee turnover and loyalty
- Management in place
- Regional demographics
- Enforceable noncompetition covenants
- Competitors
- Condition and attractiveness of the facility
- Availability of emergency and specialty services
- Average transaction charge
- Practice's gross and gross per doctor
- Level of net cash flow
- Real estate options
- Transferability of both professional and practice goodwill
- If you are buying into an existing corporation, the level of corporate indebtedness, its relationship with other shareholders, and existing commitments (retirement plans, etc.)

Thorough investigation is the key to effective due diligence. While the above list is extensive, it is not comprehensive; each practice is unique and requires a complete evaluation. If you are an associate in the practice you intend to buy, you likely already possess considerable knowledge about the practice's attributes and shortcomings. More important, you know the plausibility of effecting change.

If you are not an associate in the practice offered for sale, the investigative process is more difficult. However, with effort and persistence, you can obtain a thorough understanding of the practice.

UTILIZING THE SERVICES OF QUALIFIED CONSULTANTS

Veterinarians are intellectual islands of scientific information but are frequently ill-prepared for major business-based decisions associated with starting or purchasing a practice. For most, these decisions are some of life's most pivotal choices with long-lasting material and financial implications. Therefore, such decisions should be based on sound information and qualified advice. The use of qualified business consultants is critical. Unfortunately, while the need for counsel is great, it frequently comes at a time when your available cash to compensate such consultants is low due to educational debts, home mortgages, and the costs of raising a family. As a result, associates often decide not to engage or to minimize the use of these important advisors. Major transactions, often involving hundreds of thousands of dollars, are frequently completed with inadequate counsel.

The three most important advisors for the purchaser are an attorney trained in contract law, an experienced tax accountant, and a business appraiser.

> The three most important advisors for the purchaser are an attorney trained in contract law, an experienced tax accountant, and a business appraiser.

Legal Consultant

Critical legal decisions are made at this time, and legal counsel is strongly advised. Many legal documents, often drafted by the seller's attorney, are part of the purchase process. It is important that you obtain legal counsel to represent your interests in the purchase transaction.

320

Accounting Consultant

An accountant's advice is crucial when purchasing a practice. In many sale transactions, you must choose the new business entity (sole proprietorship, partnership, corporation). Also, in noncorporation transactions, you must make important decisions regarding the asset allocation of the purchase price. Such decisions are far-reaching and can significantly impact your future tax burden.

Business Appraiser

The professional business appraiser is a frequently overlooked member of your advisory team. Most practice offerings usually fall within one of two scenarios:

1. No appraiser has been retained by either the seller or buyer. In situations where the services of a professional appraiser are not used, the asking price is usually established by some rule of thumb. While used extensively in the 1970s and 1980s, rules of thumb are, at best, guesstimates and usually bear no relevance to economic reality. Under these circumstances, you must decide whether to hire a veterinary appraiser at your own expense.

2. The seller has retained the services of a qualified appraiser. With increasing frequency, sellers are enlisting the services of an appraiser to establish a value for their practice. Ideally, the appraiser will establish an opinion of value that is fair to both the buyer and seller. In the real world, that is not always the case. Unfortunately, since some appraisers may skew the value in favor of the party paying for their services, it behooves you to hire your own appraiser to provide a second opinion.

In the typical buy-out transaction, buyers assume significant levels of indebtedness over lengthy periods, often ten years or more. It is important to know the answers to questions like, "Is the asking price fair and based on the income-producing capabilities of the practice?" and "Will enough cash flow be produced by the practice to enable me to pay myself a fair wage and provide sufficient return on my investment to service my debt requirements and have a small cushion remaining?"

An appraiser who is knowledgeable and trained in the unique aspects of veterinary valuation can help you answer these questions. Thus, similar to the attorney and the accountant, the veterinary practice appraiser is an important and essential component of your consulting team.

FACTORS THAT DRIVE PRACTICE WORTH

You may purchase the assets of a practice, or you may purchase the stock. The stock represents the equity of the corporation and is equivalent to the assets of the practice minus its liabilities. Whether you are buying assets or stock, the value of the practice assets must be determined. Two fundamental types of assets are recognized in all successful, ongoing veterinary practices: net tangible assets and intangible assets.

Net Tangible Assets

Tangible assets are pieces of property owned by a practice that can be seen, weighed, possessed, and estimated using the physical senses. Tangible assets usually sold in practice transactions include:

- Professional equipment and supplies
- Office equipment and supplies
- Inventory

Typically, cash does not transfer in a buy-sell transaction. It is relatively uncomplicated to derive a value for the tangible assets by ascribing a fair market value for each item. From this total, any outstanding liabilities are deducted, giving a value for the net tangible assets.

Intangible Assets

The term "intangible assets" refers primarily to goodwill (also called blue sky), which consists of the value of the business's name, reputation, and location, and the value of client lists and patient medical records. In comparison to the tangible assets, the intangible assets are more difficult to value. Accurate determination of the intangible assets is critical, because in many successful practices, the value of the intangible assets accounts for 70% or more of the determined practice value.

Conceptually, buyers of veterinary practices judge the business based on its ability to earn a fair return on their investment. When purchasing a successful veterinary practice, the premium you are willing to pay in excess of the tangible assets is the value of the intangible assets, which is also called goodwill. It is critical to recognize that the intangible asset value is dependent on the earning power of the practice.

METHODS USED TO VALUE VETERINARY PRACTICES

Appraisers use several methods to value tangible and intangible assets of veterinary practices. While it is beyond the scope of this chapter to provide a detailed analysis of each method, a general discussion of the major approaches commonly employed in the veterinary industry follows. Additional resources are listed at the end of the chapter.

Guideline Company Method

A "guideline company method" of valuing a business can be a superior valuation method because it reflects what is actually happening in the marketplace. This method, like in the housing market, compares the subject property or business to a number of actual like properties or businesses that have been bought and sold in the open market in a like demographic area. The problem lies in the closely held nature of veterinary businesses; details of actual sales are often unavailable.

Rules of Thumb

Rules of thumb are formulas that express the purchase price of a practice as a percentage of gross revenues or earnings. The quest for a "quick fix" to the complex issue of determining a practice's worth has led many to base buy-sell transactions on such rules. There are many rules of thumb; the more commonly used rules express value as a percent of revenue:

- A veterinary practice's value is equal to 85% of one year's gross revenues.

- A veterinary practice's value is equal to one year's gross revenue.

- A veterinary practice's value is equal to the average of the last three years of revenue.

Theoretically, rules of thumb are based on knowledge of actual transactions that have occurred in the marketplace. The reality, however, is that such buy-sell transaction information is not readily available. These rules of thumb are actually based on tradition, word of mouth, salespersons, veterinary publications, and other non-expert information sources.

There are significant hazards in employing rules of thumb to determine practice value:

- Rules of thumb assume that all practices are homogeneous—that all practices having similar gross revenues are equally desirable to the buyer. If this were true, buyers would have no preferences to purchase one practice over another. Clearly, that is not the case.

- Rules of thumb are, at best, guesses and should be used cautiously. More than one buyer has purchased a practice based on a rule-of-thumb determination, only to find out later that the practice was not able to support the determined value because the value was not based on economic reality.

> Rules of thumb assume that all practices are homogeneous—that all practices having similar gross revenues are equally desirable to the buyer. If this were true, buyers would have no preferences to purchase one practice over another. Clearly, that is not the case.

- Rules of thumb may often ignore a practice's true economic earning capacity, which can vary remarkably from practice to practice. Rules of thumb can just as easily overstate or distort profitability.

- Rules of thumb have no provision for assessing the risk factors inherent in every practice. The absence of a knowledge base often makes for ambiguities about exactly what is being sold, what assets are included and excluded, what liabilities, if any, are included, and what the sale terms are—cash up front or long-term favorable financing.

Income- or Economic Earnings-Based Methods

The income or economic-earnings methods are more complex and more difficult to understand than the rules of thumb. Since appraisers of veterinary practices commonly use these methods, it is important for sellers and buyers to have an understanding of them.

The income/earnings methods determine value from the viewpoint of an investor. These methods assume that investors would invest in businesses that offer the greatest return on their investment. These methods determine a practice's value based on its ability to generate economic earnings or income—or the earning power of the business. In spite of being a popular methodology to value practices, you must be cognizant of the advantages and disadvantages in using such methods:

ADVANTAGES OF INCOME/ EARNINGS-BASED METHODS
A major advantage is that the determined value for a practice is based on earnings or cash-flow-generating abilities. There is a strong relationship between the practice's value and the practice's ability to generate earnings, i.e., those with higher earnings capability are worth more. Income/earnings methods place value on the intangible asset—the major component of most successful veterinary practices.

DISADVANTAGES OF INCOME/ EARNINGS-BASED METHODS
It is often troublesome to accurately predict what

an appropriate income stream is for a given practice and whether that income stream is sustainable. It is extremely difficult to develop the proper capitalization or discount rate that will be used to capitalize or discount the income or earnings stream. This is a subjective assessment of risk requiring the judgment of a knowledgeable appraiser. While there are several viable income/earnings methods that an appraiser can use to determine the value of a veterinary practice, the most commonly used method is the excess-earnings method. More recently, an alternative income-based method, the single-period capitalization method, has gained favor.

EXCESS-EARNINGS METHOD
In reviewing Table 28-1, which illustrates the excess-earnings method, it is important to note that there are two factors that determine practice value:

- The amount of excess earnings

- The capitalization rate

Even small changes in either factor can produce significant variations in practice value.

Amount of Excess Earnings. Excess earnings are those revenues that remain after paying all the customary and legitimate operating expenses of the practice and after compensating the owners for their work as veterinarians. The remaining (excess) earnings are monies owners can use as they choose. The more discretionary earnings a practice generates, the greater its value will be.

Another way to conceptualize the excess earnings is that these earnings represent the owner's return on investment (ROI) in the practice assets. Many practices provide owners with a good job and a comfortable living but generate little excess earnings. Inasmuch as these practices do not produce a fair and expected return on investment, they are of less value.

Two general areas determine a practice's excess earnings—the revenue-generating ability and the efficiency in managing the practice's operating expenses. In-depth discussions of these factors are beyond the scope of this chapter, but it is important for you, as a buyer, and your advisors to evaluate these areas thoroughly. Particular attention should be given to the stability and predictability of the future practice revenue production and to the efficiency with which management effectively minimizes expenses.

Capitalization Rate. The capitalization rate (also called the discount rate) is a measure of the risk associated with a particular investment—in this case, a veterinary practice. This rate will vary from practice to practice since practices vary in their degree of risk. Determining the appropriate capitalization rate for a given practice is very important, because small variations in this rate can cause significant swings in determined practice value.

There are factors that define the risks associated with a specific practice. Anything that can be accomplished to reduce risk lowers the capitalization rate and increases the worth of the practice. Consider the following risk factors when purchasing a practice:

- **Form of ownership of the practice entity—** The type of business entity selected for the practice (sole proprietor, partnership, corporation) can affect value. This is especially true for C-corporations. Because of double-taxation issues, C-corporation owners desire to sell stock. However, most outside buyers want to purchase assets rather than stock. There are many reasons for this, but here are two significant ones:
  - The buyer does not wish to inherit the seller's liabilities.
  - The buyer does not receive the tax advantages of asset depreciation and amortization when buying stock. The pool of potential buyers of C-corporation stock is normally limited to practice associates. When the pool of potential buyers decreases, the risk increases.

- **The consistency of historic earnings growth—** For most practices, the rate of growth of the historic revenue generation can be a predictor of the future. A history of substantial revenue growth over recent years reduces risk.

- **Expected future earnings—**What a practice is expected to earn in the future depends on many factors, such as the economic state of the region, the regional demographics, etc. The more uncertainty there is in these factors, the greater the risk.

- **Transferability of goodwill—**Two types of goodwill are generally recognized—practice goodwill and professional goodwill. Practice goodwill refers to attributes associated with the practice entity itself and includes such intangibles as location, workforce in place, client base, and operating procedures. Professional goodwill refers to the intangible attributes associated with an individual practitioner. To assess the magnitude of professional goodwill, you must consider whether there would be a major impact on income generation and practice operations if the practitioner suddenly left the practice. As opposed to practice goodwill, professional goodwill does not increase the value of the practice, because it is difficult to transfer professional goodwill to the new owner. Risk increases with professional goodwill and decreases with practice goodwill.

- **Practice size—**Larger, multiperson practices are usually less risky than single-doctor facilities, which tend to have more professional goodwill than practice goodwill.

- **Practice demographics—**Years in existence, historic trends in growth of the number of clients and revenue, location, adequacy of parking, attractiveness of the facility, and quality and adequacy of the equipment are some of the factors that affect the risk associated with a given practice.

- **Regional demographics—**Inflation expectations, population-growth dynamics, employment stability of the region, total household income, and the number of nearby competing practices are some regional demographic factors that account for a portion of the risk of a specific practice.

- **Presence of fair and enforceable noncompetition agreements—**Veterinary-practice owners who have employment agreements with their associates that contain restrictive covenants reduce the risk of having a departing associate take the practice goodwill. These agreements protect the buyer's investment by preventing associates from establishing nearby competing practices and potentially taking significant practice goodwill with them.

324

Table 28-1
CALCULATING PRACTICE VALUE WITH THE EXCESS-EARNINGS METHOD
This worksheet is also available on the companion CD.

Step #1	Determine the practice's excess earnings.		$200,000
Step #2	Determine the fair return on the tangible assets (tangible assets less liabilities).		
	Normalized net tangible assets	$175,000	
	Rate of return on investment in tangible assets	× 11%	
	Fair return on tangible assets	$19,250	
Step #3	Subtract return on tangible assets from excess earnings		($19,250)
			$180,750
Step #4	Determine the value of the intangible assets.		
	Excess earnings attributable to the intangible assets	$180,750	
	Divide by the capitalization rate (25% is an example)	÷ 25%	
	Value of the intangible assets	$723,000	
Step #5	Determine the value of the practice.		
	Value of the intangible assets		$723,000
	Value of the net tangible assets		+ $175,000
	Total practice value		$898,000

The above factors are only a partial listing of the subjective risk considerations that you and your advisory team must assess.

The income/economic earnings-based methods of valuation rely on mathematical computations called capitalizing and discounting. You can view the practice buy-sell transaction as being similar to that of making an investment. An investor desires to have an adequate return on his or her investment considering the risk associated with the particular investment. Through these processes, you seek the answers to these questions:

• How much would I pay today for a practice that is predicted to return a specific flow of dollars in the future?

• What would I pay for the capital that generated a predicted earning of "X" dollars?

• What would I be willing to pay for the bundle of assets representing a veterinary practice generating "X" dollars of predicted earnings each year?

• What level of return will I require in order to be motivated to invest in a specific opportunity, given the risks associated with that investment?

• What level of return will I require to invest in a particular veterinary practice, given the riskiness of that practice?

An example of the excess-earnings method is presented in Table 28-1. This table illustrates each of the following steps used in the excess-earnings method.

- **Step #1: Determine the practice's excess earnings**—A practice generates an earnings stream that is a direct result of investment in all practice assets, both tangible and intangible. Those assets produce revenue, and that portion of revenue which exceeds the normal operating expenses of the practice is the practice's excess earnings. These excess earnings translate into the total return on investment realized from investing in all the practice assets.

- **Step #2: Determine a fair market value for investment in the tangible assets**—In the second step, a reasonable return on investment in the more easily determined net tangible assets (tangible assets less liabilities) is subtracted from the total practice excess earnings of the first step.

- **Step #3: Subtract the return on tangible assets from the excess earnings**—The remaining earnings can be considered as having resulted from the intangible assets (total assets = tangible assets + intangible assets).

- **Step #4: Determine the value of the intangible assets**—These remaining earnings—the earnings attributable to the intangible assets—are then capitalized to arrive at a value for the practice's intangible assets. A capitalization rate of 25% is used in Table 28-1.

- **Step #5: Determine the value of the total practice**—Having at this point determined a value for each major asset class—both tangibles and intangibles—the total value of the practice is determined by adding these two assets. If any liabilities are to be transferred, they must be deducted from this total.

SINGLE-PERIOD CAPITALIZATION

A major shortcoming of the excess-earnings method of valuation is that it is heavily dependent on the accurate valuation of the tangible assets, including inventory, equipment, and drugs and supplies. The value of these tangible assets is difficult to determine without performing a true and thorough appraisal. In actuality, complete equipment and inventory appraisals are seldom done; instead their value is estimated from rules of thumb, depreciation schedules, or financial statements, none of which are indicative of fair

market value. Inaccurate assessments of these tangible assets can lead to significant misstatement of practice value.

The single-period capitalization method is often a more reliable method for determining the value of a veterinary practice. This method is similar to the excess-earnings method in that it relies on the capitalization of a practice's profits to determine value. Where it differs is that an appraiser using this method assumes that *all of the assets*, both tangible and intangible, are responsible for the profits of a practice. Consequently, this method does not require a thorough and accurate tangible asset appraisal and therefore significantly reduces the potential for error in the determination of practice value.

This theory appeals to the savvy buyer who, as long as the tangible assets are those typically owned by a modern practice, is more concerned with the income-generating capabilities of those assets than the value of the assets themselves.

The equation for the single period capitalization method is straightforward:

Value = Excess Earnings ÷ Capitalization Rate

See Table 28-2 for an example of this type of calculation.

This method is unique because the appraiser capitalizes the *entire* earnings stream (cash flow) rather than dividing it into cash flow from the tangible assets and cash flow from the intangible assets, as is done in the excess-earnings method. The capitalization rate is specific to the type of earnings stream and is different from the rate used in the excess-earnings method.

The single-period capitalization method is gaining popularity among professional appraisers of veterinary practices. It uses a direct approach, does not require a tangible asset appraisal, and produces practice values that are less subject to error.

For most associates, purchasing a practice is one of life's critical decisions. It has both financial and personal ramifications long into the future. Such a decision should be well researched and based on accurate knowledge of the many factors that, in the aggregate, create value in a veterinary practice.

Several publications offered by AAHA Press address buying or starting a practice. See the

Table 28-2
CALCULATING PRACTICE VALUE WITH
THE SINGLE-PERIOD CAPITALIZATION METHOD

Step #1	Determine the practice's excess earnings.	$200,000
		÷22.5%
Step #2	Divide excess earnings by the capitalization rate for all assets, both tangible and intangible.	$890.00
		÷22.5%
Step #3	Calculate the total practice value.	$888,890

327

Resources section on this page for more detail.

To avoid costly mistakes, use qualified business consultants, including an attorney, tax accountant, and business appraiser. With adequate knowledge and sound advice, the purchase of a practice can be an exciting venture, providing you with life-long professional, personal, and financial rewards.

RESOURCES

Books

Be Your Own Boss: Starting Your Veterinary Practice by S. Messonier.

Buying a Veterinary Practice by L. Monheiser List. Available through AAHA. Expected publication date: summer 2005.

Starting Your Own Veterinary Practice by L. Monheiser List. Available through AAHA. Expected publication date: fall 2005.

Structuring an Associate Buy-In by L. Monheiser List. Available through AAHA.

Valuation of Veterinary Practices by L. Monheiser List. Available through AAHA.

Websites

Quicken Small Business Center
www.quicken.com/small_business/
Get information on contracts, tax deductions, managing finances, and much more.

American Demographics
www.demographics.com
Online version of the magazine that includes demographic trends affecting veterinary hospitals and client bases.